PUT AWAY

*A sociological study of institutions
for the mentally retarded*

INTERNATIONAL LIBRARY OF SOCIOLOGY AND SOCIAL RECONSTRUCTION

Founded by Karl Mannheim
Editor: W. J. H. Sprott

A catalogue of the books available in the INTERNATIONAL LIBRARY OF SOCIOLOGY AND SOCIAL RECONSTRUCTION, and new books in preparation for the Library will be found at the end of this volume

PUT AWAY

*A sociological study
of institutions
for the mentally retarded*

Pauline Morris

*Foreword by
Peter Townsend*

LONDON
ROUTLEDGE & KEGAN PAUL

First published 1969
by Routledge & Kegan Paul Limited
Broadway House, 68–74, Carter Lane
London, E.C.4
Printed in Great Britain
by C. Tinling & Co. Ltd
Liverpool, London and Prescot

SBN 7100 6465 9

CONTENTS

PART ONE: BACKGROUND TO THE SURVEY

PART TWO: SURVEY FINDINGS

PART THREE: DISCUSSION

ACKNOWLEDGMENTS

THIS study was carried out at the direct invitation of the National Society for Mentally Handicapped Children, whose very real concern about residential conditions for the mentally handicapped was expressed through a most generous grant to Professor Peter Townsend, Chairman of the Department of Sociology at the University of Essex. I am greatly indebted to the National Society for making the work possible, and to Professor Townsend who entrusted me with the research, yet whose help and supervision was invaluable, particularly in the task of writing the report.

The staff of the Ministry of Health smoothed our path in every way possible and gave helpful advice at all stages of the research. But it is to the staff of all the hospitals and homes visited that we must tender our most grateful thanks; without their willing cooperation no report would have been possible, and I can only hope that the picture which emerges on these pages reflects adequately the wide variety of views expressed by them.

Discussions took place at various stages of the research with workers and practitioners in the field; they are too numerous to mention individually, but I am particularly grateful to Professor Brian Abel-Smith, Professor Alan Clarke, Professor J. Tizard, Dr. A. Kushlick, Mrs. M. Crozier, Dr. P. Mittler, Dr. F. Martin and his research team, and to my husband, for all their help and comments. If inaccuracies remain in the text, or if I have ignored their suggestions, the responsibility is mine alone, for I have not lacked advice.

For most of the duration of the research, Mr. G. Kalton of the London School of Economics, acted as statistical adviser to the project; during his absence abroad his place was taken by Miss Kathleen Gales, and to both I am very much indebted. Also to Mr. P. Wakeford of the London School of Economics computing department who sorted out so many queries so quickly and patiently, and to Mrs. Alfanday, for her most efficient typing service.

Finally, my very special thanks to the following colleagues whose work on various aspects of the project made the final report possible:

Mrs. L. Sawyer   Research Officer, February 1964 to September 1965

Mr. B. Cox   Research Assistant June 1965 to May 1966

Miss S. Mujib   Research Assistant, October 1965 to October
                     1966
Miss D. Munn ⎤
Miss C. Humphreys ⎬ Interviewers
Mrs. J. Milne ⎦
Mr. D. Walsh ⎤
Mr. P. Wiles ⎬ Coders
Miss C. Peake ⎦
Mrs. P. Corbett   Secretary, April 1964 to July 1966
Mrs. D. Wisbey   Secretary, July 1966 to January 1968

PAULINE MORRIS

March 1969

Foreword:

SOCIAL PLANNING FOR THE
MENTALLY HANDICAPPED
by Peter Townsend

DO we need to revise totally our conceptions of mental handicap
and therefore transform our methods of treating it? This is the
fundamental question which the research carried out by Dr. Pauline
Morris and her colleagues obliges us to pose. Until now we have
lacked information of a kind and range sufficient to challenge in
detail the system not just of services but of thought and belief about
handicap which has developed over the years. Valuable work has
been undertaken recently on the meaning and prevalence of handicap
(by, among others, Kushlick, Castell and Mittler), the effects upon
handicapped children of care in small residential units rather than
in large hospitals (Tizard) and the response even of the severely
handicapped to industrial and social training schemes (A. and
A. B. D. Clarke, O'Connor and Tizard). But research into mental
illness and handicap has always been starved of resources, by comparison with research into physical illness and certain forms of
physical handicap. Kenneth Robinson, the Minister of Health from
1964 to 1968, pointed out in 1958 that only 6d. in every £1 spent by
the Medical Research Council went towards research on mental
illness and handicap.[1] The Mental Health Research Fund has
difficulty in raising more than modest sums from voluntary and
private sources.

In the absence of comprehensive data about their physical and
mental capacities plainly it is impossible to obtain an intelligent
understanding of the needs of the handicapped, the conditions in
which they live, the educational, social and occupational facilities
afforded to them and the kind of skilled treatment they receive. And
since the nature of the problem, especially of needs, has not
previously been documented for the country as a whole, is is not
surprising that the most imaginative and enlightened proposals for
change, put forward by pressure-groups of parents,[2] as well as
individual specialists,[3] have lacked the persuasive force they may
have deserved.

[1] *Policy for Mental Health*, Fabian Research Series, No. 200, 1958.
[2] For an account of the activities of groups of parents see, *Parents Voice*,
Journal of the National Society for Mentally Handicapped Children.
[3] For example, Tizard J., *Community Services for the Mentally Handicapped*,
London, Oxford University Press, 1964.

Too much must not be claimed for the research in this book. Dr. Pauline Morris has not attempted in her study to explore the origins, development and prevalence of handicap, nor the problems of the handicapped who live at home with family or friends. She carefully states the limitations. Detailed studies require to be undertaken on, for example, committal procedures, diet, relations between parents and children, effectiveness of different forms of industrial training and social therapy, methods of recruitment and training of hospital staff and the social structure of both the hospital and the hostel. This research survey has concentrated upon institutional services and much of the evidence has been drawn from staff rather than from interviews with patients and their families.

Yet, when these and other reservations are expressed, the coverage of the study is still extremely wide. For the first time it is possible to comprehend the size, organization, staffing and operation of a national system of hospitals and residential services for the subnormal. For the first time it is possible for reliable estimates to be given of the scale and severity of certain problems. The basis has been laid for an evaluation of the effectiveness of hospitals for the subnormal. The basis has also been laid for rational planning of services for the subnormal, hitherto missing from the Hospital Plan of 1962[1] and the subsequent revision of 1966[2] as well as from the complementary local authority plans for community care.[3] All this has been made possible by a generous grant from the National Society for Mentally Handicapped Children to the Department of Sociology in the University of Essex upon the foundation of the University. Of course, a great deal of further research remains to be done but a preliminary network of information is now available to all those deeply concerned about the handicapped.

The study was conceived as the third in a series of national surveys of institutions[4] and although other comparative research on institutions has been done in this country and overseas, little or none of it has yet been national in range and representativeness.[5] This kind of

[1] *A Hospital Plan for England and Wales*, Cmnd. 1604, London, HMSO, 1966.

[2] The Hospital Building Programme: *A Revision of the Hospital Plan for England and Wales*, Cmnd. 3000, London, HMSO., 1966.

[3] Ministry of Health, *Health and Welfare: The Development of Community Care*, Cmnd. 1973, London, HMSO, 1963; and revisions under the same title published in 1964 and 1966. The latter (Cmnd. 3022) took the plans for the health and welfare services of the local authorities in England and Wales to 1976.

[4] The other two studies were: Townsend, P., *The Last Refuge: A Survey of Residential Institutions and Homes for the Aged in England and Wales*, London, Routledge and Kegan Paul, 1962; Benson, S., and Townsend, P., *The Elderly in Long-Stay Institutions:* A Survey of Persons aged 65 and over in Psychiatric, Chronic Sick and Geriatric Hospitals, Nursing Homes, and Residential Homes throughout Britain, London, Routledge and Kegan Paul, (forthcoming).

[5] There have been a number of comparative studies of institutions and of institutional conditions both in this country and overseas. See for example,

research offers special advantages. Knowledge about institutionalized minorities puts knowledge about non-institutionalized majorities in a new light. The connections between organizations and social structure, and between organizations and national policy, tend to be revealed. And programmes of further research can be devised more rationally and alternative policies discussed more realistically than in terms just of the information which is available in administrative reports.

In this introduction I shall try to review our conceptions and methods of treating mental handicap in the light of Dr. Morris's findings and also other recent work. I shall argue first, that the accumulating evidence of social influences upon intelligence has weakened if not destroyed the eugenic case for social segregation; secondly, that the evidence of the present survey, together with evidence from other countries, notably the Soviet Union, throws grave doubt on the hospital as the right environment for the care of the subnormal, and finally that the social, occupational and emotional needs of the great majority of the subnormal might be met better within various forms of sheltered family or community care than in existing hospitals and hostels. I shall then attempt to suggest how a phased programme of changes in policy might be introduced.

Social Structure and Mental Handicap: (i) *Subnormal intelligence*

In classifying someone as mentally retarded, defective or subnormal most societies refer, though not in so many words, to subnormal intelligence, personal incapacity and deviant behaviour. I want to consider each of these conceptions in turn, for I believe that this is essential in defining needs and finding whether they are met. From early in this century subnormal intelligence has come to dominate scientific conceptions of mental handicap, and the implications for the care of the handicapped should be considered at some length.[1] Societies find that individuals vary along a continuum according to verbal, numerical, spatial and other aptitudes. Below a certain level it is found that they make little progress at school and cannot hold any one of a range of ordinary occupations. They seem to require special schooling and occupation. But in families and neighbourhood

[1] For a particularly discerning and astringent discussion of the criteria of handicap see Wootton, B., *Social Science and Social Pathology*, London, Allen & Unwin 1959, pp. 254–67.

Wing, J. K. and Brown, G. W., 'Social Treatment of Chronic Schizophrenia: A Comparative Survey of Three Mental Hospitals, *Journal of Mental Science*, **107**, 1961; Jones, K. and Sidebotham, R., *Mental Hospitals At Work*, London, Routledge and Kegan Paul, 1963. For the United States see Ullmann, L. P., *Institutions and Outcome: A Comparative Study of Psychiatric Hospitals*, Oxford, Pergamon, 1968.

groups in Britain, many young children who would obtain very low scores in an intelligence test are not denied an ordinary upbringing or singled out for special treatment. A distinction has to be made between real and perceived ability. This suggests that the *identification* of those with low ability may depend considerably on culture.

In psychology some of the pioneering attempts to measure intelligence aimed to identify mental handicap. Early in this century Alfred Binet was asked to help the Paris education authorities to produce a scale for picking out retarded children. Later in Britain Cyril Burt and others worked on the mentally deficient and then seized on intelligence testing to show how poor but bright children might be selected to be given an academic type of education. It is ironic in present circumstances to recall that intelligence tests were originally regarded as a means of bringing about radical social reform and of establishing equality of educational opportunity. At first the results of intelligence testing were interpreted rather strictly. Educationists and psychologists believed that with few exceptions individual abilities were more or less constant from early childhood. They also assumed too readily that intelligence tests measured intelligence. The separation of mildly subnormal children from ordinary schools and communities and the creation of the tripartite education system was unjustly legitimated.

In recent years society has become very conscious of the limitations of such tests. First, although tests of varying scope have been devised they tend to measure a limited number and combination of individual abilities. They rarely reflect qualities of perseverance, creativity, and judgement, for example. And we now know that many children and adults who are classified as mentally subnormal have astonishing powers of perseverance.[1]

Second, the tests are only crudely approximate for individual persons. Results obtained from pre-school tests are extremely unreliable. Results for some children may vary by up to 10 points or more even when similar tests are carried out within a short space of time. Over a period of two or three years between tests some children's performance differs by up to 25 or 30 points.[2] It is also

---

[1] Tizard, J., *Survey and Experiment in Special Education*, London, Harrap, 1967, p. 13.

[2] Professor Vernon, an acknowledged expert on intelligence tests, is one of those whose accounts of the scope of such tests have become properly more cautious over the years. For example, 'One should never think of a child's IQ (or other test result) as accurate to 1 per cent. Rather an IQ of, say, 95 should be thought of as a kind of region or general level. For a few weeks or months to come there are even chances that it falls between 92 and 98; and the odds are about 10 to 1 that his IQ lies within the range of 88 to 102. But the possibilities of much larger discrepancies should not be forgotten. Over several years, say from 6 to 10 or from 11 to 15, the most we can say is that there is fair certainty (i.e. 10 to 1) of its lying between 80 and 110'. Vernon, P. E., *Intelligence and Attainment Tests*, London, University of London Press, 1960, p. 114.

difficult to measure intelligence when physical handicaps like deafness intrude.

Third, performance in intelligence tests often improves with practice and coaching. Simply by taking one previous test an average score can be raised five points. McIntosh found an average gain of 7·2 points among 11-year-olds at the second trial.[1] When 11-year-olds are given two complete practice tests and a few hours of interspersed coaching the average gain is about nine points. A significant minority of children gain from 15 to 25 or more points.[2] The implications are important. If this is what can be done by familiarity and concentrated practice for a few hours or weeks, how much more important may be the years of 'coaching' in a privileged social setting?

Perhaps the most important fact about intelligence tests is that they are not culture-free. Psychologists admit the great difficulties in comparing different races and ethnic groups. Some sociologists have gone on to argue, in effect, that the same difficulty arises in applying the same tests to different social classes and different sub-cultures. Middle-class children may have an unfair advantage, in the sense that the tests are usually drawn up from the vantage point of the kind of intellectual qualities shown by those in middle-class occupations and those who have had the kind of education typified by the grammar and independent schools.

The recent discussion of intelligence testing has acknowledged the many subtle ways in which society and not just environment (for that is a static concept) shapes individual ability. The impact of this idea upon education has been huge and the repercussions are still being felt. Streaming at young ages in schools and selection for secondary schooling at 11 on the basis of intelligence tests are now discouraged. Comprehensive schools are slowly being introduced and the school system is changing. Authoritative surveys, by the Crowther and Robbins committees, for example, have called attention to the wastage of ability. Few people still believe in a limited 'pool' of ability. It is possible, for example, that before long 40 or 50 per cent of each age-group in Britain will be eligible to enter higher education.[3] Any wide-ranging analysis of recent evidence must conclude that human excellence is a social product as well as

[1] McIntosh, D. M., 'The Effect of Practice in Intelligence Test Results', *British Journal of Educational Psychology*, 14, 1944.

[2] Vernon, P. E., *op. cit.*, p. 131.

[3] The Robbins Committee was unable to specify an upper limit, and although the percentage of each age-group in England and Wales with entry qualifications was likely to grow from 6·9 in 1961 to 14·5 in 1985 untapped ability was 'most unlikely to be fully mobilized within the next twenty years'. Half of each age-group in California already enter higher education, though to correspond roughly with British university entry qualifications the figure would probably be reduced to between 25 and 30 per cent. The United States Office of Education accepts an estimate that a figure of 50 per cent of each age-group entering higher education will be reached in the United States as a whole in 1970. In Oslo the

an individual quality. The kind and degree of ability may not only be shaped by the structure and organization of family, peer-group, social class and community, but also of the school and the firm as social organizations. The resources available to individuals within these settings, such as books, TV, and facilities for play, are important, as are also the type of relationships and the complicated interplay of speech, gesture and emotional expression.

The identification of mental handicap and the development of special services for handicap now have to be looked at in this new context. There seems to be wastage of ability in hospitals for the subnormal as well as in ordinary schools. Before the Mental Health Act of 1959 was passed there was keen controversy about the extent to which the classification of a person as 'subnormal' would have to depend on him being demonstrably subnormal in intelligence. Many argued that 'social competence' and 'emotional maturity' should continue to be crucial criteria. The British Psychological Society and others contended that these social and emotional criteria were imprecise and if they continued to be used it was possible for people to be treated wrongly as mentally defective instead of being treated for various forms of neurosis.[1] The eventual Act adopted a clause including subnormality of intelligence within mental subnormality.

But former practice has been maintained and there is evidence that a substantial number of people are classified either as 'subnormal' or 'severely subnormal' when their intelligence test scores considerably exceed the limits normally accepted for purposes of definition by psychologists.[2] Dr. Morris was unable to trace the scores for large numbers of a random sample of patients. For over a quarter of all patients no evidence existed that tests had been carried out and another substantial proportion were said to be untestable. Even among those for whom scores could be given around two-thirds had not been tested for at least two years, most of them not for more than five years. Ignorance and inertia in obtaining scientific information about ability seem to be poor foundations for a service

[1] See, for example, British Psychological Society, Working Party on the Report of the Royal Commission, *Bulletin of the British Psychological Society*, Vol. 35, pp. 1–26, 1958.

[2] Thus, while psychologists generally regard an IQ of 70 (on a Wechsler-type test with a mean of 100 and a standard deviation of 15 points) as the upper limit of subnormality, a quarter of a sample of adult admissions who were studied in 1961 had scores of over 80. And while they regard an IQ of 55 as indicating the upper limit of *severe* subnormality, half the sample of patients actually classified as severely subnormal had IQs of over 60. Mittler, P., 'The Contribution of Intelligence Testing to Classification', *Journal of Mental Subnormality*, Vol. XI, Part 1, December 1964.

number passing the University entrance test has reached 40 per cent. See, for example, Halsey, A. H., (ed.) *Ability and Educational Opportunity*, Paris, OECD, 1961.

which owes its legal justification to a definition of subnormality which includes subnormality of intelligence.

There is evidence, too, that severely subnormal persons improve in intelligence test scores and in other ways when given training elsewhere than in an institution. The best known example is the work of Tizard. He took a group of severely subnormal children from a large and overcrowded hospital and arranged for them to be looked after in a small, family-type unit like a Children's Home. This was the Brooklands experiment. He compared their progress with that made by a matched group of children who remained in hospital. The children in the Home made significantly greater advances than those in hospital in verbal and social development.[1] There are a range of supporting research studies, though most of them refer to children of higher grades of intelligence.[2] In a study in 1965 Stein and Stores found an intellectual improvement up to the school leaving age among a large proportion of subnormal children, sufficient in a few cases to 'lift the children well into the range of intellectual normality.'[3] In general there is more evidence of improvement in test scores for mildly than for severely subnormal people and a distinction needs to be made between the two. For the latter there are not many data on improvement in scores – except verbal IQ – but perhaps this is partly because of the difficulties of devising and applying suitable tests.

Finally, there is evidence from general studies of the distribution of intelligence in the population as well as from special studies of the prevalence of mental subnormality that there are many subnormal and even severely subnormal persons who are not known to the services supposed to be dealing with them. The most carefully devised recent study is that of Kushlick. He found a peak for the age 15–19 of 3·65 severely subnormal persons per 1,000 population in the Wessex region of England who were known to the local authorities, hospitals, and nursing and residential Homes. As in other studies the prevalence rates for both severe and mild subnormality were found to rise after infancy and during adolescence, as shown below. This phenomenon is very important and illustrates the strong social element in the identification of handicap. At the age of compulsory schooling, and then again after the end of compulsory schooling, the administrative prevalence of subnormality rises. The step to a new social milieu is one which some individuals cannot take or are prevented from taking.

[1] Tizard, J., *Community Services for the Mentally Handicapped*, op. cit., p. 85.
[2] See a review by Kirk, S. A., *Early Education of the Mentally Retarded*, Urbana, United States, 1958.
[3] Stein, Z. A., and Stores, G., 'IQ Changes in Educationally Subnormal Children at Special School', *British Journal of Educational Psychology*, Vol. 35, Part 3, November 1965.

SUBNORMAL PERSONS PER THOUSAND POPULATION IDENTIFIED
IN THE WESSEX REGION

Age	Severely Subnormal	Mildly Subnormal	All Subnormal
0—	0·52	0·18	0·72
5—	2·52	0·60	3·16
10—	3·01	0·56	3·59
15—	3·65	3·17	6·84
20—	2·91	2·98	5·91
30—	2·19	1·83	4·05
40—	1·87	1·76	3·66
50—	1·27	1·38	2·66
60+	0·52	0·63	1·11
All Ages	1·87	1·46	3·35

Source: Kushlick, A. and Cox, G., 'The Ascertained Prevalence of Mental subnormality in the Wessex Region on 1st July, 1963'. Proceedings of the First Congress of the International Association for the Scientific Study of Mental Deficiency, Montpelier, September 1967.

Kushlick and those who have studied the 'administrative' or perceived prevalence of subnormality before him consider that the rates for the mildly subnormal cannot be used to make estimates of the 'real' prevalence in the population. By the late teens there may be substantial numbers of people at work who have completed a school career and who have not been identified as requiring special education or other services and who may yet score only between 50 and 70 in a carefully applied intelligence test. The great majority of them are integrated into the community and the crucial question is why some are placed in hospitals and hostels. But by ages 15–19 most of the severely subnormal are believed to have been notified to the appropriate authorities. Kushlick uses the rates for this age-group to show how many children below this age remain undetected. For every 100,000 population in Wessex he estimates that as many as 45 of a total of 96 severely subnormal children aged 15 and under are not known to the local authority. This gives one measure of the desirable expansion in services.[1]

I have tried to establish, first in general terms and then with specific reference to the handicapped, how the concept of intelligence is much more elastic and much more open to social influences than we have supposed hitherto. A test of intelligence must not be treated as a sufficient criterion, therefore, of mental handicap or of admission to an institution. By this I do not mean to deny that it has a valuable

[1] Kushlick, A., 'A Method of Evaluating the Effectiveness of a Community Health Service', *Social and Economic Administration*, October 1967.

function as a diagnostic device. It is particularly useful for planning purposes in distinguishing between the mildly and the severely subnormal and elucidating the numbers of the latter. However, we might heed the terms in which a member of the Eugenics Society resigned from the Society. After working for six years among the handicapped and experiencing doubts about the utility of the criterion of intelligence the ex-member observed that the handicapped 'showed such a great variety of other virtues—generosity, goodwill, altruism, sweet temper—that I began to think a world peopled by mental defectives might be an improvement on the present one.'[1]

Social Structure and Mental Handicap: (ii) Personal Incapacity

A second means of understanding mental handicap in relation to the social structure is through the concept of personal incapacity.[2] Legislation in Britain and in other countries has included references to persons 'incapable of leading an independent life'. Intellectual ability overlaps with behavioural capacity but a population can be ranked according to individual incapacity to manage personal functions and undertake a range of common personal and household tasks, such as walking, running, climbing stairs, tying string, and washing and dressing. Some of Dr. Morris's most striking data refer to the low extent of physical incapacity among a large proportion of patients. It would be wrong of course, not to emphasize the dependent state of substantial numbers of patients who are bedfast, doubly incontinent and grossly disabled. But it is important to note that 83 per cent are fully ambulant; 66 per cent can both feed and dress themselves and another 17 per cent can feed although not dress themselves; 74 per cent of the adult patients are continent (and half the remaining adults only moderately incontinent); rather less than a third of all patients are said by staff to have one, two or more physical handicaps or to suffer from severe mental illness (though Dr. Morris points out that this may have been an underestimate).

Dr. Kushlick recently found in his Wessex survey that no less than 56 per cent of the severely (and 88 per cent of the mildly) subnormal adults in institutions could feed, wash and dress themselves. Nearly all of these were also continent, ambulant and free of severe behaviour disorders. He showed that over two-fifths of the severely and three-fifths of the mildly subnormal, some of them with severe incapacity, were living at home under the supervision of the local health authority.[3]

---

[1] *Eugenics Review*, October 1946, p. 115. Quoted by Wootton, B., *op. cit.*, p. 264.

[2] See, for example, Townsend, P., *The Last Refuge, op. cit.*, especially Chapter 10 and Appendix 2; Shanas, E., *et al, Old People in Three Industrial Societies*, London, Routledge & Kegan Paul, 1968, especially Chapter 2.

[3] Kushlick, A., and Cox, G., *op. cit.*

In another recent study 1,652 patients in 13 hospitals for the sub-normal in the Birmingham region were assessed by a hospital doctor and a charge-nurse. Only 7 patients required investigation or active medical treatment of a kind which would make it necessary for them to be in hospital. About half were considered to require no medical treatment of any kind. Forty per cent were believed to need mental nursing with or without basic nursing and about 13 per cent required only basic nursing.[1] These data certainly pose the awkward question whether large numbers of patients require nursing and medical treatment in hospital. The real extent of personal incapacity in a population is determined to some extent by the demands placed upon individuals by the culture. The level of incapacity accepted for special attention and care depends on the perceptions and tolerance of families, peer groups, the community and the bureaucratic institutions.

Social Structure and Mental Handicap: (iii) Deviance

There is a third means of understanding mental handicap in relation to the social structure. Sociology can help to teach that some persons are classified as mentally handicapped not so much because they are of subnormal intelligence or are incapacitated but because they are deviant. A population can be ranked according to its conformity with social norms. Norms are not minute regulations which are precisely formulated. They are standards of conduct to which people are expected to approximate in their daily activities. Again we must make a distinction between 'real' and 'perceived' behaviour. There are no distinct categories of behaviour. Just as physical restraint shades off into violence, so gossip by degrees becomes slander, or seduction becomes rape. Moreover, the exact points on this con-tinuum at which norms are offended are difficult to locate and they tend to vary from place to place, class to class or society to society. Thus a loving family may not recognize a child's backward behaviour for several years until it is pointed out to them in the child's first year at school. Alternatively, an agricultural community with small need, say, for the symbols of literacy may not find it necessary to take notice of the backward behaviour of an adult man other than to express mild reproofs, to the effect that he is a bit simple. It follows, therefore, that a 'censure-line', if it may be called such, may be drawn at one level within a sub-community of society, but at another level elsewhere. A compromise tends to be struck by the different groups in society. The norms for society as a whole may be more loosely interpreted. Difficult cases may be determined through

[2] Leck, I., Gordon, W. L., and McKeown, T., 'Medical and Social Needs of Patients in Hospitals for the Mentally Subnormal', *British Journal of Preventive and Social Medicine*, Vol. 21, 1967.

the formal procedure of the courts which apply the more stringent rules of law.

If a person behaves to others invariably with trusting obedience, makes gestures or noises inappropriate to the context, repeats statements or instructions, touches and embraces others with embarrassing familiarity or affection, he is liable to be assigned to a social category of 'simple fool' and perhaps soon of 'imbecile', 'moron', or 'mentally subnormal'. He runs the risk of becoming a deviant with inferior status. As Dr. Morris reminds us, strong views are held even among psychiatric and nursing staff as well as the public about the supposed inability of many mentally handicapped persons to observe social norms. In particular there are fears and prejudices about violence and promiscuity, which are as difficult as racial fears and prejudices to allay.[1] On the one hand we must ask coolly for statistical evidence of assault and violence, and of promiscuity, to compare with that for comparable age-groups in the ordinary community. It is difficult to obtain suitable evidence, but certain data are on the whole reassuring. For example, Kushlick finds only about 14 per cent of severely subnormal and only 5 per cent of mildly subnormal persons in Wessex with behavioural disorders, though an additional small percentage have mild disorders.[2] On the other hand, one has to investigate carefully the ways in which the organizational communities within which handicapped persons live oblige them, as much as any other persons who might be placed in such conditions, to react stridently. A bleak and overcrowded environment, together with the denial of certain physical and occupational outlets, seems likely to induce occasional frustrated behaviour of extreme forms. So we need to introduce the idea that organizational form may reinforce if not actually cause 'handicapped' behaviour. A person tends to adopt the role expected of him. Some families impose handicapped roles upon their members. And in their structure and operation hospitals may steer individuals into performing more exaggerated versions, including more limited versions, of the handicapped roles they have played in outside society. Behaviour adapts, in short, to social form, and is causally connected.

There is a tendency for society to separate people into strictly distinct categories of deviant and non-deviant, incapacitated and

[1] Under former legislation there was a category of moral defective, in addition to the categories of idiot, imbecile and feeble-minded. In 1960, 73 moral defectives were admitted to hospitals for the subnormal in England and Wales, all but a few to two hospitals in the Sheffield region. Although this category is now in disrepute, social deviance is undoubtedly an important influence in determining admissions and, indeed, the pattern of hospital management. General Register Office, *Registrar General's Statistical Review of England and Wales for the Year 1960, Supplement on Mental Health*, London, HMSO, 1964, p. 37.

[2] Kushlick, A., and Cox, G., *op. cit.*

non-incapacitated, subnormal and normal, irrespective of the graded differences of degree revealed in any objective study of behaviour. In one psychiatric study a research team found that although a majority of people in a community could accept a proposition that mental illness could be cured they found it hard to stomach a proposition that abnormality and normality were not distinct and shaded into one another.[1] It seems that people are prepared to ignore mental illness as far as possible and tolerate a wide range of behaviour. But once this tolerance is exhausted and illness recognized people at once wish a patient to be segregated and sent off to hospital. A potential danger to the community is removed, and a sick person is symbolically identified as different, going through all kinds of 'stripping' or 'degradation' procedures, and being deprived of common rights and resources. If people admit that abnormality is just one end of a continuum then they might have to admit that a sick or handicapped person might not be different from themselves, and segregation might not be the obvious solution. So are different beliefs linked in a system of belief.

Explaining Variations in the Prevalence of Mental Handicap

There are a number of implications of this approach for the study of mental handicap. One is that a society may go through a cycle of identifying relatively large and relatively small numbers of mentally handicapped persons, even though the prevalence of handicap, when measured according to *objective* criteria of subnormal intelligence, personal incapacity and behavioural deviance, may remain constant. Or again, its mode of treating them may depend on the relative weight attached socially to each of these three criteria. The development in the late nineteenth century of a national school system brought to light those who could not be accommodated, or accommodated only with difficulty, in that system. So occurred an expansion in the proportion in society who were identified as mentally handicapped and this was reinforced by the rigid and punitive trends in the moral code of society during the Victorian period. Custodial values were extolled by eugenicists who claimed that the subnormal would reproduce their kind disproportionately and contribute to a decline in national intelligence.[2]

Although from the fourteenth century a legal distinction was drawn between 'lunatics' and 'idiots' most persons with mental disorders were in practice housed indiscriminately in workhouses

---

[1] Cumming, J., and Cumming, E., 'Mental Health Education in a Canadian Community', in Paul, B., *Health Culture and Community*, New York, 1955.

[2] These claims were confounded by measures over time in the distribution of national intelligence and by studies of the handicapped. Penrose for example, found that over 90 per cent of the mildly subnormal in his hospital survey had parents of normal or dull average intelligence. Penrose, L. S., *A Clinical and Genetic Study of 1280 Cases of Mental Defect*, HMSO, 1938.

and, later, asylums. It was only in the middle of the nineteenth century that the first 'idiot asylum' was opened by a voluntary society, and later still before such asylums added the term 'institution for the feeble-minded' to their title.[1] I am therefore arguing that as time went on the demands of the educational system, together with the imposition of a stricter moral code, increased the proportion of persons with mildly subnormal intelligence or mildly deviant behaviour who were institutionalized. It was the incursion of many 'feeble-minded' persons without personal incapacity but with supposedly fixed low intelligence which caused institutions independent of asylums to be set up. The system of mental deficiency hospitals evolved. More recently, there has been a tendency for the rates to diminish, partly because intelligence is now seen to be more complicated and adaptable than formerly supposed, and partly because punitive controls on individual departures from moral conformity is thought to be less necessary.

It is within some framework such as this that the prevalence of mental handicap in different societies, and the division between institutional and community care, has to be explained. In appreciating what the imprecise criteria of subnormal intelligence, personal incapacity and deviance contribute to our concept of mental handicap we can perhaps see the need to revise our standards of humanity and justice. For the significance of this analysis is much more than semantic. It implies that there may be persons who are deprived of full civic rights and responsibilities and even in some cases of their personal freedom because their ability to read and write has not yet been perceived, their relatively adequate intelligence has not been measured (or has not been measured efficiently), their behaviour is found to be morally repugnant or they are an embarrassment in school. It also implies that *any* physical segregation, even of people of extreme handicap, may be improper.

The Unsuitability of Hospitals

To what extent are hospitals for the subnormal the right setting for the patients in them? What sort of facilities do they provide? Theoretically the needs of the patients can be explored first in relation to the formal or agreed purposes of the hospitals; we can show how far clinical, nursing, occupational and welfare purposes are actually fulfilled. Second, we can compare the patients with the population outside (or with patients in other hospitals or in hostels), we can show the space they occupy, the resources they command, the diets they consume and the number of close friends and relatives to whom they have access, and we can go on to apply objective criteria of deprivation, such as the prevalence of infectious disease

[1] *Report of the Royal Commission on the Law Relating to Mental Illness and Mental Deficiency, 1954–57*, Cmnd. 169, London, HMSO, 1957.

correlating with degree of overcrowding. The first is primarily organizational and the second comparative in method. Sometimes standards of comparison may be indirect rather than direct.

The quality of any hospital service varies and Dr. Morris studiously avoids laying undue emphasis on either end of the continuum. She pays tribute to the nursing staff and goes to considerable lengths to place data which might be interpreted as critical of individuals in a context which makes us aware that it is the organization that is at fault. Since her report follows hard on the heels of the report of an inquiry into a Welsh hospital,[1] which has provoked public anxiety, this approach is most important, for it helps us to concentrate attention on the fundamental issues rather than embark on a self-righteous search for scapegoats.

A depressing picture emerges from the national survey. There is considerable personal, environmental, occupational and social deprivation among the hospital population, and no good purpose can be served by concealing this fact. This can be shown either by reference to a memorandum circulated to all hospitals by the Ministry of Health in 1965[2] or to what is known about facilities and resources enjoyed by individuals in the outside community. I shall select just a few indicators. Sixty-one per cent of patients are in hospital complexes of more than 1,000 beds each, and a third are in annexes which are often isolated from the main buildings, themselves sometimes remote from urban and shopping centres. Only 1 per cent of patients are in single rooms; 38 per cent are in wards with 60 beds or more. The Ministry of Health recommends, 'A ward should not normally accommodate more than 30 adult patients or 20 children'. Sixty-nine per cent are in dormitories with only two feet or less space between the beds. Nearly 60 per cent are in dormitories with only one or two amenities or none at all among a list including lockers, bedside chairs, bedside mats, pictures and ornaments. Nearly 60 per cent are in dormitories where no personal possessions are displayed on beds, tables or window-sills and many of the others are in dormitories where personal possessions of only *some* patients are found. The Ministry states, 'Each patient requires a measure of privacy and at least a locker in which to keep his private possessions and in the case of a child, his toys.' Only 21 per cent have their own toothbrushes, shaving kit or hairbrushes. Most of the clothing is communal in the sense that it is not retained by the individual after being laundered. And brassières and corsets, for example, are not generally supplied to women. The Ministry states: 'All patients, adults and children, must have personal marked clothing, including

---

[1] *Report of the Committee of Inquiry into Allegations of Ill-Treatment of Patients and Other Irregularities at the Ely Hospital, Cardiff*, (The Howe Report) Cmnd. 3975, London, HMSO, 1969.

[2] Ministry of Health, *Improving the Effectiveness of the Hospital Service for the Mentally Subnormal*, HM(65)104.

underclothing, which they can regard as their own'. In 1966–7 the average cost of food and drink per patient per week was only £1 19s. 10d. compared with £2 4s. 6d. in mental illness hospitals £2 10s. 4d. in chronic sick hospitals and much larger amounts in general hospitals. There is insufficient variety in meals, and there is doubt, because of the patience and time required to feed them, whether all are adequately fed.

The majority of children either have no toys or the toys tend to remain shut up in cupboards. The Ministry recommends:

> Each child needs to have toys and possessions of his own. There should also be a large stock of playthings which can be used by all the children on the ward. Simple, solid, play equipment of a semi-permanent or permanent nature should be provided, e.g. swings, climbing frames, chutes, roundabouts, and toy trucks and push carts in which children can sit. (HM(65)104).

All these provide some measure of the barren conditions in which many patients live and of the meagre resources available to them.

Large proportions of the patients have little to occupy them in the day and few social relationships. Just over a tenth of patients are of school age. About 43 per cent of them attend the hospital schools, though measured intelligence seems to have only a little bearing upon whether or not a child attends school, and there are children who could attend school who do not. Facilities for part-time adult schooling exist for only a third of the patients in hospitals and only 12 per cent of them actually attend classes. The proportion of adult patients attending for occupational therapy or industrial training fluctuates from about 3 per cent in some hospital units to over 60 per cent in others. The average in any particular week appears to be about 22 per cent, though a further 24 per cent work in the hospital or its grounds and a small population outside the hospital on daily licence. However, nearly half the patients either have no occupation or only domestic work or occupational therapy on their own ward.

Contacts with family and community are relatively few. Dr. Morris points out that the failure to look upon admission as being of concern to the family as a whole sets the seal upon the patients' isolation. The staff assume parental roles without actually fulfilling them. Forty-three per cent of patients are not visited in the course of a year and only a third as often as once a month. Seventy-five per cent have never gone home. Forty-two per cent are confined to the ward in which they live, even though this figure far exceeds the proportion limited in mobility by physical handicap. Wards are locked for 14 per cent of patients. (The worst and very exceptional instance was a hospital in which 41 per cent were in locked wards. Many adults and children were netted into their cots, a practice which has mostly disappeared from Britain.) Eighteen per cent are allowed to go unaccompanied outside the hospital. Few patients go on holiday for as much as a week, whether organized by the hospital, relatives or voluntary associations. In most hospitals the figure varies between 10 and 25 per cent. Though there are many institutionalized relationships with voluntary associations, raising funds, holding religious services, celebrating Christmas and birthdays and so on, the fostering of personal relations—through invitations to visit clubs or houses in the community, or call regularly on particular patients—is not highly developed. They are better developed in medium sized hospital units than in those with 1,000 beds or more. Some of the biggest hospitals have no Parents' Association.

Perhaps the most serious findings of all for policy are those which show that medical treatment and skilled nursing are not the predominant functions of the hospitals. Medical staff are in practice concerned with the supervision of hospital organization, the introduction of occupational therapy, the provision of a sheltered environment and the treatment of those temporary illnesses and disabilities such as colds and minor injuries, which afflict any population. Only with a relatively small proportion of patients suffering from illness, including mental illness, are they immersed in questions of specialist medical care. Some medical staff have launched positive programmes of rehabilitation. They are concerned constantly to improve the specialized facilities of the hospital and they run extremely efficient, and sometimes modern, units. Yet few of these leadership activities are specifically medical in content. And at the other extreme there are medical staff who seem to avoid medical involvement in the hospital and become engrossed with solely administrative duties and outside conferences. Significantly, few medical staff are involved in research. Some of the hospital annexes are rarely visited.

Nursing roles tend to be confined to dressing, washing and feeding patients, supervising occupations on the ward and accompanying patients outside the ward. It must be remembered that 83 per cent of patients are fully ambulant and only 9 per cent bed-fast. The high proportion of domestic work tends to reduce morale, particularly among nurses who are trained. Some say they are not nurses but glorified domestic workers or, alternatively, jailers.

Yet, because these institutions are hospitals, with medical and nursing staff in charge, the expansion of specialized services needed by subnormal persons is discouraged. The services are felt by medical and nursing staff to be a threat to their interests. Dr. Morris calls attention to the conflict between medical and nursing staff, on the one hand, and specialized staff, on the other. Only 2 per cent of the patients receive physiotherapy; and many more than an average of 12 per cent could receive occupational therapy. Only a quarter of the hospitals employ a speech therapist, inadequately in most even of these. Only half the hospitals employ social workers, most of whom are untrained. There is insufficient provision for psychopaths, epileptics, spastics, and autistic and psychotic children. There is, in short, a gross lack of basic professional services of various kinds.

Future Policy

Even when every account is taken of the immense variety of need and of quality of service, and the devoted efforts on behalf of subnormal patients made by many of the staff, the disturbing conclusion has to be faced, that the wrong system of care has been developed over the years for this minority of the population. What can now be done to remedy the system? Drawing upon the evidence so far available, the long-term purposes or objectives must first be defined, and the strategy to achieve those purposes then devised.

Useful lessons can be learned from some other countries. In the Soviet Union, for example, there seem to be only about a third as many mentally handicapped persons in hospitals and welfare institutions as in Britain and the United States, proportionate to population. That group of severely subnormal children who are 'imbecile' rather than 'idiot' fall under the administrative care of the Ministry of Education. Craft states, 'it seems that far more imbecile children are both afforded a chance of state schooling in the USSR, and are persisted with, than in the UK'. They are taught by special teachers, with high status and extra pay, in day or boarding schools. These schools lay emphasis on self-help rather than adult protection but by Western standards are generously staffed. After school all are expected to work in the home district.[1]

Britain may now be embarking cautiously on this path. In November 1968, following various pressures,[2] the Government announced that legislation would be introduced transferring responsibility for education of all subnormal children from health authorities to education authorities. Until now relatively fewer children in Britain than in the United States, though more than in the Soviet Union, have been a responsibility of health authorities.[3] Compared with many areas

[1] It is difficult to be sure how well the system works throughout the USSR, and how many gaps there are, but the major difference in the stress on education seems genuine enough. Craft, M., 'A Comparative Study of Facilities for the Retarded in the Soviet Union, United States and United Kingdom', in Freeman, H., and Farndale, J., (eds.) *New Aspects of the Mental Health Services*, Oxford, Pergamon, 1967.

[2] The Seebohm Committee had recently recommended that 'the local education authority should become responsible for the education and training of all subnormal children and take over the junior training centres'. *Report of the Committee on Local Authority and Allied Personal Social Services*, London, HMSO, 1968, p. 116.

[3] Kety, S. S. (Chairman), *Report of the Mission to the U.S.S.R.*, President's Panel on Mental Retardation, Washington, United States Department of Health, Education and Welfare, 1962.

of the United States, hospitals for the subnormal are more advanced in Britain. Services are more plentiful and ward organization more varied and idiosyncratic, in keeping with the rather piecemeal accumulation of different buildings over the decades. In most of them standards of care seem to be higher than in certain other industrial societies—than those, for example, in Austria and Hungary, which I visited recently. Yet the care is not only deficient. It is inappropriate. The problem is not simply one of finding more money and more staff, putting up new buildings and introducing comprehensive training schemes. It is one of reconstructing the system.

The evidence collected by Dr. Morris, and by others, such as Dr. Kushlick and Professor Tizard, justify a much more dramatic shift from custodial and institutional to community care than has so far been proposed.[1] And the evidence on mental nursing and residential Homes, (or hostels) does not really suggest that, at least in their present form, they are a suitable stopping-point. Dr. Morris shows that they provide a much more homely environment and are less isolated from the community. For example, proportionately more of the residents go home or go on holiday for a week or more than do patients in hospital. But by the criteria of occupation and social relations those who live in them are not dramatically better off than persons in hospital. Few are employed in the community and though many are engaged on domestic work few have occupational therapy. As many as 27 per cent (compared with 42 per cent in hospital) are not visited at all in the course of a year and only 18 per cent (the same figure as in hospital) are allowed out, despite fewer being severely subnormal. Few of these half-way institutions have Parents' Associations and they can be very isolated from a range of psychiatric and other professional services.[2]

The long-term aim should be to allow the great majority of persons with the same handicaps as those in hospitals for the subnormal to live in sheltered housing or small family homes in the community— when they can no longer be cared for by their families. Sheltered housing is being provided on an increasing scale for old people and the disabled, and could be planned to accommodate the subnormal. There might be family homes for the severely subnormal run in the same way as small group homes for 6 to 10 children, with housemothers and housefathers. Private housing for groups of 6, 10 or 15

[1] By community care I mean living in a private household, not a hospital or a residential Home, and receiving a range of medical, social and occupational services, which may include attending a day school or day hospital.

[2] See also, Apte, R. Z., *Halfway Houses: A New Dilemma in Institutional Care*, Occasional Papers on Social Administration, No. 27, London, Bell, 1968. Mittler points out that 'Small hostels are not necessarily superior to hospitals: there is always the danger that, unless well run, they may be unstimulating and remote places in which too little is done for the children educationally or socially.' Mittler, P., *The Mental Health Services*, Fabian Research Series, No. 252, 1966, p. 23.

less severely subnormal adults could be provided in clusters of bungalows, ground floor flatlets or even converted flatlets in ordinary houses in all localities. Subnormal persons with really severe psychiatric illnesses or multiple disabilities who require constant nursing and medical treatment would be cared for in units attached to district general hospitals.

The tenants of this sheltered housing would be able to take advantage of certain communal facilities, and there would usually be a resident housekeeper in one of the flatlets, or an adjoining house. In the day children would attend the local school, and adults would go to ordinary employment, sheltered workshops, day hospitals or day centres. In each local authority area Community Boards would be set up to manage a number of sheltered housing units, appoint staff and safeguard the tenants' welfare. These Boards would consist of three equal groups of people: lay representatives of the local community, representatives of parents or other relatives, and specialists, such as doctors, social workers, physiotherapists and occupational therapists. Associations of parents and of local residents would have specific functions. For example, they might staff a person-to-person visiting service for subnormal persons lacking relatives, organized by a full-time social worker. They might organize regular outings to shops and holidays. The social integration of the handicapped depends on two principles—the continuity of relationships with family and locality and the supervision and organization (under the Community Boards) of all community services by full-time paid specialist staff. A network of professional services—medicine, nursing, physiotherapy, occupational therapy, speech therapy and the rest—has to be provided in health centres, day hospitals and day centres, rather than in long-stay institutions. Consultants might be appointed to serve groups of health centres. A strong independent inspectorate covering community services as well as hospitals should also be created. Minimum standards of care and education should be laid down nationally.

Work in sheltered workshops and in ordinary employment would be a necessary part of this plan. The derisory and degrading system of 'rewards' for those in hospital would be replaced by a wage-structure worked out nationally. People with an intelligence quotient of between 25 and 50 have been shown not only to respond to training but to become so enthusiastic that in one case, for example, they broke into their workshop on Sundays to do extra work.[1] The best known workshop is one run at Slough, first by the National Society and then by Buckinghamshire Council, which has shown the possibilities of industrial training even for the severely subnormal. The employment services provided by the Department of Employment for all kinds of handicapped people need to be overhauled.

---

[1] For example, Clarke, A., and Clarke, A. D. B., *Mental Deficiency: The Changing Outlook*, London, Methuen, 1966.

In particular, strong placement services and properly conducted schemes for workshop instructors need to be introduced.

This entire pattern would require new legislation, together with a deliberate and massive redirection of resources, in money and manpower, from hospitals to community care. In 1966–7 about £128 million was spent on hospitals for the mentally ill and subnormal, compared with only about £17 million on all local authority mental health services.[1] The actual distribution of resources should be explored further but these figures give a rough indication of the relative value we actually place on institutional care as compared with community care. Only when this ratio is reversed will the distribution of services begin to represent the distribution of need. All this is conditional too on a drastic change in public attitudes.

What can be done in the meantime? While preparing legislation the Secretary of State for Social Services should invite local authorities and Parents' Associations in conjunction with Hospital Management Committees, to set up *ad hoc* Community Boards of the kind outlined. He should urge local authorities to review their plans for sheltered housing, training centres and mental health workers, in advance of legislation which introduces special government subsidies and perhaps percentage grants to expand facilities for community care. He should at the same time give them guidance about the assumptions on which planning might be based and also bring the Hospital Plan of 1962 up to date.

As sheltered housing and other services expand it will be possible to divert persons who would formerly have been admitted to hospital to the community. Some long-stay patients might also be encouraged to live in group homes. Some of the smaller hospital annexes could be transferred to the local authorities for use temporarily as residential hostels and overcrowding in the large hospitals could be reduced. Dr. Morris pays particular attention to the problem of the physical and professional isolation of many of the hospital units and argues that as well as turning some of them into hostels other units should progressively be staffed by autonomous groups of training staff and social workers. She also stresses the desirability of patients going out to schools, workshops and centres in the day, and of living in mixed units in the hospital. She rightly perceives that improvements in the quality of care depend on changes in social and professional structures.

Throughout this period staff should be encouraged to recognize that they are participating in a planned reform of benefit to the subnormal. Some of them might take part in training programmes for mental health workers or welfare assistants in the community services and be transferred at the appropriate time. Others might prefer

---

[1] *Annual Report of the Ministry of Health for the Year 1967*, Cmnd. 3702, London, HMSO, 1968, p. 147 and estimate of costs of psychiatric hospitals made on basis of weekly costs and numbers of patients on pp. 189 and 201.

to transfer eventually to other parts of the hospital service, and should be given the chance of working for spells at general hospitals.

From the start, Regional Hospital Boards should be committed to finding the resources so that the environment and facilities of the hospitals can be improved immediately. A few million pounds a year represents a tiny fraction of expenditure on the National Health Service and yet if devoted to furniture, carpeting, clothing, toilet requisites, toys, partitions and so on could transform the wards and raise the morale of both patients and staff. With the help of social workers attached to the local authority, associations representing parents and local residents should be made responsible for organizing person-to-person visiting services, play groups, shopping expeditions, hair-styling, holidays and so on. A local authority social worker should be temporarily attached to each hospital for this purpose. Meetings should be encouraged between groups of parents, local residents and staff on wards to discuss measures that might be adopted. Patients themselves should be persuaded to play a part in improving and furnishing the wards.

The general direction taken by these proposals is not original. The Royal Commission on the Law Relating to Mental Illness and Mental Deficiency of 1954–7 foresaw that the admission to hospital at least of the subnormal rather than of the severely subnormal would become unnecessary in the future. The Hospital Plan of 1962 tried to suggest dividing the subnormal from the severely subnormal, so that the former would be cared for in smaller units of not more than 200 beds—a proposal which has shown no signs of coming into being—and recognized that community care services would continue to expand. A memorandum issued by the Ministry of Health in 1965 stated,

> In the absence of complicating conditions, such as severe physical disability or disturbed behaviour, the severely subnormal patient who has been adequately investigated and treated ought not to be primarily the responsibility of the hospital service for long-term care. Ultimately, when facilities outside hospitals are fully developed, continued hospital care will be necessary only for patients who require special or continuous nursing and for those who, because of unstable behaviour, need the kind of supervision and control provided by a hospital.[1]

And independent specialists have sometimes elaborated the compelling arguments for a transfer of resources to the community services.[2]

[1] *Improving the Effectiveness of the Hospital Service for the Mentally Subnormal, op. cit.*

[2] In particular, Tizard, J., *Community Services for the Handicapped, op. cit;* Kushlick, A., 'A Community Service for the Mentally Subnormal', *Social Psychiatry*, Vol. 1, No. 2, 1966; and Mittler, P., *The Mental Health Services, op.cit.*

There are grounds then, for believing that the Government would not be opposed to changing policy so as to favour community care. But whether it could be persuaded to move far enough and fast enough is another thing. The difficulties of achieving a dramatic change should not be underrated. A much more serious approach to planning is required. Expressions of good intent in Ministers' speeches and exhortations in Government circulars, though perhaps necessary, do not penetrate very far into the system. What is lacking is a leadership strategy, worked out in fine detail with the co-operation of the hospital management committees, local authorities, staff and parents. Reform does not consist just in releasing more government money for staff and new buildings, important as these additional resources are. Nor does it consist in sitting tight and acting only when public attitudes soften. A structural change must be started which will ramify the length and breadth of society. There must be a complete reorganization of services—so that subnormal persons are no longer isolated in hospitals remote from the community and can be accepted into ordinary schooling and employment. They should have access as easily to family or locality and as easily to the professional services of physiotherapists, occupational therapists, psychotherapists and social workers as to the professional services of hospital doctors and nurses. For it is in a different structure of relations that the best hope lies of protecting their rights. The interests of parents, community and professions can be given a new, and more balanced, representation.

It is only in this different structure of relations that the punitive attitudes of some sections of the public and, indeed, of some professional staff can be modified. The present system of hospitals for the subnormal has been created very largely, I have tried to show, by social conceptions of low intelligence, personal incapacity and deviant behaviour. The isolation, cruelty and deprivation of the hospital organization, as it must be seen to be, is of our own making.

Disturbing accounts of conditions at individual hospitals have recently been described in the press[1] and in a Blue Book presented in Parliament. It would be wrong in such instances to assume that all we must do is apportion blame among individuals, discipline those who are narrowly responsible, and set up an inspectorate. The Committee inquiring into irregularities at the Ely Hospital, Cardiff, were not to know that the overcrowding and many of the deprivations, such as the shortages of toothbrushes and dentures, did not apply just to that hospital but to many other hospitals in Britain, as Dr. Morris now shows. The Committee concluded, 'the trouble has arisen not from any lack of [staff] good-will . . . but more than anything else, from a lack of awareness of how far Ely has lagged

---

[1] See, for example, Shearer, A., 'Dirty Children in a Locked Room: A Mental Hospital on a Bad Day', *The Guardian*, 28 March, 1968, (and subsequent correspondence).

behind what ought to have been, and can be, achieved.'[1] This conclusion could be applied more generally. Because almost everyone—hospital management committees, staff and public—regards the poor conditions of these hospitals with comparative equanimity and because almost everyone adopts an attitude of untutored pessimism about the possibilities of educating and occupying the handicapped, unjustifiably low standards of care are tolerated. The hospitals have been gripped with a kind of creeping organizational sickness, within which the handicapped have little chance either to fulfil themselves or enjoy the rights available to other citizens. This is the tragic problem we must try to understand and to solve.

PETER TOWNSEND

Colchester,
   April 1969

[1] *The Howe Report (op. cit.),* p. 115.

C

Part One
BACKGROUND TO THE SURVEY

INTRODUCTION

THE object of this study has been to examine the range and quality of institutional provisions made in England and Wales[1] for that group of handicapped individuals who are broadly known as mentally deficient. The term mental deficiency is not the only one in use, as will be seen from later discussion of the whole problem of defining the limits of mental subnormality, but it will suffice for this present introduction.

The study was undertaken in the belief that the objectives of social research within organizations are three-fold. The first is to discover what are the stated objectives of policy, both deriving from within and beyond the organization, and where there *are* no such explicit statements, to find out what the objectives are thought to be.

The second objective is to examine the extent to which aims are being fulfilled, and the third relates to the dichotomy of latent and manifest function first suggested some thirty years ago by Robert Merton in his classic article 'Social Structure and Anomie'.[2] The significance of this dichotomy is that from the distinction between the subjective purposes of action and the objective consequences of behaviour which may not be perceived, important practical considerations follow for the day to day patterns of action within all structured organizations. Thus in studying the mental subnormality institution, we are concerned to discover what is *actually* happening in a given situation as well as what is *said* to be happening, or what is thought *ought* to be happening.

Any plans for the future must be based upon the realities of the present situation, and this report attempts to present a comprehensive range of factual data about the conditions prevailing in a representative sample of hospitals and homes for the subnormal.[3]

[1] Some information was obtained for hospitals in Scotland, but the information can in no way be regarded as representative for that country (see Chapter 2).

[2] Merton, R. K.: *American Sociological Review*, 3, 672–82 (1948).

[3] It had originally been intended to include a sample of local authority hostels, but in view of the limited resources available, it was felt that our efforts should be concentrated on hospitals and homes. The inclusion of local authority hostels would have involved considerable additional expense in terms of travel and subsistence, as well as the design of different questionnaires. For information purposes it should be noted that in March 1965, the number of hostel places

To do so, we visited nearly half the hospitals for the subnormal in the country. Usually two interviewers spent between one and two weeks at the hospital, depending upon the size and dispersion of units. A considerable number of voluntary hospitals and homes were similarly visited, but being both smaller in size and situated on a single site, the time spent at each was usually no more than one or two days.

We sought to discover what facilities – physical, occupational and educational there were for patients, and to learn more about their social environment. We sought to learn the extent to which both staff and patients are affected by their social environment, and by administrative action. And we sought to learn something of the relationship between the hospital as an institution and the outside community, as well as between the patients and the outside world.

Further we aimed to examine the extent to which the provisions and facilities available met the needs of the patients in relation to their physical and mental handicaps. But evidence suggests that factors other than 'need' may determine whether or not a patient receives a particular service; furthermore the concept of need is an extremely nebulous one which does not lend itself easily to statistical analysis.[1] As will be seen in subsequent chapters when discussing the provisions and facilities available, we have in most cases been able to relate these to the proportion of patients receiving such services, but it becomes much more problematic if one tries to assess how many more people would benefit from such services were they available. Furthermore the range and quality of services varies greatly, as we shall hope to show, so that mere quantification of data is somewhat unsatisfactory and there are very real dangers in attempting to 'rate' hospitals in an overall sense.

Nevertheless in a descriptive survey such as this, the application of statistical techniques for quantification is essential if we are to have an overall view of the provisions available in the country, as well as an over-view of the type of patients in the institutions. In order, therefore, to minimize the possible distortions resulting from quantitative analysis, a more intensive sociological study of the structure and functioning of two hospitals, one urban, one rural, was carried out.

Finally it was our intention to interpret the data in sociological terms; most research carried out in the field of subnormality in this country has been either medically or psychologically orientated. Where relevant we have tried to incorporate the findings of such

[1] This will be discussed more fully in Chapter 2 when dealing with problems of analysis.

---

for subnormal adults was 1,466 and for children 900. At that time out of 174 local health authorities, 123 had no adult hostel provision and 134 had no such provision for children. (*Health and Welfare: The Development of Community Care*, HMSO Command 3022, 1966.)

research, but we feel that sufficient data exists in relation to other types of institution, in particular prisons and mental hospitals, to indicate that a sociological approach has an additional and important contribution to make in understanding the world of the subnormality institution.

In the last fifty years an extensive literature has emerged, not only about the incidence and aetiology of mental deficiency, but about the range of social arrangements for the care of individuals who are handicapped in this way.[1] There has also been a growing, though still very inadequate, amount of research and from this, together with the experience of practitioners in the field of subnormality, certain propositions are gaining currency, paramount amongst them being the view that environmental factors are important in producing certain types of mental retardation. Further, it is now recognized that adequate social and educational provisions play an important part in preventing deterioration; experiments carried out by Tizard, Gunzberg, Gordon, Loos, Clarke and Hermelin, to name but a few, have made it clear that certain subnormal patients are capable of increased efficiency and improved literacy, given suitable supervision and stimulus.

Research on the implications of residential care, and on the education and training of subnormals, has so far involved quite small numbers. The question then arises – how realistic is it to extend such programmes and what are the factors that prevent their widespread acceptance in practice? Are the hospitals using their existing resources in the best possible way; is lack of money and/or staff the stumbling block; is it a question of size; or is the problem one of inertia both within the institution and in the field of public policy as a whole?

Much has been said and written about the desirability of caring for an increasing number of subnormal patients in the community, but as Mittler and Castell[2] point out, although the Ministry of Health plans are in their general formulation often praiseworthy, 'the regional and local proposals for carrying out these intentions are more doubtful'. Any study of institutional care must bear in mind in a realistic manner the available community provisions. It will serve no useful purpose to empty our hospitals on the grounds that they are outmoded and unsatisfactory, if the alternative provisions for care simply do not exist. There have already been difficulties of this nature in respect of mental illness. 'A determination

---

[1] For a full discussion of the problems of mental deficiency and its treatment the reader is referred to the work of Tizard and O'Connor (1956), Tizard (1964), Tizard and Grad (1961), Clarke and Clarke (1965), Susser and Kushlick (1961), Martin (1966), Penrose (1963), Tredgold and Soddy (1963), Lewis (1929) and others too numerous to mention.

[2] Mittler and Castell: "Hospital and Community Care of the Subnormal" in *The Lancet*, 18 April, 1964.

to keep a patient out of hospital at all costs cannot be accepted as a positive indication for community care'.[1]

In order to provide a meaningful framework for our own survey findings, Chapter 1 will attempt to give a brief outline of four important features of the background to subnormality:

The meaning of subnormality and the ways in which various definitions and classifications have developed in Britain; how a system of institutional care has developed in relation to changing public attitudes; popular conceptions about subnormality; and information regarding prevalence.

Chapter 1

SOCIAL ASPECTS OF SUBNORMALITY

Historical development

THE problem of mental subnormality is not new, for history and literature are full of references to individuals who were considered incapable of participating in ordinary life on account of their 'dull wits'. Before the advent of modern medical science, medical abnormalities of all kinds were explained in terms of the intervention of supernatural forces, this being particularly true in the case of what would now be termed psychotic illness. But epilepsy was also interpreted as spirit possession, whether by good or evil spirits depending upon the social context, and gross physical deformities such as dwarfism or hydrocephalus could be explained in folk law by the activities of witches and demons in working spells or leaving changeling children in the night.

From what we now know about the physiological states associated with the most acute forms of mental subnormality, it seems likely that the problem of the grossly subnormal was taken care of by the high rates of infant mortality that affected the population as a whole. In the absence of medical care, only the fittest babies survived beyond the cradle; moreover it is quite likely that children born with gross physical deformities were less seriously cared for. But this is not to say that empirical distinctions were not made between 'idiots' and 'lunatics'. O'Connor and Tizard[1] note that in the early fourteenth century a distinction was drawn for the purpose of deciding whether a person could be allowed to inherit property and manage it. A man who had lost his reason through madness was presumed to be capable of recovering it, whereas 'born fools' were believed never to have had any understanding, and could therefore be properly deprived of their legal rights to manage their inheritance. The corollary of this was for the King as *parens patrie* to assume rights over the fool and his property as if he were an 'infant' – that other legal category of person who is deemed incapable of managing his own affairs. This principle, whereby the Crown assumed legal responsibility for persons considered to be socially incompetent has come down to the present day in the form of guardianship by the State. It also explains in part the view that socially incompetent people are to be regarded as *children*, a view which is perhaps understandable in the case of the grossly

---

[1] O'Connor and Tizard: *The Social Problem of Mental Deficiency*, Pergamon Press (1956).

subnormal who are unable to acquire the most basic skills such as speech, or the capacity to feed and dress themselves, facilities which children normally develop in the first few years of life.

But only a minority of those who are mentally defective are grossly subnormal, and therefore by no means all of them require the kind of physical care and attention that is normally lavished on very young children.

It is important to recognize that the demands made upon the intellect in pre-industrial society were not, comparatively speaking, very great. In the days when the bulk of the population worked on the land, it was not necessary to read and write. Thus those individuals who nowadays have great difficulty in becoming literate and numerate, and who present a problem in a society that demands basic educational skills of all its members, would, in former years have been a little more easily accommodated in an occupational structure that depended very largely on manual dexterity and simple reasoning powers.

Historically then, it was the grossly subnormal who were first recognized. Those who survived infancy yet still required physical care were, until the eighteenth century, dealt with either in the family or in the various charitable institutions for the care of the chronic sick. The eighteenth century saw, however, the beginning of the movement to train the mentally deficient, essentially in terms of the psychology which was accepted at that time.

Reason was regarded as the mainspring of human behaviour, and it was assumed that people behaved as they did on the basis of the sensations they experienced, either of pleasure or of pain, of satisfaction or discomfort. The first known attempt to train defectives appears in the work of Pereire who developed his technique out of his experience in training the deaf. In France, J. M. Itard discovered a 'wild' boy in the woods near Aveyron, whom he attempted to train in the ways of civilization. Itard's method, like that of Pereire, was based on the theory of sensationism and he managed to teach the boy, known as Victor, certain skills, even the use of words. By giving him hot baths, Itard claimed to have developed his sensory perception of warmth, and therefore stimulated him to wear clothes. In 1801 Itard published his *Wild Boy of Aveyron*, which was translated into English in 1932, and has recently (1962) appeared in a second edition. Commenting on the experiment, O'Connor and Tizard[1] write:

> His final state was very different from that of the normal adolescent, but the changes achieved by education are a remarkable testimony to the value of the training and treatment of grossly backward people. (p. 3)

Itard's contemporary, Pinel, took a contrary view to sensationism, namely nativism, by which he meant that knowledge, or the capacity

[1] *op. cit.*

to acquire it, was not the result of learning but of heredity. In his *Treatise on Alienism* (1806) he argued that the fundamental principles of the institutional care of both defectives and lunatics was a constant round of mechanical work, both to train the faculties and to prevent the recurrence of disturbing thoughts. As far as defectives were concerned, the training could relate only to those faculties that the patient already possessed; nature could not be improved upon. Pinel's theory of nativism was accepted by his successor in France, Seguin, who in 1846 published his *The Psychological Treatment, Hygiene and Education of Idiots* as a handbook for institutional care. He had been responsible for the establishment of a training centre in Paris in 1837. Seguin appears not only to have been concerned with teaching patients to eat, dress, and keep themselves clean, but also to perform work tasks. In 1848 he went to the United States where he was responsible for laying the foundations of institutional care for defectives in that country.

In the latter years of the nineteenth century an important distinction came to be made between the severely subnormal and those who were markedly less so, and the terms 'idiot' and 'imbecile' on the one hand, and 'feeble minded' on the other came into use. Bearing in mind what has been said earlier about the relatively undemanding nature of agricultural and unskilled employment, it is scarcely surprising that the growth of industrialism began to reveal a group of mentally subnormal individuals whose presence had not been previously apparent, in contrast to the obvious handicaps of the grossly subnormal. The operation of the labour market in the nineteenth century effectively depressed handicapped people of all kinds to the bottom of the market, and it is clear that among the legions of the destitute and vagrant who existed in the cities of Victorian England, there were many who fell into the category of feeble-minded.

Although around the turn of the century educational psychologists, notably Binet, began to make it possible, through the perfection of intelligence testing, to distinguish between various grades of mental subnormality, the concepts employed by the legislators were very confused. Until the Report of the Royal Commission on the Care and Control of the Feeble-Minded in 1908 the terms 'idiot', 'imbecile' and 'feeble-minded' were often employed as if they were synonymous, and to confuse matters even more, the Lunacy Act of 1890 used the term 'idiot' in its definition of certain classes of lunatics.

The development of mental tests, in particular the Binet-Simon test, had social effects which extended far beyond the sphere of technical diagnosis. As early as the 1870s, the Italian criminologist Lombroso had put forward theories of degeneracy as accounting for the behaviour of the criminal and the socially incompetent, and had conducted a great deal of observation on institutional populations, arguing that amongst other things, social atavism was correlated with physical abnormalities. Although Lombroso's theories underwent very considerable modification, the concept of 'degeneracy' with all its eugenic connotations, was one that engaged an enormous amount of attention among those who were concerned with the problems of the socially incompetent, whether their incompetence took the form of poverty or crime, or as was often the case, both. Given a lack of adequate provisions for the care of the mentally handicapped, especially the feeble-minded, it is not surprising that many of them found their way into work-houses and prisons. Although Charles Goring[1] in his study with Karl Pearson found no evidence to support the original Lombrosian thesis about crime, he did find a number of severely handicapped criminals, a substantial proportion of whom were almost certainly feeble-minded. Later he added moral defectiveness as a constitutional factor in order to account for the conduct of some serious offenders who were neither physically nor mentally inferior. The eugenics movement however was probably more concerned with the possible proliferation of mentally subnormal (and therefore socially incompetent) people who would contribute increasingly to such problems as poverty and illegitimacy. The work done in the United States by Dugdale (1910), Estabrook (1916) on the Juke family and by Goddard (1912 and 1914) on the Kallikak family and the Vineland Training School for Defectives, had the effect of giving a scientific *imprimatur* to the belief that mental defect was, *and could only be*, inherited. If this was so, and defectives were allowed to marry and procreate in large numbers (as it was feared they would) then pauperism, crime, and illegitimacy would increase, and the quality of the race go into a progressive decline. The extent to which the anxiety of the eugenicists developed can be judged by a statement made by Fernald in 1912:[2]

> The feeble-minded are a parasitic, predatory class, never capable of self-support, or of managing their own affairs. The great majority become public charges in some form. They cause unutterable sorrow at home and a menace and danger to the community. Feeble-minded women are almost invariably immoral and if at large usually become carriers of venereal disease or give birth to children who are as defective as themselves. Every feeble-minded person, especially the high grade imbecile, is a potential criminal, needing only the proper environment and opportunity for the development and expression of his criminal tendencies.

In this climate of opinion, it is hardly surprising that it was widely held that defectives ought to be controlled as far as possible and prevented from reproducing at all costs. Tredgold (1909) wrote an article in the *Eugenics Review* entitled 'The Feeble-Minded: A Social

---

[1] Goring, C.: *The English Convict: A Statistical Study*, London HMSO (1913). See also Mannheim, H. (ed.), Driver, E.: in *Pioneers in Criminology*, Stevens and Co. Ltd. (1960).
[2] Quoted by Tizard in Clarke and Clarke (1965), p. 16.

Danger', and argued the case for segregation in his *Textbook on Mental Deficiency* (1908) a view held right through to the eighth edition of this book, as late as 1952. A Statutory Instrument was added to the Mental Deficiency Act of 1913 aimed at preventing the attachment of any defective on licence to a person of the opposite sex, and the Criminal Law itself made it an offence for any male person to have carnal knowledge of a female certified as defective. The most effective way of controlling defectives was to keep them in institutions, and according to O'Connor and Tizard[1] sterilization continues to be carried out in certain American states.

Contemporary writing about mental defect is highly critical of the studies of half a century ago that gave such apparent scientific validity to the fear that mental defectives were a parasitic menace to society. Within a few years it became apparent that Goddard's early reliance on the Binet-Simon test, without standardizing it on a normal adult population, had led him erroneously to believe that vast numbers of criminals were defective, and therefore all defectives were potential criminals.

Improvements in the tests themselves brought about a change in the alleged proportion of defectives among the delinquent and criminal, and as Cressey[2] has shown, the proportion shrank by fantastic amounts in studies between 1915 and 1930.

As for those frequently described as socially incompetent, the large families in poverty and in constant receipt of welfare benefits, it appears from recent work that the role of low intelligence is by no means as paramount as formerly thought, and that psychopathy and psychosis are also features of problem families (*vide* Blacker 1952). Moreover, it is now increasingly recognized that social factors can in some circumstances, restrict the expression of intelligence. Whilst genetic factors may be of considerable importance at the lowest level of intelligence, people with IQ 70 and above vary greatly in the extent to which their intellectual potential has or has not been stultified by their environment. According to Penrose,[3] whereas idiots and imbeciles suffer primarily from handicaps which are biological, the feeble-minded suffer largely from handicaps which are socially determined.

Large scale studies of intelligence in recent years have not substantiated the fear that the intellectual quality of the population is declining[4] and research in the whole field of mental defect has established that although genetic factors are responsible for some

---

[1] *op. cit.*

[2] Sutherland and Cressey: *Principles of Criminology*, Lippincott Co., Chicago (1960).

[3] Penrose, L. S.: *The Biology of Mental Defect*, London, Sidgwick and Jackson (1963).

[4] See for example, Maxwell, J.: *The Level and Trend of National Intelligence*, University of London Press (1961).

forms of mental subnormality, there are other strictly environmental factors that are no less important.

Changing concepts and definitions

As has been indicated already, our society has not found it easy to identify those who are mentally handicapped. Scientific knowledge about mental processes and human development remains, even today, more limited than knowledge in other fields of scientific enquiry. Mental abnormality and mental subnormality tend to be confused in the mind of the layman, and in the last century, the attempts of legislators to provide for the mentally subnormal were confused by the vague and ill-defined terminology that was employed by doctors, laymen and legislators alike. Moreover, the criteria employed by medical men tends to change at a different rate from that used by lawyers, a situation only too clearly illustrated in the misunderstandings in the forensic field where the Courts found the greatest difficulty in understanding that mental states cannot easily be considered as distinct phenomena in water-tight classificatory compartments.

The Idiots Act of 1886 did however make a distinction between lunatics and mental defectives, and distinguished a further category of defectives less handicapped than the idiot, namely the imbecile. By the time the Royal Commission on the Deaf and Dumb had been set up in 1889, it was recognized that in addition to 'educable imbeciles' there was another category, the 'feeble-minded', who needed to be separated from ordinary children and given special educational care. The Departmental Committee of 1897, charged with enquiring into the educational facilities for subnormal children, came to the conclusion that idiot and imbecile children could not be educated to become wholly or partially self-supporting while the feeble-minded could be so trained. By the time of the Report of the Royal Commission on the Care and Control of the Feeble-Minded in 1908, a clear continuum of mental subnormality was beginning to emerge, with a good deal of interest being concentrated on the upper levels, that is the feeble-minded, who, because they were more likely to be 'at large' in the community, were seen as constituting the most immediate social problem.

The Mental Deficiency Act of 1913, which, as amended in 1927, was to provide the legislative criteria of subnormality until it was repealed by the Mental Health Act of 1959, defined mental defectiveness as:

> ... a condition of arrested or incomplete development of mind, existing before the age of eighteen years, whether arising from inherent causes or induced by disease or injury.

This legal definition gives no exact criteria of the condition, leaving a wide margin for interpretation, and it is interesting to note that with a passage of time, legal draftsmen have become no more enamoured of precision than they were. The Homicide Act 1957, in setting out the criteria of diminished responsibility in Section II, employs strikingly similar terminology referring to an accused person as possibly:

... suffering from such abnormality of mind (whether arising from a condition of arrested or retarded development of mind or any inherent causes or induced by disease or injury) ...

This definition was intended to get away from the absurdly archaic definition of responsibility in criminal cases embodied in the M'Naughten rules of 1843, in particular to cover the psychopath who did not fit neatly into the dichotomy of sane/insane, but a future historian of forensic medicine might be pardoned for confusing a definition of mental deficiency made in 1913 with a definition of diminished responsibility made in 1957.

The Mental Deficiency Act of 1913 identified four categories of person as 'defectives' within the meaning of the Act as follows:

(i) *Idiots* that is to say, persons in whose case there exists mental defectiveness of such a degree that they are unable to guard themselves against common physical dangers.

(ii) *Imbeciles* that is to say, persons in whose case there exists mental defectiveness which, though not amounting to idiocy, is yet so pronounced that they are incapable of managing themselves or their affairs, or, in the case of children, of being taught to do so.

(iii) *Feeble-minded persons* that is to say, persons in whose case there exists mental defectiveness which, though not amounting to imbecility, is yet so pronounced that they require care, supervision and control for their own protection or for the protection of others or, in the case of children, that they appear to be permanently incapable by reason of such defectiveness of receiving proper benefit from the instruction in ordinary schools.

(iv) *Moral defectives* that is to say, persons in whose case there exists mental defectiveness coupled with strongly vicious or criminal propensities and who require care, supervision and control for the protection of others.

Clearly this classification was based upon implied degrees of social competence increasing from the first to the third category; moral defectiveness was however something new and provided a useful way of disposing of those mentally abnormal offenders who could not be judged guilty but insane. Because of its concern with cognition as an essential element in criminal responsibility, the law still made heavy weather in some cases. John Thomas Straffen a 'high grade' defective, when first charged with child murder in 1952 was found insane and unfit to plead, the assumption being that his mental and intellectual state precluded his comprehension of the proceedings.

After he had escaped from Broadmoor and committed murder again, he was adjudged fit to stand trial, and was indeed sentenced to death. At the time, great play was made of the fact that he had learned to play bridge in Broadmoor, which was variously cited as evidence that he could be neither insane nor defective! Although it is not easy to prove, the chances are that those certified as moral defectives in the earlier part of this century may have included a substantial number of subnormal persons whose sexual promiscuity was socially problematic,[1] together with some whom we would now consider as psychopathic rather than defective, notwithstanding their low level of intellectual ability.

There can be little doubt that the work of the Royal Commission on the Law Relating to Mental Illness and Mental Deficiency which reported in 1957, bore substantial fruit in the form of the Mental Health Act of 1959. The last complete review of the Law Relating to Mental Illness had been the Lunacy Act, 1890, and that relating to Mental Deficiency in 1913. The Royal Commission noted that not only had the law become extremely complicated by virtue of the extensive amendments that had been made over the years, but that it embodied concepts and attitudes that were obsolete, both in the light of modern knowledge and articulate public opinion. Section 4 of the Mental Health Act 1959 sets out a series of definitions which are in most respects a distinct improvement on what had gone before. The five subsections of Section 4 are as follows:

(i) In this Act 'mental disorder' means mental illness, arrested or incomplete development of mind, psychopathic disorder, and any other disorder or disability of mind; and 'mentally disordered' shall be construed accordingly.

(ii) In this Act 'severe subnormality' means a state of arrested or incomplete development of mind which includes subnormality of intelligence and is of such a nature or degree that the patient is incapable of living an independent life or of guarding himself against serious exploitation, or would be so incapable when of an age to do so.

(iii) In this Act 'subnormality' means a state of arrested or incomplete development of mind (not amounting to severe subnormality) which includes subnormality of intelligence and is of a nature or degree which requires or is susceptible to medical treatment or other special care or training of the patient.

(iv) In this Act 'psychopathic disorder' means a persistent disorder or disability of the mind (whether or not including subnormality of intelligence) which results in abnormally aggressive or seriously irresponsible conduct on the part of the patient and requires or is susceptible to medical treatment.

[1] See Tizard in Clarke and Clarke: *Mental Deficiency: The Changing Outlook*, Methuen (1965).

(v) Nothing in this Section shall be construed as implying that a person may be dealt with under this Act as suffering from mental disorder, or from any form of mental disorder described in this Section, by reason only of promiscuity or other immoral conduct.

The most important aspect of the 1959 Act has undoubtedly been to make it possible for all kinds of mentally disordered people, whether mentally ill, mentally deficient, or psychopathic, to enter hospitals and other institutions for care and treatment informally, and so avoid the social stigma which was an invariable concomitant of the old procedures of certification. Although some patients must clearly be detained compulsorily, either for their own good or that of society, in the past certification was a barrier to treatment simply because it was so like a sentence of imprisonment. In practice very few patients of any kind need to be physically detained, although the criticism has been made by Dr. Ann Clarke[1] that the Act makes it easier compulsorily to detain patients over the age of twenty-five if they are severely subnormal.

There is an obvious temptation, therefore, to use this category in the case of difficult patients – a temptation that is apparently not always being resisted. (p. 52)

It still remains true that the term 'subnormality of intelligence' can be defined in a variety of ways, and it is therefore essential, in order to be more specific, to study the problem in more precise behavioural terms. We need to have data about personal, occupational, and social activities in order to select individuals for specific forms of treatment and care, and we need to be able to measure the effect of rehabilitation and to relate the activities of subnormal to normal people.

At this point it is perhaps useful to turn towards consideration of the various attempts that have been made to provide *clinical* measures of subnormality that are capable of quantification as a means of modifying the less well-defined *social* criteria that have been the basis of legal classification throughout this century.

The terms 'mental defective' and 'mental deficiency' have been used for many years to describe the mentally subnormal as a whole, irrespective of the extent of their subnormality, but they are tending to fall into disuse. The Act of 1959 refers to 'subnormality' and in the United States the term 'mental retardation' is widely used. Other synonyms are oligophrenia and amentia. According to Tizard[2] deficiency or subnormality begins at two standard deviations below the mean for intelligence, at 70 IQ. There are, of course, many problems raised by the testing of intelligence, in particular the variations that may result from the use of different tests, and the fact that there are distinct problems in the testing of children as opposed to

---

[1] Clarke and Clarke: *op. cit.*
[2] In Clarke and Clarke, *op. cit.*, p. 7.

adults.[1] The term mental retardation places stress on backwardness in intelligence as a necessary feature in subnormality and Tizard notes that an IQ of 85 is used to define the limit of 'sub-average intellectual functioning'. But, as he points out, whereas only about 2 per cent of the population have IQs below 70, about 16 per cent have IQs below 85. Tizard appears to prefer, on grounds of utility, the traditional method of employing *grades* of defect, that is idiots, imbeciles, and feeble-minded (or in American terminology, morons). Idiots and imbeciles are therefore referred to as low-grade defectives and the feeble-minded or moronic as high-grade defectives. Defective patients are usually classified as idiots if they have an IQ of less than 20 or, in the case of adults, test ages of less than three years.[2] E. O. Lewis (1929) placed the IQ limits of imbecility as between 20 and 45–50 in the case of children and 40 in the case of adults. Whereas few children with IQs around 50 are taught to read, there is some evidence that most *could* be taught simple reading; older imbeciles are now taught a few rudimentary things, and Tizard suggests that Lewis was unduly pessimistic about their social prospects. His argument is that the majority of imbeciles cannot survive in open employment, not because their general behaviour is unsatisfactory, but because they are 'too simple, and very frequently, too physically handicapped'. Above 50 IQ, subnormal individuals are regarded as feeble-minded or moronic. The great majority in this group (50 to 70 IQ) never come to public notice, except in the educational field where they may be defined as educationally subnormal, unless their low intelligence is coupled with physical disability, troublesome behaviour, or lack of a proper home. As has been suggested earlier in this chapter, the use of intelligence testing has a number of drawbacks when used as the sole criterion of mental deficiency. Quite apart from the intrinsic limitations of the various tests, there is a far from perfect relationship between social behaviour and IQ. Tredgold[3] rejects the use of intelligence tests as a criterion, just as he rejects the use of scholastic tests, and advocates what he calls a biological and social criterion, based on the notion that the essential purpose of mind is to enable the individual 'so to adapt himself to his environment as to maintain an independent existence'. Given that his contribution to the subject has spanned most of the period under discussion in this chapter it is not surprising that he has been criticized for basing his views on Mc-Dougall's theory of instincts and sentiments which, as Dr. Ann Clarke suggests '. . . few scientists today would accept as being either valid or useful'. The use of social criteria for the definition of mental deficiency has, it has been argued, resulted in the population of institutions containing a substantial number of patients with IQs

[1] See O'Connor and Tizard, *op. cit.*, pp. 12–13.
[2] For a further discussion of the use of IQ tests in practice see Chapter 4.
[3] Tredgold, A. F.: *A Textbook of Mental Deficiency*, Bailliere, Tindall and Cox, 8th edition (1952).

above the figure of 70.[1] According to Clarke,[2] something like a quarter of all mentally deficient patients confined in institutions in the mid nineteen-fifties had IQs of 70 or above. The inference to be drawn from these data is that the population of institutions contains a number of patients whose social rather than intellectual incompetence is the impediment to their re-absorption into the community and who might well be the subject of intensified training programmes.[3]

Popular conceptions about subnormality

It is not easy to generalize about public attitudes towards social issues, and such evidence as is presented here is based not on the conclusions of any surveys of opinion, but rather upon inferences drawn from the nature of the social techniques that have been employed to deal with the problem. If one notes a change in legislative language between the very titles of the Idiots Act of 1886 and the Mental Health Act of 1959, one can gauge something of the changes that have occurred in the most articulate sector of public opinion that has a direct influence on the formulation of social policy.

We know very little about how people actually felt about the mentally subnormal as distinct from the mentally ill in pre-industrial England, and from contemporary accounts it is reasonable to suppose that although they might be treated with public derision, in their families they were the objects of love and care. Wordsworth's Idiot Boy is movingly described as the object of his mother's affection, although he appears to have needed a great deal of supervision. Poor Barnaby Rudge on the other hand is caught up by the gin-soaked London mob of the Gordon Riots. Before this century the conditions of life, particularly for the poor, were such that the sufferings of most handicapped people were blurred by the all-prevailing poverty, disease and destitution that was the stuff of life for the majority of town dwellers. In terms of Christian charity the handicapped were the objects of compassion; in practice their submergence in the process of social Darwinism left them and their families no alternative but to survive as best they could.

Perhaps it is useful to point out at this stage that one of the handicaps experienced by the mentally subnormal, and one which they may have even yet to shake off, is their misfortune in having a mistaken identity. At various times they have been confused with the indigent poor, the criminal, the promiscuous carriers of venereal disease and the mentally ill. Where mental handicap has been aug-

---

[1] O'Connor and Tizard: 'A Survey of Patients in Twelve Mental Deficiency Institutions' in *British Medical Journal*, I, 16–18 (1954).
[2] In Clarke and Clarke, *op. cit.*
[3] See also Doll's 'Six Criteria of Mental Deficiency: The Essentials of an Inclusive Concept of Mental Deficiency' in *American Journal of Mental Deficiency*, 46, 214–19 (1941).

mented by physical handicap, they have been regarded at times as inferior stock, as if they were no better than some poor breed of cattle. Pauperism, quite apart from crime and delinquency was regarded as a self-evident evil by nineteenth-century middle-class society, and researches first of Lombroso and his pupils, and later the work of Dugdale and Goddard gave an air of scientific legitimacy to the beliefs of those who had earlier been attracted by the social implications of biological inferiority and superiority – a compassionate attitude towards the mentally subnormal could be decried as mistaken idealism. The perversion of Darwinian concepts in the field of social and political theory was as damaging as it was prolific.

Evolutionary theory was claimed as an explanation for the superiority of European civilization over the primitive and coloured peoples of the world; the primitives themselves were regarded as atavistic, and degeneracy was seen as a threat to progress. Worse than this, it was a charge on the Exchequer and the local rates. Hence in the eyes of the eugenic enthusiasts, the presence of the subnormal was a threat in economic and social terms. The whole question of mental development was, in some intellectual circles, bound up with the notion of evolutionary differences and thus with the relative inferiority of certain groups of mankind. It was widely assumed that primitives had the mentality of children and that they were an inferior species.

Whether seen as a danger, or merely an expensive social inconvenience, the view was held that society was wasting its efforts in preserving the grossly subnormal and ought to recognize that while the less severely subnormal might with some effort be accommodated for a period of their lives, they should as a group be guided towards extinction by setting every obstacle in the way of breeding. If physical sterilization was unpalatable, and euthanasia ethically intolerable, then the next best thing was the device of social euthanasia – the incarceration of the mentally subnormal in institutions where they would be unable to get into mischief and be for the most part out of sight. It is not without significance that the term 'Mental Defective *Colony*' was widely used to describe these institutions; for more than a century our society had exported its awkward members to penal settlements far beyond the seas, and the classic solution to the problem of the late Victorian or Edwardian misfit was for him to seek a new life 'in the Colonies'.

Although the eugenicists' fears that were widespread among the intelligentsia half a century ago are no longer voiced, and certainly play no part in the making of contemporary social policy, the filtration of their views to those unable to examine them critically has left a residue of folk belief about subnormality.[1] Goddard's work formed

---

[1] It is not suggested that all beliefs about subnormality derive from such a process of filtration. It is conceivable that other beliefs may be culturally transmitted from generation to generation and may be equally effective in reinforcing the stereotype of the subnormal.

the basis for the first article on mental defect to appear in the *Encyclopaedia Britannica* in 1919, and Murchison's *Handbook of Child Psychology* (1933) contained statements to the effect that feeble-mindedness was due almost exclusively to heredity, and that it was incurable. To identify a condition as 'incurable' is unlikely to encourage efforts to ameliorate the handicaps of the subnormal, let alone to enable them where possible to become self-supporting members of the community. Whereas the early and mid-nineteenth century was a period of comparative optimism concerning the subnormal in so far as the emphasis was upon training, the first half of this century has been characterized by varying degrees of pessimism, and it is only in very recent years that the public mood has swung towards a more positive view. However, there were signs of slow improvement in the inter-war years. For example Occupation Centres were founded, mainly by voluntary bodies, to provide an alternative to institutional care; between 1928 and 1954 the number of defectives in this kind of extra-mural care increased from some fourteen hundred to almost eleven thousand. But even this number is not large in relation to total population and the capacity of these individuals to be economically self-sufficient was limited, particularly during the depression years, by the state of the labour market.

Probably the most widespread belief about the mentally subnormal or defective relates to their lack, in varying degrees, of the basic social skills. Most people think of them as children; this is understandable in that the grossly defective may not be able to speak or communicate even as well as nursery school children, nor to wash or dress themselves, nor use cutlery. The feeble-minded, even though they are far more skilled than this, may still appear to react to external stimuli much as children do, and may be less competent in the management of everyday matters than are some children. This child stereotype has undoubtedly been reinforced to a very considerable degree by virtue of the fact that the uncovering of the problem of feeble-mindedness came about very largely through the introduction of compulsory education. From 1870 onwards the State became responsible, not only for providing schools for all, but for seeing that children attended them, and it was only a matter of time before the dimensions of the problem of educational subnormality began to be revealed.[1] Faced for the first time with having to educate large numbers of children, more often than not in large classes, public authorities soon became aware of the need to identify levels of ability and to separate out those who were dull or ineducable. For this purpose, intelligence testing was of considerable use, and over fifty years the use of the intelligence test has reached a point where it has become one of the most formidable mechanisms of social selection known to man.

[1] See the terms of reference of the Royal Commission on the Blind, Deaf and Dumb of the United Kingdom, 1899, and the Report of the Departmental Committee on Defective and Epileptic Children, 1898.

Quite apart from the profound effect testing has had on normal children in the allocation of educational and therefore social opportunity, it has, by identifying certain children as educationally subnormal, succeeded in excluding them in yet another way from normal society. This is not to say that special educational provision for such children is not desirable, although whether their segregation in special schools, as opposed to special classes, is desirable, is another matter. The folk term 'Dippy School' though less commonly used in the vernacular of school children than a generation ago, has not disappeared. Moreover the provision of special schools for the educationally subnormal has been lamentably inadequate,[1] and many ESN children have had to manage as best they could in ordinary schools. The problems involved in the education of normal children have been such that, in Tizard's words:

> ... from the time of the First World War the primary concern of teachers and educational psychologists with imbeciles and idiots has been that of excluding them from school. (Clarke and Clarke, 1965, p. 19)

Most educational efforts have, not surprisingly, been concentrated upon the dull and educationally subnormal rather than upon the severely subnormal. Nevertheless the resources for special schools for the ESN have to some extent been limited by the need to provide other forms of special school, for example for the emotionally maladjusted, and for the delinquent. Many maladjusted children are academically backward not through mental defect but through emotional disturbance, but the pedagogic problems they present may be equally acute. In the allocation of educational resources, therefore, the mentally subnormal have not been the only group with special needs.

The Report of the Royal Commission on the Law Relating to Mental Illness and Mental Deficiency (1957) went a great way to providing a new charter for the treatment of the mentally handicapped, but clearly there are still vast areas of misconception, prejudice and even fear about the problem. A doctor in one subnormality hospital visited told the research worker that members of his golf club admit to driving faster as they pass the entrance to the hospital. Nor are such views confined to laymen; a consultant psychiatrist in charge of a mental subnormality hospital has strong misgivings about Local Authority Rehabilitative Hostels and in an unpublished paper (1964) writes:

---

[1] We are not here arguing the case for separate schools as opposed to separate classes, since the writer does not feel competent to pronounce on that matter – we simply make the point that so long as it remains government policy to provide such schools, we feel that they should be adequate to meet the needs of the population.

These hostels should in every case be separated, for sexual problems loom high in the lives of these patients; homosexuality, child assault, rape, exposure with the men and prostitution and some perversion with the women. Ideally the men's hostel should be in one town and the women's in a neighbouring one. They should be at least two or three miles apart. Social contacts between the two hostels should be discouraged to prevent illicit 'affairs' and marriages among the subnormal'.[1]

The development of institutional care

How did the mentally subnormal come to be accommodated as they are now? First, it should be pointed out that institutional care is one of the means whereby society controls what are, in the most general terms, socially pathological phenomena. Because of behavioural peculiarities or the existence of special problems, certain individuals cannot easily be contained within the framework of society. Some of them are mentally ill, some are delinquent and criminal, some are physically handicapped, some are intellectually handicapped, yet others are aged or senile. It might be thought unreasonable to lump together people with such a wide variety of handicaps, because they differ very widely in terms of the extent to which they can be held personally and morally responsible for their condition. Moreover the situation is confused in that there is sometimes an overlap between behaviour which is seen as culpable and that which is not; the cruel parent who is also mentally deficient is a case in point.[2] The anger of the community has to be tempered by a recognition of a morally neutral handicap. But it remains true that one of the most common ways in which industrial societies like ours have come to deal with problematic individuals, whether they be mongols or alcoholics, schizophrenics or persistent thieves, is to contain them within institutions which, although they vary in the degrees of freedom permitted to the inmates, possess in common the characteristics of what Goffman (1961) has termed *total institutions*.[3] These characteristics are more than social, they are often given highly concrete physical reality in the form of their all too solid buildings. One has only to look at an Ordnance Survey map for the words 'prison', 'asylum', 'mental defective colony' in order to see the similarity of their ground plans. Furthermore, the presence of a building set apart from the rest of human settlement gives some substance to the vague folk beliefs concerning the individuals who spend their lives in comparative isolation from their fellows.

---

[1] Compare this with Fernald writing in 1912 (see p. 10 *supra*). It should be noted, however, that the views expressed by this psychiatrist appear to be atypical of consultants in the field of subnormality.

[2] See Gibbens and Walker: *Cruel Parents*, I.S.T.D. (1956).

[3] This will be discussed in greater detail in Chapter 13.

Secondly, there is internal variety within the system; because of the differential evaluation of problematic behaviour, whether it be the incontinence of an idiot, or the violence of a psychopath, different instutitions will have different systems of recognition of patient rights – or social 'charters'. The nature of the 'charter' will vary; it may be primarily punitive, educative, custodial or curative – undoubtedly there will be considerable overlap – but whatever the 'charter' of the institution, it is likely to possess in common with other total institutions certain organizational features which will have a fundamental bearing on life within the institution for both the inmates and the staff. There will be lines of command and chains of responsibility; there will be a social gap between those who control and those who are controlled. There will be a staff culture and an inmate culture in varying degrees of sophistication. And the institution will have meaning and purpose, not only within its own frame of reference, but for the community outside.

The first institutions for defectives in England were established in the 1840s – O'Connor and Tizard[1] give the date as 1847. Certainly by the time of the passing of the Idiots Act of 1886 there were four large hospitals which had been in existence for some years. However, the kind of regime established by Seguin in France and America and by his followers in this country in the early and middle parts of the nineteenth century, should not be confused with the institutional practices which developed in the later years of the century. Here there are parallels with both prisons and mental hospitals, both of which went through a vigorous experimental phase around the middle of the century and then settled into a largely negative and custodial inertia as it became administratively popular to build large barrack-like institutions.

The provision of institutions for the grossly subnormal that had preceded the 1886 Act had been due to the efforts of the same general charitable movement that had also provided reformatory and industrial schools and orphanages, but the emphasis had been on helping those individuals whose handicaps were extreme. As the rest of the picture came into focus, so another sector of voluntary effort turned its attention to the feeble-minded in which two bodies played a notable part, the National Association for Promoting the Welfare of the Feeble-Minded, founded in 1895, and the Lancashire and Cheshire Society for the Permanent Care of the Feeble-Minded, founded in 1902. In the years between 1906 and 1914, when the attention of the government of the day turned to a whole range of issues in the field of social policy, the mentally subnormal in general, and the feeble-minded in particular, gained serious attention and this led to the Mental Deficiency Act of 1913. The effect of this Act, in providing additional accommodation, resulted in the numbers in

[1] *op. cit.*

institutional care increasing by nearly a third within a year.[1] Between 1916 and 1950 the numbers of patients in institutions rose from about 6·5 thousand to about 57·5 thousand. However in the short run the Act undoubtedly contributed to a general reduction in the *prison* population, and to the numbers of prisoners with severe mental and physical handicaps in particular.

Estimations of the prevalence of subnormality

Some of the problems involved in deciding just what is implied by the concept of subnormality and how it may be measured and defined in its various degrees have been indicated in the foregoing discussion, and it can be argued that for administrative and legal purposes there has been a heavy reliance on functional social definitions which accord more or less with prevailing social concepts and conditions. These in turn have tended to define the social status of the subnormal in the same way that they have contributed towards the definition of the status of other handicapped members of society. As the social and economic integration of the handicapped becomes more feasible, so the social relevance of being handicapped diminishes. Thus the blind, because of their tendency towards alternative sensory compensation, have been able to do a large number of jobs and lead remarkably normal lives. Those suffering from other physical handicaps have only very recently been able to enjoy sheltered employment through such organizations as Remploy and the legal obligation on firms and organizations above a certain size to include a quota of handicapped persons on their pay-rolls. Formerly such individuals would have been relegated to the category of unemployable. As we have noted earlier in this chapter, industrial technology, educational provisions and the labour market itself, each affect public awareness.

Estimating the prevalence of subnormality depends however, not merely on *definition*, which enables the researcher to know what he is looking for, but on social, administrative, and economic factors which result in focussing public attention upon the problem. Such factors may equally well, at certain times, combine to obscure such public awareness.

Surveys of subnormality began in the early years of this century, as a result of public concern focused on the issues of education and control. The study made by Binet and Simon in France in 1907 was contemporaneous with the work of the Royal Commission on the Feeble-Minded which began in 1906. The Commission took its task seriously and conducted a Census from a large number of sources ranging from educational authorities and Poor Law institutions, to the police, the Prison Commission, and homes for inebriates. Bearing in mind the relative lack of sophistication of survey techniques at

[1] *Board of Control Annual Report* (1914), quoted by O'Connor and Tizard (1956), p. 8.

that time, and the considerable possibilities of error at certain of their sources, the findings of the Commission have to be interpreted with a good deal of caution.

In the total population the Commission estimated that 4·6 per thousand were mentally deficient 'apart from certified lunatics'. The 'certified lunatics' would almost certainly have included some who were mentally subnormal, and conversely, some classified as mental defectives were probably mentally ill. But given these qualifications, it is interesting to note that they found wide variation in the prevalence of deficiency between different areas of the country. In some they found a figure of 1·35 per thousand while in others the figure was as high as 4·68 per thousand. Figures of over 4 per thousand were most common. They estimated the national distribution of idiots, imbeciles and feeble-minded persons as 6 per cent, 18 per cent, and 76 per cent respectively of the total population of defective persons. Most of the American surveys conducted at about this time reported similar prevalence rates of about 4 per thousand.

The most thorough survey of mental deficiency was carried out by E. O. Lewis for the Inter-Departmental Committee on Mental Deficiency (the Wood Committee) and published in 1929. The Wood Report indicated that there were almost twice as many defective persons in England and Wales in 1929 as there were some 20 years before. It was suggested that this increase might well be more apparent than real, in that survey methods had considerably improved in the intervening period. It is also the case that reporting is not merely a function of the adequacy of diagnostic criteria, but of local variations in awareness of the problem. Commenting on a Ministry of Health survey in 1951, where the rates varied from 0·040 per cent in Carmarthen and Merthyr Tydfil to 0·579 per cent in Sunderland, O'Connor[1] expresses the view that these variations reflect local health policy. When he correlated the rates with the expenditure on the Care of Mothers and Young Children he found a coefficient of +0·40, suggesting that those local authorities who spent most on the care of mothers and children would also be those most likely to ascertain more cases of defect. Since the provision of health and welfare services was more advanced in 1928 than it had been in 1908, it is perhaps not surprising that the Wood Report gave a figure of 8·57 per thousand, nearly twice that reported by the Royal Commission in 1908. The proportion of idiots, imbeciles and feeble-minded were however remarkably similar, being 4 per cent, 18 per cent and 78 per cent respectively.

Two important points made by the Wood Report were the association of defectiveness with social class and the differences in ascertainment noted by age. Whereas the latter is likely to be related to the educational situation, class differences are important with respect to the eugenic controversy that was by no means dead at the time of the

[1] In Clarke and Clarke, *op. cit.*

Report. Given a greater prevalence of mental deficiency among the poorer sections of the community, the pattern of differential fertility between rich and poor which was established some forty years before would, it was argued, result in a decline in national intelligence. Tredgold[1] had forcefully put the point that if society decided to prolong the existence of the unfit, then it had the duty to see that they 'did not propagate their kind'. The period between the two wars was, however, a rather exceptional one in demographic history in that the rate of population increase fell back to its lowest point since the beginning of the Industrial Revolution and the pattern of differential fertility was defined with exceptional sharpness. These were the years, *par excellence*, of the childless or one child middle-class family.

Although the suggestion of a decline in national intelligence is now to all intents and purposes discredited, the problem of social class differences in the incidence of various forms of handicap remains. In industrial societies parents of severely subnormal children are evenly distributed among all the social classes, whilst those of mildly subnormal children come mainly from the lower social strata. In the absence of abnormal neurological signs, almost no children of higher social class parents have IQ scores of less than 80. There is new evidence to suggest that class differences in IQ reflect cultural differences as well as the social and material disadvantages of the lower social classes resulting from lack of access to, or use of, medical and educational services[2].

The most important question that tends to be asked is whether the incidence of mental subnormality has increased over the years. It is not by any means easy to answer, in view of the variations in the criteria of definition that have been employed in the last forty or fifty years, and the fact that social and administrative factors play such an important part in the identification of the problem, factors which themselves vary not only over time, but from place to place. Furthermore trends in the prevalence of severe subnormality are not necessarily the same as those for mild subnormality. Thus amongst children there appears to be a decrease in severe subnormality, except in cases of mongolism, but if adults as well as children are considered, there appears to be an increase, possibly due partly to the increased survival of hydrocephalic children as well as mongols. On the other hand trends in the prevalence of mild subnormality suggest that the numbers may be decreasing, certainly the number of such patients who are hospitalized has fallen since 1938.[3] Tizard examines the possibility that any change may be due to an artifact, or to different criteria being employed. Alternatively it may be due to the existence

[1] Tredgold, A. F.: 'The Feeble-Minded: A Social Danger', *Eugenics Review*, 1, 100–103 (1909).

[2] See Kushlick, A.: 'A Community Service for the Mentally Subnormal', *Soc. Psychiatry*, Vol. 1, No. 2, 1966, pp. 73–82.

[3] See Kushlick, *op. cit.*

of confusion in the 1920s between mental retardation and certain forms of physical handicap. The implication is that the earlier estimates may have been in the pessimistic direction. On the other hand, the improvement in training facilities, in the light of the knowledge that the early education of educable mentally retarded children can raise their test intelligence, may mean there are fewer classified imbeciles.

The incidence of certain specific forms of defect, for example those resulting from congenital syphilis, has certainly decreased, and the changes in general health and welfare that have been associated with the decline in infant mortality have also resulted in changes in morbidity. Tizard also takes the view that the close association between biological and social factors ought not to be overlooked. The mothers of mentally handicapped children have a high incidence of obstetric abnormalities, and these are paralleled by a low birth weight for mentally retarded children. Fairweather and Illsley (1960) note the association of these factors with poor maternal health and physique, which in turn are related to poor social conditions and low IQ. Although the socio-economic differences still exist, the first half of this century saw substantial improvements in nutrition and in ante-natal and post-natal care. It is also possible that changes in the pattern of fertility may have had some effect, in that the number of very large families has declined and women are completing their families at an earlier age. Older mothers, and mothers of large families are more likely, according to Tizard, to have children with physical defects and possible mental defects.

Tizard's general conclusion is that there has been a decline of about a third in the 'administrative prevalence' of severe subnormality which may be due entirely to artifact, but it is possibly due to the decline in the true prevalence brought about by better medical care and better nutrition at source. On the other hand, mongolism, according to data prepared by Carter[1] and Goodman and Tizard[2] appears to have increased about four-fold. This is due almost entirely, not to changes in the proportion of mongols among live births, but to increased chances of survival. About 50 per cent of all mongol children die before the age of one, most of them within a few months of birth. However between the ages of 5 and 40 the mortality rate is only slightly above that of the normal population (i.e. only 3 to 7 per cent higher) and only after the age of 40 does the survival rate drop sharply.[3]

On the basis of present information it is still only possible to

[1] Carter, C. O.: 'A Life-Table for Mongols with the Causes of Death', *J. Ment. Defic. Res.*, 2, 64–74 (1958).

[2] Goodman and Tizard: 'Prevalence of Imbecility and Idiocy among Children', *Brit. Med. J.*, 1, 216–19 (1962).

[3] Forssman, H. and Akesson, H. O.: 'Mortality in Patients with Down's Syndrome', *J. Ment. Def. Res.*, Vol. 9, 146–50 (1965).

hazard guesses of varying degrees of reliability about the prevalence of *all* forms of mental retardation in the absence of adequate survey data based on national samples, and not confined (as most recent studies have been) to severe subnormality. Perhaps only one thing is certain, as O'Connor and Tizard (1956) remark:

> Prevalence surveys of mental deficiency have differed in many ways. They are alike in one respect: all have revealed a much higher prevalence of subnormality than any society is known to make provision for. (p. 27)

Chapter 2

THE DESIGN OF THE SURVEY

PRELIMINARY discussions and a survey of the literature, started in February 1964.[1] A small pilot study was carried out between May and July of that year when periods of between one and four weeks were spent in three large hospitals,[2] in one of which the researcher worked as a nurse in an attempt to ascertain some of the nursing problems peculiar to subnormality. In addition, some days were spent visiting residential homes for the subnormal. Much later in the research, when the hospital visits had been completed, the additional information available about the nature of the research problem prompted us to pilot the homes more systematically and further visits were paid by those interviewers who had been involved in work in the hospitals.

Between August 1964 and March 1965 lists of hospitals and homes were prepared and preliminary questionnaires drafted.

Sampling procedures

From a combination of the Hospitals Year Book for 1964 and the Registrar General's Statistical Review (1960) Mental Health Supplement, it was relatively easy to devise a list of National Health Service Hospitals for the subnormal. A letter was sent in October 1964 to all Regional Hospital Boards, requesting information about the number of beds and details of the units and annexes under each Medical Superintendent. From this information a list of hospitals and available beds was prepared from which the sample could be drawn. It was decided for the purpose of this research to define a hospital as a group of patients and staff, whether housed together in a single complex or not, under the charge of a single Medical Superintendent or his representative. Such complexes will be described in greater detail in Chapter 5 when discussing the physical setting of the hospitals, but the kind of complex we found to exist most frequently comprised an administrative block (usually an old mansion) with a number of villas and various outbuildings all on one site, with six or seven other

[1] Preliminary discussions and pilot visits were carried out by Mrs. Lucianne Sawyer before the present writer was engaged on the project.

[2] After initial appoaches had been made to a fourth hospital, they declined to allow us access in order to carry out a pilot enquiry.

mansions, large Victorian houses, or old workhouses on different sites, often separated by many miles. By these criteria seventy-eight such complexes were identified.[1]

To obtain a satisfactory list of registered homes and nursing homes[2] did not prove so easy: information regarding the names and addresses of these homes, as well as the number and type of patients in their care was obtained from lists provided by the National Society for Mentally Handicapped Children, the National Association of Mental Health, and local authority returns to the Ministry of Health. No central register of such homes appears to exist, and the lists from which we worked were often out of date. This is no reflection on the organizations concerned, but is thought to arise largely because of frequent changes of use occurring in the homes.[3] Furthermore, the Ministry of Health's figures for those in homes do not differentiate between the mentally ill and the mentally subnormal, and in view of the wide discrepancies between the anticipated number of subnormal persons and the actual number found, we think it likely that homes vary the use to which they put their beds and do not make a clear distinction between the two groups.

Selection of National Health Service hospitals

The sample design is described in detail in Appendix A. As hospitals varied greatly in size, four size strata based on number of beds, were used in drawing the sample of hospitals. Within the strata hospitals were arranged in Regional Hospital Board areas before selection and random selection methods were used in the four strata. This design was based upon the proposition that the appropriate unit of analysis would nearly always be the patient rather than the hospital, that is, how many patients were living under various conditions.[4] No weighting has been necessary when describing *sampled* patients, but any discussion of the *total* patient population in the sampled hospitals has involved weighting. Four hospitals were excluded before the sample was selected, three because they were used in the pilot survey, and one which had refused permission. Two hospitals in the sample, both in the West Scottish Region, declined to co-operate with

---

[1] The Hospital Year Book for 1966 indicates that on 31 March, 1964, there were 195 subnormality hospitals in England and 12 in Wales. This discrepancy with our figure arises because the Year Book uses the words 'subnormality hospital' to comprise a hospital unit under a single *Management Committee*. Furthermore these figures do not include Scotland. The Registrar General's Statistical Review lists 147 subnormality hospitals.

[2] Also included in this sample were residential communities and schools run by voluntary organizations, as well as voluntary hospitals.

[3] In 1965 there were 22 new registrations of homes and 22 dropped out. This involved the provision of 533 new beds and the cancellation of 344, an overall gain of 189 beds. (Ministry of Health Report, 1966, Command 3039.)

[4] See Kish, L.: *Am. Soc. Rev.*, Vol. 30, No. 4, August 1965, pp. 564–72

the research.[1] In one instance it was claimed that a considerable amount of research work was already being carried out in the hospital, and in the other case the Superintendent expressed the view that it 'might disrupt the normal routine'. He also pointed out that major structural alterations were being undertaken and the information collected would be out-of-date by the time of publication.[2] As a result, Scotland was represented in the sample by only two small hospitals.

In retrospect, there is some doubt as to whether the size of the administrative unit was a meaningful criterion for examining these hospitals. At the time the sample frame was drawn up we did not fully appreciate the extent to which patterns of care would vary even within hospitals of approximately the same size.[3] For example one hospital complex with over 2,000 occupied beds comprised a main unit of over 1,500 beds and eleven ancillary units radiating to a distance of some 52 miles, and with the number of occupied beds for subnormal patients ranging from 12 to 202; nor did all units share the same management committee. The staff of some of these units did not see themselves as in any way connected with the parent hospital, except in so far as their consultant psychiatrist was a member of the hospital's staff. It is difficult, therefore, to justify any direct comparison between conditions existing for the patients living in the above-mentioned complex, and the 2,000 patients in another hospital who all lived in close proximity in wards or villas, and formed part of a single community. Nevertheless in terms of *medical* care each of these complete hospitals is the responsibility of one person.

Selection of residential homes and nursing homes

We have referred above[4] to the difficulty of preparing a satisfactory list of homes. The procedure for sampling these homes was to divide them into five strata according to size, classification and type of patient. Within these five strata homes were selected by a random method,[5] and from each selected home a random sample of patients was selected, the number of patients being intended to be such that the sample would be self-weighting for patients, and the sampling fraction being one in eight. Appropriate weights were allocated to the

---

[1] Permission was given by the Scottish Home and Health Department, but the Medical Superintendents of the hospitals concerned felt unable to allow us access.

[2] It should be noted that instances of structural alteration were in fact taking place in many hospitals visited and we have tried to make allowance for this in our analysis.

[3] This will be discussed more fully in Chapter 3.

[4] See p. 29, *supra*.

[5] A more detailed discussion appears in Appendix B.

different homes for use when discussing the homes as distinct from the patients in them.

For the reasons mentioned earlier, the sample had to be considerably modified in practice. Twenty-seven homes were originally selected, one declined to co-operate on the grounds that they felt it necessary to contact parents individually in order to obtain their permission for our visit, and since many were abroad this was considered by the Principal to be impracticable. Of the remaining 26 homes approached, five had either closed or no longer took mentally subnormal patients, and in a further eight, the actual number of patients was very greatly discrepant from the anticipated number. In order to maintain roughly the same number of patients in our final sample, substitute homes were included.

In view of these difficulties, the original intention of making the sample of patients self-weighting had to be modified, and some adjustment was necessary when analysing the data from patients in 12 homes, in addition to weighting the actual homes (see Appendix B).

It is important to remember that since many of the homes sampled had closed or changed their function after our lists were prepared, this may well have been the case for those not originally selected. Equally, we have no way of knowing how many additional homes had opened since the lists were prepared. We are, therefore, unable to claim that our sample is truly representative in statistical terms; all we can say is that it certainly covers a wide cross-section of homes actually in operation at the time of our survey.

The final sample consisted of 24 homes which had at the time of our visit a total population of 1,697 and of these we sampled a population of 511. The Ministry of Health Annual Report (1966) shows a total of 3,526 patients in receipt of residential care at the expense of Local Health Authorities as at 31 December, 1965, but since some of the homes sampled took patients privately, we consider this figure must be an under-estimate of the total population in residential homes and nursing homes.

Making contact and visiting institutions

In the case of the National Health Service hospitals the Ministry of Health wrote on our behalf to all Regional Hospital Boards requesting that permission be given to carry out the research at the relevant hospitals in their area. We then wrote directly to the Superintendent or Medical Director of the hospitals concerned, requesting permission to start work on a given date and enclosing a plan of work.[1]

In general the response was immediate and helpful. With the exception of the two hospitals referred to earlier who refused to allow us entry, only in two others did we need to use persuasive

[1] See Appendix C.

E

powers to be allowed in! In both cases once the necessary consent had been given we received every possible co-operation. Occasionally there was some difficulty in relation to visiting ancillary units whose administrators felt that they should have been consulted direct about the research rather than through the Medical Superintendent at the parent hospital. Usually such instances arose where there was a different Hospital Management Committee involved, or where relationships between the hospitals were already somewhat tenuous.[1]

So far as the homes were concerned, letters were sent direct to the person in charge,[2] and no difficulties were encountered in obtaining permission to carry out the work, except in the one case of refusal previously mentioned.

Visits to hospitals Before visiting each hospital a short questionnaire was sent to the Medical Superintendent with the request that it be completed by either himself or the hospital secretary and returned to the office before our visit. We asked, amongst other things, for information about the type and age of buildings, the numbers of patients and the extent to which specialist facilities and nursing administration were shared between the various units. From this information it was hoped that we should be able to estimate the amount of time we should require to spend at any one unit, since this would depend not only upon the number of patients, but also on the number of people to interview, the number of wards to visit, and the travelling distances involved.

Visits took place over the period May 1965 to January 1966 inclusive. The work was carried out by a team of six interviewers (including the present writer); two interviewers normally visited all the larger hospitals and remained for a period of approximately ten working days. Work was usually carried on through the weekend and during some evenings, in order to obtain an overall picture of the institution at all times. In smaller hospitals only one research worker was used and the period of time spent at the hospital varied, depending more upon the number of subsidiary units involved than upon the total size of the hospital.

We had, in our initial request to hospitals, asked to meet not only the senior staff members, but also the staff in charge of all wards, as soon as possible after arrival, in order to tell them about the research, to ask for their co-operation, and to answer their questions. Only in two hospitals was such a meeting held, and elsewhere this often resulted in our having to spend a great deal of time explaining the purpose of the research on each ward and in each department. In the

---

[1] See further reference to this in Chapter 3, p. 44. However, by no means all linkage hospitals shared this view, as the lay superintendent of one such unit commented: 'I have no axes to grind, no chips on my shoulders, and I don't want to create problems, just to help fill in your papers'.

[2] See Appendix C.

great majority of hospitals a meeting had been arranged with the medical staff, all administrative nursing staff, all heads of specialist departments, such as psychology, physiotherapy, social work etc., and usually the hospital secretary. Such a meeting, though more limited in scope than we had hoped for, proved extremely helpful, noticeably so by comparison with those few hospitals which had made no such arrangements and where our presence was never fully understood.[1] Where the Superintendent (or hospital secretary in two instances) had sent round a memorandum to all wards and departments, as an alternative to holding a meeting, the extent to which this proved satisfactory appeared to depend largely upon general feelings about staff communication within the hospital. Thus in those hospitals where the staff felt consulted and generally involved in the overall work of the hospital, written communication appeared to be more acceptable.

The meeting with senior staff referred to above was important in so far as it gave us an idea of how to plan our work with the least possible disruption to existing routines. It was interesting that hospitals should vary so widely in their views about, for example, the hours we should work, or the extent to which plans for visiting ancillary units should be left to us to make, or were highly organized for us. An amusing but nevertheless important clue to the administrative organization in the hospital lay in the question of where the research team should eat! Chaperoned or unchaperoned (and if so by whom?), with the medical staff, with nurses, or alone in the Board Room? To pay, or not to pay?[2] These were vital questions which we were soon to learn to recognize as indicative of senior staff attitudes towards the research. If the Superintendent and the hospital secretary disagreed, the significance of the outcome was not so unimportant as might at first seem. Nor was the situation without humour, as in the case of the hospital official who told us the price of meals in a letter before our arrival. Or the unit many miles from the main hospital where the bill for one day's lunch was sent by special messenger when the research worker was having a meal with the Chief Male Nurse in his office. His confusion and embarrassment was the greater and he insisted on paying himself!

Visits to homes These took place in the period December 1965 to February 1966 inclusive. Only one of the homes was so large as to require more than one day's work, though in a few instances two interviewers went to the same home. Arrangements were usually quite informal, a meal was generally offered and taken with the staff, though in religious homes it was the practice to serve the meal to the

[1] For similar problems in a prison, see Morris, T. and P.: *Pentonville: A Sociological Study of an English Prison*, Routledge & Kegan Paul, 1963.

[2] Many Superintendents said they felt embarrassed that no entertainment allowance was available.

research worker who ate alone. The person in charge was normally interviewed on arrival, and the interviewer taken by him/her and introduced systematically to other members of the staff as required.

Selection of patients

Since the number of patients to be sampled in each hospital was known in advance, it was theoretically a simple matter to select these from the hospital register. In practice there were many difficulties, in view of the diversity of methods of record keeping employed in the institutions. Some main units had a list of the names of all patients in all ancillary units, in others each unit kept its own list and there was no central register. Some hospitals kept the information in alphabetical order, others by date of admission. Sometimes male and female patients were kept in separate registers, sometimes jointly. By no means were all registers up to date, and discharges and deaths had not been recorded (possibly admissions too, but we had no way of checking this). The facility with which it was possible to locate the relevant ward for each patient also varied greatly; in some hospitals a good deal of time was wasted in this kind of administrative congestion.

The complicated and unsystematic nature of some methods of recording used seemed surprising, since it undoubtedly resulted in considerable delay when information was required about a particular patient whose number and ward location was unknown. Only on one occasion was this actually observed to have had an unfortunate result: this occurred when a husband was called to the hospital on account of the alleged severe illness of his wife, only to find that it was another patient with the same name. In another instance, as a result of our endeavours to trace the record of a patient whose name was drawn in the sample, the staff decided by a process of elimination rather than direct information, that the patient must have died! It may be worth pointing out that in this respect the administrative organization on the male side was generally better than on the female side.

In homes the sample selection presented no problems since these were much smaller units and a central register was always kept by the person in charge.

Interview schedules

In hospitals a series of structured interviews were carried out with the superintendent, senior nursing staff, heads of all specialist departments, nurses in charge of wards and hostels wardens (where applicable). In addition questionnaires were completed on the ward regarding the sample of patients. It had been our intention to leave these on the wards for completion by the nurse in charge, but after

making some attempts to do this it was found generally more satisfactory to complete the form with the nurse in order to ensure that
the questions were fully understood and no gaps left in the information. Although more time-consuming, this method had the additional
advantage of assessing the extent to which nursing staff were knowledgeable about individual patients. Similarly it had been our original
intention to examine the physical conditions on the wards unaccompanied by a nurse. We found that by doing so we missed a great deal
of useful comment and information, so that the procedure was
changed.

Since most of the hospitals visited were situated well away from
towns, and opportunities for commercial entertainment were limited,
interviewers spent long hours in the hospitals, attending social
functions, discussing informally with staff, trying to communicate
with patients and generally observing the life of the hospital. Careful
notes were kept of all observations of this kind, in addition to the
recording of structured interviews.[1]

Many of the schedules used in hospitals were inappropriate for use
in homes, and they were therefore redesigned to include similar data
to that obtained in hospitals, as well as additional information more
applicable to the different setting. In general the methods used for
interviewing and observing were similar to those used in hospitals,
but naturally the period of observation was much shorter and it was
consequently more difficult to assess such matters as interpersonal
relationships and communications. There was also much less to
observe in terms of extra-curricular activity.

Analysis of data

After the data had been collected it was coded on to transfer sheets by
five coders working in pairs.[2] Constant discussion took place between
teams of coders in order to minimize discrepancies arising from
different interpretations of the data. Since two of the interviewers
were also involved in the coding process (though not directly responsible for coding the hospitals they visited), any doubts about
interpretation could be thoroughly discussed.

These data were then transferred to punched cards and the analysis
was conducted on an IBM 1440 computer. Frequency distributions
were obtained on all counts and tables constructed in order to
provide a descriptive picture of the life led by patients in hospitals
and homes. This information forms the basis of Chapters 4–9 and 11.

It would have been inappropriate to analyse certain of the data
relating to hospitals or homes using punch cards, and in such cases
information was transferred to manually prepared charts from which
it was processed. This method was feasible in view of the relatively

---

[1] For instructions to interviewers see Appendix D.
[2] Copies of coding instructions available on request.

small number of hospitals and homes (fifty-eight) concerned, and it was particularly useful in respect of the views expressed by Superintendents and heads of specialist departments.

Staff attitudes to research

In general staff at all levels were extremely co-operative once they had discovered 'what it was all about'.[1] In most hospitals the nursing staff formed a very parochial community and there was little opportunity for informal contact outside the hospital setting. Some of the older nurses said our visit reminded them of the old days of the Board of Control visits. They expressed the view that it was a pity no alternative to these visits existed under the 1959 Act: the Board's visits had given them something to work for, and a feeling that someone was interested in their work.[2]

At senior level, attitudes to the research varied largely in terms of the administrative structure of the hospital; this seemed to arise partly because medical staff appeared to feel less threatened by, and more involved with, the research than did the lay administrators. As a result, in hospitals where medical staff were very much 'in control', acceptance of the research and a general attitude of friendliness was more likely to prevail in the hospital as a whole. This was also observable in terms of the facilities offered to the research workers for office accommodation, use of telephone and the availability of general information so essential to the smooth running of a project of this kind.

Patients' attitudes to research

A great many patients could not communicate in any meaningful way with the research workers.[3] Where they were capable of so doing, patients talked readily, eagerly showed their possessions and made considerable demands for attention, particularly at a physical level. They appeared to see the research worker as being someone between a member of staff and a casual visitor. Subnormality nurses frequently alleged that patients do not respond to strangers. We found no evidence for this view, and it may be that it reflects *staff* attitudes towards outsiders, and where it does occur, it may be a question of patients imitating the reaction of staff.[4]

[1] Only at one hospital were the staff passive and somewhat unco-operative towards the research.

[2] For similar views see McCoull, G.: 'An Integrated Service', in Symposium on the Hospital Service for the Mentally Subnormal, *J. Ment. Sub.*, 18, 23–8.

[3] Had we been able to spend longer on individual wards this difficulty would have been overcome, since it was often *our* inability to understand them which made for failure in communication.

[4] Bettelheim, B.: 'Individual and Mass Behaviour in Extreme Situations', *J. Ab. & Soc. Psych.*, Vol. 38, 1943, discusses the way in which long-term prisoners in concentration camps adopted the behaviour of their Gestapo guards.

The intensive study

As mentioned earlier,[1] it was decided to make a more detailed study of two subnormality hospitals. The aim of this part of the research was to examine:

(a) the formal objectives of the institution as perceived by the various levels of staff;
(b) the influence of external formal agencies on the functioning of the hospitals (i.e. Ministry of Health, Regional Hospital Board, Hospital Management Committee, Local Health Authority, etc.)
(c) the formal aspects of the social organization of the hospitals;
(d) the social structure of the hospitals;
(e) formal and informal patterns of communication;
(f) the influence of informal agents, groups and individuals.

The hospitals were selected from amongst those already visited in the extensive survey. We sought two hospitals of comparable size, one rural, one urban, where some conscious policies and programmes were adopted which might be considered 'progressive'. Thus one of the hospitals had an international as well as a national reputation, in particular in relation to patient training, and the other had a systematic programme of short-term care, a special unit for severely disturbed children, and a habit-training programme.

Each research worker was attached to one particular hospital where they spent a period of approximately sixty working days. Although not sleeping on the premises they spent most of their time in the hospital, and in addition to informal interviews, observation, attending committee meetings and social functions, they were encouraged to spend some time actually helping the ward staff with their duties. A limited amount of information was also obtained about a ten per cent sample of patients in each of the hospitals and records were made available to us regarding staff turnover, qualifications and experience.

A daily diary was kept by each worker and sent to the present writer weekly for comment and discussion. Meetings took place at regular intervals to discuss progress and the two workers were responsible for submitting a final report on their work.

Reliability

It seems probable that despite frequent explanation, the scope of the research was not completely understood by most of the staff (particularly in the case of the extensive study), with the result that they tended to interpret it in terms of their own particular role or function, be it nursing, medical or specialist. The project was usually treated with some deference, presumably because it had the backing of

[1] See Introduction, p. 4.

'authority' in the form of the Ministry and the Regional Hospital Board, as well as senior staff. As the survey progressed, hospital staff seemed to be impressed by the fact that interviewers had been to so many other subnormality hospitals, and they were probably credited with a great deal more knowledge than they actually had!

One of the most frequent criticisms made of the survey was that sources of information would not necessarily be either valid or reliable.[1] Almost certainly some staff were biased, or deliberately concealed facts; others may have over-emphasized or exaggerated a point made. Usually we were in the hospitals long enough to enable us to check replies through cross-questioning, particularly where observation led us to believe that information given was inaccurate, or the result of distorted perception. As will be discussed in later chapters, there are many clashes of personality and professionalism among staff and these naturally led to prejudiced or inaccurate responses.

However, it is extremely difficult for an institution to maintain a façade over a longish period and at all times. The system is too unwieldy and too much geared to providing for the daily needs of its inmates (staff and patients) to allow for a 'special performance'. The research workers pass the same wards and departments so frequently, they talk to so many people upon identical topics, so that provided they remain interested but not personally involved, they soon become part of the scenery, and learn to sort the wheat from the chaff.

Research workers in an institutional setting are also faced with the problem of 'involvement'. It is very easy to align oneself with particular groupings within the institution, and to find one's views being biased accordingly.[2] Regular discussion amongst the research team can help to reduce this danger and instructions were given that interviewers should not live in the hospital other than under the most exceptional circumstances. The opportunity to get away from the hospital environment and influence was particularly important in relation to the intensive study. Furthermore, the fact that in the majority of cases two interviewers went to each hospital and wrote individual reports, allowed for some check on reliability.

In order to increase reliability, in addition to using the pre-codes, interviewers were asked to record as much information as possible verbatim; nevertheless at the analysis stage the problem is one of interpretation – inflections of the voice cannot easily be recorded and

[1] It is interesting that a similar fear was expressed at a meeting of parents of subnormal patients who were afraid that we would not penetrate the surface and that hospitals would maintain a façade in our presence.

[2] It can be argued that 'involvement' may be a useful method by which one begins to perceive phenomena from the point of view of the group one is studying. This method demands a high degree of skill on the part of the research workers and has serious limitations in large-scale surveys which are heavily dependent upon questionnaire techniques and where the data collectors are not themselves directly involved in the interpretation and writing up of material.

the vast amount of paperwork completed each day by all the interviewers made it impossible for the writer to carry out a detailed and immediate check on every schedule and every report.[1]

With regard to the homes, whilst our information about the physical structure and about educational and occupational opportunities is probably quite accurate, information about relationships is likely to be less reliable since we were there for such a short period, and in most cases only one worker visited the home.

General problems of analysis

The sociologist has the responsibility of analysing and reporting research findings without regard to personal prejudices or value judgments[2] a task which is not always easy particularly when, as in this survey, the work is directly concerned with human beings whose situation and inability to communicate may make them appear more deprived than they actually are, or who may equally be unable to express the full extent of their deprivation.

Nevertheless it is important to recognize that the evaluation of social facts can only take place against a background of changing social policy. We believe that in the present state of our knowledge both about institutional care and about the suitability of available measurement techniques, the concept of 'good' and 'bad' institutions is an over-simplified one; institutions are either more, or less adequate when measured against the standards set by the community, by those in charge who make explicit their goals, or against some 'ideal' type.

Townsend[3] makes a case for devising standards of comparison between different types of residential home. Furthermore, Barton[4]

---

[1] From a methodological point of view we would in retrospect have wished to spend more time on piloting. Had this been possible we should doubtless have had a better understanding of the complexity of the administrative structure of the hospitals and this might well have enabled us to rationalize the research design, and in particular to have concentrated the work of the main survey on certain more specific areas of investigation.

[2] It is recognized that this is a controversial viewpoint. C. Wright Mills for example, *The Sociological Imagination* (NY Grove Press, 1961) complains that most social scientists conform to a prevailing fear of passionate commitment, and he believes that this lies behind the avoidance of value judgments rather than, as they claim, scientific objectivity. Similar views about ethical neutrality are expressed by Alvin Gouldner 'Anti-Minotaur: The Myth of a Value-Free Society', in Stein and Vidich: *Sociology on Trial* (Englewood Cliffs, NJ, Prentice Hall, 1963). It might also be thought that what is and what is not objective may vary according to the values held within particular professions as well as particular cultures. Value-freedom is essentially relative rather than absolute.

[3] Townsend, P.: *The Last Refuge* (Routledge and Kegan Paul, 1962). Professor Townsend agrees that his rating was not evaluative nor 'ideal' but rather a rough 'community' rating. Each of the items was satisfied by some of the Homes in the sample.

[4] Barton, R.: 'Proposed Scale for Rating Psychiatric Hospitals' in *Psychiatric Hospital Care*, ed. Freeman, Bailliere, Tindall and Cassell (1965).

has made preliminary suggestions for rating psychiatric hospitals, and Brown and Wing[1] have also attempted to do this, though in respect of a limited number of criteria. In the present study some scaling has been carried out in relation to physical structure and material comforts, but at the time when our data were collected, so little information about *subnormality* hospitals was available, that any attempt to build up extensive rating systems would, we believe, have been inappropriate. We hope, nevertheless, that our findings will suggest suitable items and means of scoring them in any subsequent scales which might be developed by other workers.[2]

It might be suggested that simply by virtue of having similar kinds of inhabitants, with similar needs, it should in practice be possible to find criteria which could be applied to all institutions, and a single rating scale devised to measure them. We can only say that, as the research proceeded, the disadvantages of any single rating scale which embraced too many aspects of the hospital provisions became increasingly apparent. This danger is referred to by Forsyth and Logan[3] who devised a model for measuring the quality of care in a casualty department. They refer in particular to the countervailing nature of some topics. For example they ask: is a department with poor medical staff able to attract efficient, capable and dedicated nursing staff? Does a 'poor' doctor remain 'poor' despite good physical amenities and *vice versa*? In our opinion sophisticated rating scales, of the kind currently being developed, will be necessary to overcome this kind of dilemma. As Forsyth and Logan say, measurement of quality is only possible 'in certain specific areas and situations to indicate certain concrete things which ought to be done in given circumstances and then ascertain whether they are being done or not'.

In order to overcome some of these difficulties, we have, therefore, used a variety of scales, each one covering only those aspects of the hospital which we feel are genuinely comparable, and where possible we have avoided incorporating too many widely differing factors in the same scale. Thus we have a scale measuring what we term the physical structure of the hospital, and another measuring the degree of 'homeliness'. As will be illustrated in subsequent chapters, there are wide variations between different areas of the same hospital: some patients live in stark comfortless wards and yet others in the

[1] Brown, G. W. and Wing, J. K.: 'A Comparative, Clinical and Social Survey of Three Mental Hospitals', in Sociology and Medicine, *Sociological Review Monograph*, No. 5, ed. Halmos (1962).

[2] Since writing King, R. and Raynes, N. have devised a scale for measuring practices adopted in the management of children in residential institutions. See *Soc. Sci. and Med.*, 1968, Vol. 2, pp. 41–53.

[3] Forsyth and Logan: 'Studies in Medical Care: An Assessment of Some Methods' in *Towards a Measure of Medical Care: Operational Research in the Health Services, a Symposium*, OUP for Nuffield Provincial Hospitals Trust (1962), and also Forsyth and Logan: *Casualty Services and Their Setting: A Study of Medical Care* (1960).

same hospital live in 'homely' wards, with no sign of institutional atmosphere. Or again, a ward might be well decorated and physically pleasing, but have no 'homely' touches and *vice versa*.

Furthermore, interpersonal relationships were as important as physical conditions in determining the kind of care given to patients; the significance of this lies in the fact that our findings suggest that there was not necessarily any direct connection between the quality of nursing care given to patients and the physical setting.

This raises the difficult problem of measuring the quality of services, which in turn must be related to the concept of *need* to which reference was made earlier in this chapter. In considering the investigation of medical care, Brotherston,[1] discussing definitions of need writes:

> The most difficult area with least agreement is in the field of mental health, where one man's criterion of medical need may be another man's conception of original sin . . . the areas of need move with medical knowledge and social ideology. Even when definitions are agreed, we are up against technical difficulties in achieving assessment.

The difficulty of measuring the provision of services is illustrated by the following example: hospital A had no physiotherapist on the staff, but an exceptionally experienced practitioner came over weekly from another hospital, quite informally, and trained the nursing staff in this type of work. Many nurses were extremely enthusiastic and used his techniques between visits so that a relatively high proportion of patients really appeared to benefit from physiotherapy. Hospital B, on the other hand, had a full time physiotherapist but he was given no facilities for treating patients; he had no equipment and had to work in a corner of an enormous children's day room surrounded by all the other children who constantly jumped on him, and pushed and punched those receiving treatment. The hospital had a number of ancillary units, some at quite a distance away, but the physiotherapist was not entitled to a petrol allowance, though in order to avoid wasting too much time he used his car rather than wait for infrequent buses in country districts. As a result of this situation the number of patients receiving treatment in hospital B amounted to only a handful. This example is one of many that could be used to illustrate the fact that a purely statistical approach may give a quite false impression if used as an indicator of satisfactory service. The most that can be claimed is that if statistically the indicator *usually* reflects efficiency or adequacy there may be justification for using it.

Again much emphasis is laid upon industrial training in some hospitals and there is often a rather general and nebulous assumption

---

[1] Brotherston, J.: 'Medical Care Investigation in the Health Service' in *Towards a Measure of Medical Care: Operational Research in the Health Services*, a Symposium, OUP for Nuffield Provincial Hospitals Trust (1962).

amongst certain medical superintendents and training staff that this kind of treatment is preferable to other forms of work and that it can be termed 'rehabilitative' if it is carried out in a workshop. But this may well be an over-simplification, since it will certainly depend more upon the type of training, and its relationship to employment prospects outside, than upon the mere fact of having an industrial workshop. Even for those patients who will never leave the hospital it would be difficult to compare the training value of patients employed, for example, on tearing up paper bags, and those working in, say, the laundry.

Finally, in discussing the use of research data, there is the problem of presentation. Whilst the social scientist might be interested in rigorous research design and scientific method, as well as the clarification of theoretical concepts, hospital administrators, politicians, the staff of the institutions studied and the 'informed' public are likely to be primarily interested in the clarification of administrative problems and in the factual results of the survey. Yet another group, the parents, may be more interested than others in the accurate and systematic documentation of the availability and quality of the services provided for their handicapped children. We were frequently asked to discuss our findings with hospital staff, and the fact that we felt unable to do so certainly caused some dissatisfaction. Nevertheless whilst carrying out a field survey of this kind, it is extremely easy to leave a particular institution with a series of faulty interpretations of observed situations. For this reason we considered it essential to wait until we were able to look much more closely and intensively at the data before venturing an opinion.

Unfortunately there is a very real danger that a survey of this nature can do harm as well as good, since it may alienate the staff of the institutions instead of fostering in them the wish to involve themselves in improving the service offered. Few of those to whom we spoke were satisfied with the *status quo*; it is not our intention to allocate blame, nor to criticize individuals or groups, but rather to try to sign-post where the roots of the problem lie, so that administrators and staff may be better equipped to bring about changes. More money and more staff are certainly urgent necessities, but unless those working in the field understand the need for change, they may well throw good money after bad. The problems of institutions – be they for criminals, the mentally ill, or the mentally subnormal – are more complex than the mere provision of additional finance.

In this chapter we have attempted to outline the objectives of the research and to indicate the methods used. Before setting out our findings in relation to a specific sample we feel it would be helpful to give some idea of the overall hospital provisions for the subnormal, as well as an indication of the way in which such hospitals are administered.

Chapter 3

HOSPITAL PROVISION FOR
THE MENTALLY SUBNORMAL

ANY attempt to present a meaningful statistical picture of the current hospital provisions in Britain for subnormal patients is frustrated by two factors. The first results from the inadequacies of the statistical returns: the Annual Report of the Ministry of Health for the year 1965[1] devotes only two of its seventy-two pages of text to the psychiatric services, and only one paragraph relates to subnormality hospitals. The information for Scotland is even more sparse. Furthermore, subnormality is dealt with under the umbrella heading of psychiatric services, and the distinction between the mentally ill and the mentally subnormal is not always clear. Nor is it possible to estimate from the statistics how many of the population of subnormal patients are also mentally ill, though considerably more information is available in the Registrar General's Statistical Review, Supplements on Mental Health. At the time of writing the latest figures available in the Supplement are those for 1960 and in view of the fact that the Mental Health Act (1959) was brought into effect on 1 November, 1960, this information can throw no light on any changes which may have resulted from the new Act.

The second problem arises from the wide diversity of settings in which the mentally subnormal are cared for, even within the hospital service.[2] In the previous chapter we expressed some doubt about the meaningfulness of the concept of administrative size in relation to the study of these hospitals and as an example we considered two two-thousand bedded hospitals operating under very different organizational systems. Size is not the only misleading aspect of the situation, for there exist a wide variety of structural forms: there are hospitals where the Medical Superintendent[3] is administratively centred on the local mental hospital which may, or may not, house subnormal patients. In most such cases he is also medically responsible for at least some, if not all, the mentally ill patients in the mental hospital, but in at least two instances known to the research this is not the case,

[1] Command 3039, HMSO (1966).
[2] Voluntary hospitals have not been included in this section but will be discussed in Chapter 11, dealing with registered nursing homes and residential homes.
[3] Throughout this report the term 'Medical Superintendent' is used for purposes of simplification, it covers Medical Directors, Physician Superintendents, Clinical Directors, etc.

and it is difficult to see any administrative advantage in such an arrangement.

There are also a considerable number of subsidiary or ancillary units where the subnormal patients constitute a small minority in a hospital which caters largely for mentally ill or geriatric patients; alternatively subnormal patients may be housed in one ward or villa of a general hospital. Whilst we have observed instances where this worked relatively well, in the great majority of cases observed, the unit housing the mentally subnormal patients was very much the 'Cinderella' of the hospital. Such a situation is clearly not inevitable, but it seems likely that these are matters which have received little attention in discussion about the future of subnormality hospitals; yet the experience of such units is particularly important now that increasing consideration is being given to the setting up of district general hospitals absorbing all specialist units.[1]

Then again there is the question of Management Committees. We have already referred to the fact that units under the direction of the same Medical Superintendent may have different Management Committees, or they may have the same Management Committee but a different House Committee. In some areas the significance of these situations is obscured by the fact that the smaller hospitals may have Lay Administrators or Matron Superintendents who are administratively responsible to the Management Committee for the running of the unit. Nevertheless the *medical* responsibility for the patients rests with a psychiatrist of consultant status, who may be based on a hospital with a different Management Committee. It can arise that the dispersion of patients in a large number of units may result in a Superintendent having dealings with three or four different Management Committees. From a purely practical point of view the only matter which is likely to produce any disagreement centres round the question of patient transfers, which have to be agreed by the Management Committee, but problems of relationship are likely to be more frequent than in the case of a Superintendent having dealings with only one Management Committee.[2]

Distribution of hospitals

We have attempted to give on the attached map (see p. 46 below), a rough idea of the distribution of all the main subnormality hospitals; inevitably many of the smaller units to which reference has been made above cannot appear on such a small scale map.

The Hospital Plan (1962)[3] provisionally accepted the existing bed

[1] In his address to the NAMH Annual Conference in February 1968 the Minister of Health said it was not the intention to provide for subnormal or severely subnormal patients in district general hospitals (see 'What's Wrong with the Mental Health Services?' report of proceedings published by NAMH).

[2] See, for example, attitude to research (Chapter 2, p. 32, *supra*).

[3] Command 1604, HMSO (1962).

ratio for subnormal patients of 1·3 beds per thousand of the general population. This was based on the view that an expansion of community services and the prevention of some forms of subnormality would off-set the waiting lists, the greater expectation of life, and what was thought to be a trend towards greater public acceptance of admission to hospital. The Plan stated that subnormal and severely subnormal patients should be cared for separately, and advocated small units of not more than two hundred beds. Mittler and Castell[1] point out that according to the published plans of the fifteen Regional Hospital Boards, the tendency appears to be to close the smaller hospitals and centralize services: the projected number of subnormality hospitals per region is smaller (14·2 in 1960 and 11·2 in 1975) and the number of beds per hospital is larger (437 in 1960 and 477 in 1975).

The Revision of the Hospital Plan (1966)[2] commented that 'there is no reason yet to adopt this estimate as a firm basis for long-term national planning, or to propose a different ratio'.

Number of beds

Table 3.I sets out the provision of beds by region as at October 1965:

Table 3.1
NUMBER OF STAFFED BEDS PER REGION

Regional Hospital Board	Pop. of catchment area (millions)	No. of staffed beds allocated to subnormal and severely subnormal patients (per thousand pop.)
Newcastle	3·09	1·23
Leeds	3·19	1·26
Sheffield	4·55	1·10
East Anglia	1·62	0·97
North West Metropolitan	4·20	1·38
North East Metropolitan	3·40	1·03
South East Metropolitan	3·46	1·30
South West Metropolitan	3·27	2·16
Wessex	1·88	1·04
Oxford	1·77	3·49
South Western	3·00	0·96
Birmingham	4·98	1·12
Manchester	4·55	1·52
Liverpool	2·20	0·65
Wales	2·69	0·62

Information calculated from Revision of Hospital Plan (1966) and Annual Report of the Ministry of Health (1966).

[1] Mittler and Castell: 'Hospital and Community Care of the Subnormal', *The Lancet*, 18 April, 1964, pp. 873–5.
[2] Command 3000, HMSO (1966).

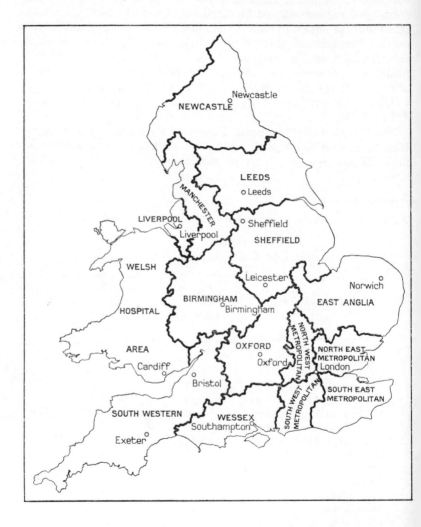

These wide variations are difficult to explain; normally variations in provision between different Local Authorities can be explained in terms of (a) available financial resources and (b) the political control and consequent nature of social policy. However the Regional Hospital Board areas do not conform to such boundaries and variations cannot therefore be explained in these terms. To some extent historical accident may account for the discrepancies, but as Rehin and Martin[1] suggest, variations in housing conditions, in the physical environment and in the socio-economic composition of the population, all affect the regional pattern of disease.

Patient statistics

In 1965 the average daily number of beds occupied by the mentally subnormal accounted for approximately 14 per cent of the total daily number of occupied beds in the hospital service as a whole. Table 3.2 sets out information relating to admissions and discharges between the years 1960 and 1965: it also shows the daily average population and the size of the waiting list.

The overall picture between 1961 and 1965 is, in general, one of stability, there being virtually no increase in admissions following the Mental Health Act of 1959. As might be expected, the number of *severely subnormal* patients in every year exceeds the number of subnormal patients, the ratio varying from 3:1 to 2:1.

Calculation of admission rates is confused by the fact that the data available cannot discriminate between *admissions* and individual *patients*, who may have been admitted more than once in a single year. In 1965, of a total of 8,849 admissions, 4,101 were first admissions and readmissions accounted for 4,748.[2]

Just as the size of the patient population has altered very little, so too has the average number of available beds. The size of the waiting list has declined from almost 8,000 in 1960 to just under 5,000 in 1965, that is by 37 per cent, but this is a particularly unreliable statistic in view of different interpretations about the use of waiting lists. Unfortunately the Ministry of Health's Statistics[3] do not differentiate between discharges and deaths and we cannot therefore say with certainty how many deaths occurred in this period. On the assumption that the figure approximates the years 1957 to 1960, we would estimate it to be in the region of 800 to 1,000 per annum.[4]

[1] Rehin, G. and Martin, F. M.: *Psychiatric Services in 1975*, PEP Planning, Vol. xxix, No. 468, 4 February, 1963.

[2] Not all of these, of course, were necessarily admitted more than once *in 1965*, but are readmissions over a period of the indefinite past.

[3] See Registrar General's Statistical Review for 1960, Supplement on Mental Health, 1964.

[4] Ibid.

F

Table 3.2

HOSPITAL STATISTICS 1960–1965

Year ending 31st December	Admissions						Total all admissions	Discharges and deaths	Average daily no. of occ. beds	Waiting list at 31st December
	Subnormal			Severely subnormal						
	Informal	Compulsory	Total	Informal	Compulsory	Total				
1960*							4,071	7,614	57,186	8,289
1961†	2,131	724	2,855	5,492	342	5,834	8,689	9,841	56,930	7,566
1962	1,832	674	2,506	5,271	310	5,581	8,087	8,809	56,958	5,512
1963	2,961	802	3,763	6,575	381	6,956	10,719	9,692	57,367	5,350
1964	2,130	773	2,903	5,690	326	6,014	8,917	9,838	57,529	5,312
1965	2,010	694	2,704	5,902	243	6,145	8,849	11,624	57,815	4,938

Source: Ministry of Health Annual Reports.

* The Ministry of Health did not publish these figures because of the introduction of the Mental Health Act. The total number of admissions for 1960 has been obtained from the Registrar General's Statistical Review.

† Because of a change in the collection of data resulting from the introduction of the Mental Health Act, these figures cover an additional two months as compared with figures for 1962 onwards. The Act was introduced on 1 November, 1960, and the 1961 figures date from then.

One other point that might be made is that over this five year period, the number of compulsory admissions has declined in the case of the severely subnormal, although it has fluctuated where the subnormal are concerned. The year 1963 appears to have been somewhat unusual in that the figures for admissions of both subnormal and severely subnormal, compulsory and informal, were the highest for the five year period. As the figure given for the waiting list at 31 December, 1962 was not unusually high, it is impossible to suggest a reason for this abnormal fluctuation except in terms of chance.

Detailed demographic data in relation to admissions is very limited. The most recent published figures with regard to age and grade of defect do not go beyond 1960. Table MD 1 in the Registrar General's Statistical Review[1] indicates that between 1957 and 1960 admission rates per million home population have consistently been highest for both males and females in the fifteen to nineteen years age group, which group also shows the highest actual number of admissions of any five-year age group.

With regard to the distribution by grades of subnormality, the greatest caution needs to be used in interpreting the figures in view of the variability in grading criteria that may be applied by the wide range of diagnostic personnel involved. Doctors vary not only in their interpretation of classifications, but also in their methods of recording such information. One of the categories employed in the Registrar General's Tables, for example, is that of 'moral defective', one no longer having any legal meaning under the terms of the 1959 Mental Health Act. Table MD 2 indicates that the great majority of admissions under the age of fifteen are imbeciles (approximately 57 per cent), about 28 per cent are idiots, and only approximately 13 per cent are feeble-minded. The position is, however, reversed amongst patients of fifteen years and above, where the greatest number (approximately 63 per cent) are feeble-minded, approximately 32 per cent are imbeciles, and about 4 per cent idiots. As will be mentioned later when discussing data from the hospitals sampled, staff at all levels share the view that the number of low grade patients is increasing; the figures for the years 1951 to 1960 certainly show no change in overall average IQ and mental age of admissions,[2] but the impression of a wide difference may be related to the fact that more of the *children* coming in are severely subnormal. At the same time the increase in the number of untestable cases *may* indicate that such patients should be included among the low grades. Alternatively staff may need to hold this view in order to explain the inadequacy of institutional performance.

[1] Mental Health Supplement, 1964.

[2] This fact should be interpreted with caution in view of the fact that since 1957 an increasingly large proportion of cases have been excluded from the table because they are untestable or because no test result is stated. In 1960, 20 per cent of admissions were untestable and for over 41 per cent no result was stated.

Social class

Information about the social class of patients in institutions is virtually non-existent. The Registrar General's statistics give no information on this subject, nor do many previous surveys. Berg[1] suggests a social class differential amongst a group of 800 children admitted to the Fountain Hospital between 1949 and 1960. However most of the information about the relationship between intelligence level and socio-economic status refers to the population of retarded persons living in the community. O'Connor and Tizard[2] found that the distribution of grades in hospitals differs from their distribution in the community, so that we cannot assume that the socio-economic status of patients in institutions is comparable to that found amongst retarded persons in the community. However, Penrose[3] in his Colchester survey does refer exclusively to patients in institutions and his figures show very clearly that high grade and low grade defect are differentially distributed in the occupational grades of patients.

Staff

It is perhaps significant that the majority of writings about hospital provision for the mentally subnormal do not mention the staff in any detail,[4] yet it is frequently said that our subnormality hospitals are not only overcrowded but understaffed. Table 3.3 shows a comparison of medical staffing in subnormality hospitals between 1962–1965:

Table 3.3

MEDICAL STAFF IN SUBNORMALITY HOSPITALS

	1962	1963	1964	1965
Consultants	76	75	76	93
SHMO/SHDO with allowance	17	13	13	5
SHMO/SHDO without allowance	38	36	33	26
Senior Registrar	10	8	10	7
Registrar	8	31	15	19
JHMO	43	45	45	41
SHO	2	—	2	2
GP	30	30	36	36
TOTALS	224	238	230	229

Source: Annual Reports of the Ministry of Health for 1963 and 1965, HMSO Command 2389 (1964) and Command 3039 (1966).

[1] Berg, J. M.: in *Proceedings of London Conference on Scientific Study of Mental Deficiency*: eds. Richards, Clarke and Shapiro (1962).

[2] *op. cit.*

[3] Penrose, L. S.: 'A Clinical and Genetic Study of 1280 Cases of Mental Defect', *Sp. Rep. Ser., Med. Res. Council*, No. 229, London, HMSO (1938).

[4] A notable exception being Cross, K. W.: 'A Survey of Mental Hospitals and Mental Deficiency Institutions in the Birmingham Region', *Brit. J. Prev. Soc. Med.* (1954, 8, 162–71).

This table indicates that despite a gradual but steady increase in the daily average number of occupied beds, the total number of doctors has changed very little, although the decline in the number of registrars since 1963 is very marked. The number of GPs increased noticeably in 1964, as did the number of consultants in 1965.[1] Assuming all regions to be equally well staffed this would provide a ratio of approximately one doctor to every 250 patients, and one consultant to every 621 patients.[2]

The situation with regard to nursing staff for recent years as compared with 1949 is set out in Table 3.4:

Table 3.4

NURSING STAFF IN SUBNORMALITY HOSPITALS

Date	Registered nurses		Student nurses	Enrolled nurses		Pupil nurses	Other nursing staff		Total	
	F/T	P/T		F/T	P/T		F/T	P/T	F/T	P/T
31 Dec. 1949*	2,613	250	1,135	—	—	—	1,800	1,522	5,548	1,772
30 Sept. 1962*	3,628	450	1,335	—	—	—	4,330	2,538	9,293	2,988
30 Sept. 1964	3,805	485	1,432	48	19	—	4,490	2,621	9,775	3,125
30 Sept. 1965	3,868	553	1,517	1,197	398	33	3,593	2,431	10,208	3,382

Source: Ministry of Health Reports: they point out that the figures for 1964 and 1965 are not entirely comparable with 1949.

* The figures for enrolled nurses are not shown separately in these years, but are included in Other Nursing Staff.

[1] This increase in consultants resulted from the implementation by the Regional Hospital Boards of the recommendation of the Joint Working Party on the Medical Staffing Structure of the Hospital Services (HMSO, 1961). The Working Party recommended that SHMO's with allowance holding posts which the Minister had approved as consultant posts should be upgraded.

[2] In an address to the Royal Medico-Psychological Society, Dr. R. Wilkins, SMO Ministry of Health, estimated that in 1966 each consultant had approximately 620 beds under his supervision. An average of 120 such patients were new admissions – roughly 2 per week. In addition each consultant saw about 18 new and about 46 old patients per annum in out-patient clinics. Other commitments included approved schools, remand homes, prisons and domiciliary consultations. The Platt Committee on Medical Staffing recommended one consultant to 300 patients.

These figures show an overall increase of 4·4 per cent full time and 8·2 per cent part time nursing staff between 1964 and 1965.[1] Although in this table for purposes of simplification we have not shown separate figures for male and female nurses, the Ministry of Health sets out this information in 1965 'because of the high incidence of male nursing staff in these hospitals' (4,729 full time males as compared with 5,479 full time females).

The great rise in state enrolled nurses is accounted for by the introduction of this grade in 1964 and a special allocation of revenue funds made to Regional Hospital Boards in September of that year which enabled the number of appointments to increase rapidly. The system of promotion from assistant nurse to state enrolled nurse by virtue of experience as distinct from training was a matter which caused very considerable comment and dissatisfaction at all hospitals included in the survey and this will be discussed in a later chapter.

Since we have no information about the hours worked by part time staff, we cannot give an accurate assessment of staff/patient ratios, but on the assumption that on average part time nurses work half time, the ratio of all nursing staff to patients for the year 1965 would be roughly 1 : 4·8 and the ratio of trained staff would be 1 :14.[2]

Clearly, however, any evaluation of total nursing staff to patients is misleading, since at any one time only approximately one-third of the total is likely to be available for duty, and a distinction should be made between day and night availability. These matters will be dealt with in greater detail when discussing our survey data.

Administration

Prior to 1948 subnormality hospitals were governed by the legal provisions of the Lunacy and Mental Treatment Acts, and the Mental Deficiency Acts. Authority was vested in the Visiting Committee appointed by the Local Authority. The Visiting Committee could appoint and discharge officers, and made the rules governing the staff, which were in turn ratified by the Board of Control (the specialized Government Department responsible for administering

---

[1] The overall increase of all full-time nursing staff for England, Wales and Scotland at 31 March, 1966, was 3·1 per cent and for part-time staff was 10 per cent. (*The Lancet*, 10 December, 1966, p. 1322.)

[2] In 1951 the ratio of nurses to patients in subnormality hospitals was 1 : 5·75 and in 1955 it was 1 : 6·9 and the ratio of trained staff was 1 : 17 (see Ministry of Health Annual Reports for 1952 and 1956, Command 8655 and 9857). The fact that our figure for 1965 shows a slight improvement *may* be due to a general increase, but may only be due to the uncertainty regarding the average number of hours worked by part-time staff. Worked out on a similar basis (i.e., from the Ministry of Health Report for 1966) the ratio of all nursing staff to patients in hospitals for the chronic sick for 1965 was 1 : 3·9 and for psychiatric hospitals 1 : 4·1.

the legislation). These Acts required the Visiting Committee to appoint a Superintendent, and the Board of Control through its power of sanctioning rules, insisted that he be in complete charge of the hospital. Provision was also made for a clerk to the Committee, a clerk to the hospital and a treasurer.

The effect of the National Health Service Act (1948) was to break up the separate administrative system of the psychiatric and mental subnormality hospitals (although retaining in a somewhat changed form the role of the medical superintendent) and thus to bring them into line with the general hospitals. The administrative functions of the Board of Control were transferred to the Minister, leaving the Board with certain quasi-judicial functions in relation to the care and custody of patients. The Visiting Committees were dissolved and Hospital Management Committees acting for the Minister, were substituted. The appointment of senior doctors became a function of the Regional Hospital Board, not the Hospital Management Committee.

Important changes in relationships were produced by administrative action. In the first place the Medical Superintendent was no longer the head of the clinical hierarchy, but a colleague *primus inter pares* who had additional administrative responsibilities carrying additional pay.

The Ministry of Health issued a memorandum[1] outlining the staffing of Hospital Management Committees and their functions. A full-time secretary was to be appointed for each Committee, who would be its principal administrative officer, and responsible for the administration of the Group as a whole and for one hospital in it. It will be observed that such a situation could produce particular problems of relationships in those hospitals where a number of Hospital Management Committees were involved in a hospital complex under one Medical Director.

The Hospital Management Committees could be appointed to include general or mental hospitals as well as mental subnormality ones, or alternatively each hospital could have its own individual Committee. In the smaller units this latter step was considered impracticable and they became members of composite groups under one Hospital Management Committee. Where this situation occurred, a subordinate of a *group* administrative officer could conceivably find himself working under conflicting instructions from the Superintendent.

Difficulties arose early on as a result of the fact that many of the secretaries appointed to Hospital Management Committees were the same people who had previously been clerks to the old Visiting Committee. As such they had experience, but usually little formal training in hospital administration, and they were projected into a situation

[1] HMC, 48 (2).

where they had potentially considerably more responsibility and authority.[1]

Needless to say the professional organizations disagreed about the extent to which the proposed changes in the administrative system would be workable in a mental subnormality hospital. The medical organizations supported the retention of the Medical Superintendent in these hospitals in view of their special nature. They considered that the whole life of the hospital was the concern of the psychiatrist, and that he should have the controlling voice in the day-to-day running of the hospital. Nevertheless they recognized that each department should have autonomy as far as practicable, and that they should be able to present their views direct to the Committee.

The Association of Hospital Management Committees and the Institute of Hospital Administrators were equally concerned about the problems of authority. The latter thought that the administration should be in the hands of a person trained in administration, whether or not they also possessed medical qualifications. They considered the characteristics of the mental subnormality hospital did *not* warrant a special organizational regime. The Association of Hospital Management Committees preferred to rely on one principal officer appointed by them, and responsible only to them for the administration of their hospital or hospitals. They considered that the Statutory Instrument (SI, 1948, No. 419) issued by the Ministry of Health (which established the position of the Medical Superintendent in relation to the other staff of the Committee) interposed between themselves and the hospital secretary, a person charged with the general management of the hospital and enjoying some degree of independence of the principal officer. This was felt to be particularly threatening since Superintendents, being of consultant status, were appointed by, and under contract to, a superior body – the Regional Hospital Board.

The official view of the Board of Control and the Ministry of Health appeared to be that the work of a lay administrator might well be essential in safeguarding patients, but that vital decisions regarding the care of such patients should be made by doctors. They maintained that authority in medical hands was necessary, in order to deal with day to day emergencies, and that the Medical Superintendent should be in a position to intervene on any matter affecting a patient. Consultant colleagues were to be allocated beds with full consultant responsibility.

The administrative changes also included the nursing staff, who

---

[1] At the time of the research in the 34 hospitals visited 15 secretaries were Fellows of the Institute of Hospital Administrators (3 of these had additional experience in a limited liability company and 1 had a Diploma in Public Administration). Ten secretaries were Associates of the Institute of Hospital Administrators (4 of these with experience in limited liability companies). Eight secretaries had no formal qualifications and one hospital had no secretary. We have only included the secretaries of the main units of the hospitals.

became the third prong in the tripartite system. However, whereas the controversy in relation to medical versus lay administration has been relatively continuous, problems of authority arising between nursing and medical administration have been minimal, and they have been relatively minor between nursing and lay administration.

In 1950 the Central Health Services Council set up a committee to examine the internal administration of hospitals (the Bradbeer Committee) and they reported in 1954.[1] They made a number of recommendations from which the following excerpts have been selected and shortened; they are included as being particularly relevant to the field of mental subnormality:

1. The special nature of the mental hospital[2] demands the concentration of a considerable degree of authority in the hands of the Medical Superintendent (para. 135).
2. Model Standing Orders for the government of mental hospitals should be circulated, defining the function of the Medical Superintendent (paras. 135 and 136).
3. Major mental hospitals require the services of a resident psychiatrist of consultant status; problems of patient management are too complex to be effectively handled by a lay officer on medical advice (para. 137).
4. The Medical Superintendent's power of suspension in relation to senior officers should be used only after consultation with the Chairman or Vice-Chairman of the Governing Body (para. 141).
5. Measures should be adopted to give Hospital Management Committees a more effective voice in the appointment of Medical Superintendents (para. 142).
6. There exist insufficient inducements to attract adequate numbers of experienced medical men to the post of Medical Superintendent (para. 143).
7. Medical Staff Committees should be set up (para. 137).

With regard to nursing administration in mental hospitals, the Committee thought that there was some justification for the belief that the status of the Matron (and Chief Male Nurse) was lower than is the case in general hospitals, and they recommended that 'although the Medical Superintendent must exercise supervision over all matters concerning patients, his supervision over matters within the Matron's jurisdiction should be discreet and minimal'.

The evidence of the Royal Medico-Psychological Association and other bodies had expressed some anxiety at the removal from nursing administration in some hospitals for any concern in maintenance departments such as laundry, sewing room, farms, gardens, etc. The

[1] *Report of the Committee on the Internal Administration of Hospitals*, HMSO 1954, reprinted 1961.

[2] In these recommendations the term 'mental hospital' includes mental subnormality hospital.

Committee recommended that where such work was part of therapy, the decision should be a medical one, but that 'it should be possible for Matron, in the interests of patients, to have considerable influence in the day-to-day running of the departments'.

There was a general feeling amongst Committee members that the sense of isolation of nursing staff in a tripartite system was more acute in mental than in general hospitals.

The Committee discussed the relationship between the Matron and Chief Male Nurse and although it was recognized that the Matron was normally 'supreme' in questions of training, and that such a situation perpetuates 'the inferior position of the Chief Male Nurse', they added a rider that despite this, the co-ordination of male and female staff under a Principal Nursing Officer was seen as 'unsuccessful'.[1]

Most of the recommendations in relation to Matrons (and Chief Male Nurses) lay in the direction of making them directly responsible to the Governing Body of the group, and giving them direct access to it. In her non-professional functions (that is when acting as Chief Resident Executive, or when responsible for domestic staff), the Matron's responsibility was to be to the Chief Administrative Officer in the first instance, rather than the Governing Body direct. The Committee recommended the setting up of various nursing committees, and consideration was to be given to recognition of joint responsibility between Matron and Chief Male Nurse for nurse training.

The Committee's recommendations regarding lay administration are important only in so far as, unlike recommendations relating to medical and nursing administration, they do not differentiate between general hospitals and mental hospitals. They set out the responsibilities and duties of different types of administrative officer: Group Secretary, Finance Officer, Supplies Officer, etc.

The degree to which the Ministry of Health's views should be 'imposed' upon Regional Hospital Boards and Management Committees has always been open to disagreement, or at best uncertainty. Certainly the situation regarding the administration of subnormality hospitals appears to have remained a very tenuous one; the direction of change, if any, depended chiefly upon the individual personalities involved and their ability to win support for their point of view.[2]

In July 1960 a further circular was issued by the Ministry of Health[3] revoking the regulations of the NHS (Superintendents of mental hospitals, etc.) Regulations, 1948. As from 1st November 1960:

a psychiatric hospital will be in the same position as any other hospital in that, although a Superintendent may be appointed for

---

[1] These findings are not shared by the *Report of the Salmon Committee* (1966).

[2] For a more detailed discussion of the results of administrative change see in particular Chapters 10 and 13.

[3] HM (60) 66.

the hospital, there will be no obligation for this to be done. As and when Superintendent posts at psychiatric hospitals become vacant, it will be for the hospital authorities to decide whether or not the hospital should continue to be administered by a Superintendent, *and if one is appointed what his precise duties should be*.[1] Before coming to any decision, Regional Boards will no doubt seek and give much weight to the wishes of the individual Hospital Management Committees concerned.

The circular then goes on to indicate ways in which the lay administration might be constituted in order to allow due weight to medical considerations.

In many ways this circular did little more than give official blessing to a confusion which already existed, and which continues to exist today.

It might be felt that undue attention has been given in this chapter to the question of administration, but our evidence suggests that by virtue of Circular HM (60) 66, the Ministry of Health gave to the Regional Hospital Board and Management Committee the task of deciding upon the administrative organization of any particular hospital. But since the Medical Superintendent and the Group Secretary both attend meetings of the committees concerned in making the decision, the uncertainty and dissatisfaction arising from this ambiguous situation have created major problems affecting not only the organization of the hospitals, but through this, the treatment that patients receive. We shall hope to give evidence of this in subsequent chapters.

Costs

The Ministry of Health Annual Reports (1962–7) set out the average national weekly cost of maintaining in-patients in various types of hospital. Table 3.5 (page 58) has been prepared from this source since it might be thought to represent types of patient requiring roughly parallel expenditure.[2]

In general yearly increases in the average amount spent per patient per week have been considerably smaller in subnormality institutions than in other types of hospital. Between 1961 and 1967 there has been an increase in in-patient cost per week in subnormality hospitals of only approximately 44 per cent, whereas in mental illness hospitals the increase is approximately 48 per cent.

Figures for the mid-nineteen-fifties are not published in strictly comparable form, mainly because no separate costing was carried out as between mental illness and mental subnormality hospitals.

[1] Author's italics.
[2] The difference between long-stay and chronic is not made clear in the Ministry of Health Report.

Table 3.5

NATIONAL AVERAGE COST PER WEEK (IN-PATIENTS)

Type of hospital	1961–2			1963–4			1964–5			1966–7		
	£	s.	d.	£	s.	d.	£	s.	d.	£	s.	d.
Mental Subnormality	8	2	0	9	1	8	9	17	6	11	11	7
Mental Illness	9	2	10	10	9	5	11	5	11	13	11	1
Long-Stay	13	16	4	13	12	1	16	17	0	20	9	7
Chronic	12	17	4	14	9	5	15	9	5	18	6	2

Source: Annual Reports of the Ministry of Health.

The Report of the Committee of Inquiry into the Cost of the National Health Service[1] stated 'in 1953–4 the mental illness and mental deficiency hospitals which cared for over 40 per cent of the in-patients absorbed only 20 per cent of the cost of the hospitals'.

The fact that the cost of maintaining a patient in a subnormality hospital is lower than in any other type of hospital[2] may be surprising in view of the fact that there are very heavy laundry costs arising from a high incidence of incontinence, as well as the fact that a high proportion of clothing is supplied by the hospital. Unfortunately detailed expenditure is not readily available, but it is certainly true that these averages obscure wide differences from one region to another,[3] particularly in relation to the distribution of expenditure, i.e. how much is spent on food, clothing, drugs, etc.

In this chapter we have attempted to portray a general picture of hospital provisions for the subnormal in the hope that this will provide the reader with a background against which the research data can be examined. The next eight chapters, forming Part Two of the report, will be concerned with the empirical findings of the survey.

[1] HMSO Command 9663 (January 1956).

[2] It is also worth noting that the cost is lower than in all penal institutions. The average cost in these for the year 1965 was £13 5s. 8d. (Report on the Work of the Prison Department, 1965, HMSO, Command 3088 (1966)).

[3] Although separate figures are not given for mental illness and mental subnormality hospitals, the Ministry of Health Report for the year ending 1955 (Command 9857) shows that in certain regions, notably Newcastle, North-East Metropolitan, Oxford and South-Western, there were marked increases in the share of total capital expenditure in hospitals, whereas in other regions, such as Sheffield, North-West Metropolitan, South-East Metropolitan and Manchester there was little or no such increase. These regional differences affect not only subnormality hospitals: in 1965 and 1966 the Oxford region had the highest patient-week costs, but the lowest patient-treatment costs of all 15 regions. (*The Lancet*, 10 December, 1966, p. 1322).

Part Two
SURVEY FINDINGS

Chapter 4

THE PATIENT POPULATION

Background characteristics

MANY of the recent studies of populations of subnormality hospitals have concentrated primarily on age and grade of defect, and the emphasis has been on establishing the extent to which training and education are important in bringing about improvements in patients' mental and physical capabilities.[1] In this chapter we shall attempt to give a picture of the social background and degree of physical handicap among the 3,038 patients in our sample.

Table 4.1

SEX AND AGE DISTRIBUTION OF PATIENTS IN HOSPITAL SAMPLE
(PERCENTAGES)

Age group (years)	Male	Female	Total	Estimated total population England and Wales 1964*
0 – 4	1·1	1·1	1·1	8·4
5 – 9	4·5	3·8	4·2	7·2
10 – 15	7·3	6·1	6·8	8·5
16 – 19	8·5	6·8	7·7	6·3
20 – 29	19·5	15·6	17·7	12·9
30 – 39	16·7	13·9	15·5	12·7
40 – 49	16·3	17·4	16·8	13·0
50 – 59	15·4	17·9	16·5	13·1
60 and over	10·7	17·4	13·8	17·6
TOTAL	100·0	100·0	100·0	100·0
No information	16	14	30	—
No. of persons	1,664	1,374	3,038	47,511,000

* *Source:* Registrar General's Statistical Review of England and Wales for the year 1964.

[1] See for example Castell and Mittler 'Intelligence of Patients in Subnormality Hospitals: A Survey of Admissions in 1961' in *Brit. J. Psychiatry*, Vol. III, No. 472, March 1965; also *British Psychological Society Report* on 'Children in Hospitals for the Subnormal' (1966). However, two noticeable exceptions are Cross, K. W.: 'A Survey of Mental Deficiency in Institutions in the Birmingham Region', *Brit. J. Prev. Soc. Med.* (1954, 8, 162–71) and O'Connor and Tizard, *op. cit.* (particularly Chapter III).

It will be seen from Table 4.1 that by comparison with the total population of England and Wales as at 30 June, 1964, children between the ages of 0–16 are under-represented in hospitals for the subnormal, whereas adults from the age of 20 are markedly over-represented, except in the upper age bracket, by which time many subnormal persons will have died and others may be in mental hospitals or geriatric units. The possible reasons for the preponderance of adults will be discussed later in the chapter when it will also be shown that a high proportion of patients enter hospital as adults.[1]

Table 4.1 shows that the number of children in the population sampled totalled 12·1 per cent; this compares with a figure of 12·33 per cent obtained by O'Connor and Tizard in their Home Counties study.[2] However these authors found almost no difference in the daily population as between the sexes, whereas our own study shows that 54·4 per cent of the patients were male, although in the case of those aged 60 and over, the distribution follows the normal demographic pattern, with females exceeding males. Penrose,[3] who also found a preponderance of males, suggests that this may be due to a form of social selection operating against boys, society being less able to tolerate inadequate role performance amongst males.

Table 4.2 shows how long the patients had been in the particular hospital he or she was in at the time of our visit. Whilst a few patients may have spent a period in another hospital on a previous occasion, we found that transfers were, in general, quite infrequent. Furthermore, when looking at this table, it should be borne in mind that in those cases where patients had on some occasion been discharged and then readmitted, we counted the time from the most recent date of admission.

Clearly a high proportion of those entering hospital at the present time do so as adults (i.e. from the age of 16); thus 28 per cent of sampled patients who had been in hospital for less than one year, were over the age of 16; the point is further illustrated by the fact that over 55 per cent of sampled patients aged 20 to 29 came into hospital between four and ten years ago, that is when they were between the ages of ten and 19. This tendency for patients to be admitted in late childhood and early adulthood may be due to the fact that social pressures on the family become more acute once the patient ceases to be a 'child', or alternatively it may reflect past as well as present shortage of places in senior training centres in the community.[4] The former suggestion confirms views expressed in-

---

[1] For an interesting discussion of the factors involved in parents seeking admission to hospital for their handicapped child see *Mental Subnormality in London: A survey of community care*; a PEP Report (1966).

[2] *op. cit.*

[3] *op. cit.*

[4] The number of places in training centres for adults in 1965 was 15,348, representing 0·32 places per 1,000 population. There are wide regional differences varying from 1·08 to 0 per 1,000 population. Although there are plans to increase

Table 4.2

AGE BY NUMBER OF YEARS IN HOSPITAL (PERCENTAGES)

Number of years in hospital	Age									% of sampled patients
	0–4	5–9	10–15	16–19	20–29	30–39	40–49	50–59	60 and over	
Under 1 year	57·6	18·7	5·9	9·9	5·3	4·5	3·4	2·6	2·3	5·5
1 – 3 years	36·4	60·2	27·5	22·4	14·9	12·3	9·3	6·6	5·1	14·4
4 – 9 years	6·0	21·1	53·9	41·8	35·3	20·9	25·2	18·2	14·4	26·6
10 – 19 years	—	—	12·7	25·9	35·6	34·8	20·9	20·6	14·9	23·5
20 or more years	—	—	—	—	8·9	27·5	41·2	52·0	63·3	30·0
TOTAL	100·0	100·0	100·0	100·0	100·0	100·0	100·0	100·0	100·0	100·0
No information	—	2	—	—	—	3	2	1	5	—
No. of patients*	33	125	204	232	533	465	505	497	414	3,008

* Excluding 30 patients about whose age we have no information.

formally by both doctors and parents to the effect that siblings and friends or neighbours are able to tolerate a defective child, but not a defective adolescent or adult. In an unpublished survey of families with retarded children carried out by the present writer in San Francisco, parents found it extremely difficult to manage their children once they reached the age of 15 or more, often because siblings were embarrassed to bring home their friends, and chances of 'dating' were felt to be reduced by having a mentally subnormal brother or sister.[1] Similarly the problem of what to do with an adult in terms of occupation becomes more acute; there is considerable tolerance in the community for a child who plays or does nothing, but such tolerance is rarely extended to an adult, except possibly within a limited social network.

Marital status and social class Of those aged 16 and over in our sample only 1·2 per cent had at any time been legally married. At the time of the research 23 of the 33 still were married, two were separated, four divorced and four widowed.

In the extensive survey no attempt was made to obtain information about the social class background of patients. Such an attempt was made, however, in connection with the intensive sample, and this revealed a preponderance of patients coming from the families of manual workers.[2]

Family status The nurses in charge of wards were asked whether the sampled patients were known to have parents, siblings, and/or other relatives. Nurses often experienced considerable difficulty in answering this question, though the existence of parents and siblings was usually recorded somewhere in the case notes.[3]

A total of 12·4 per cent of patients, one-third of them being under

[1] See also Adams, M.: *The Mentally Subnormal, the Social Casework Approach*, Heinemann (1960), who noted that those who were admitted to institutions were not necessarily more handicapped, but were those who had failed in their social adjustment to adult life, and the majority of them had adverse family backgrounds.

[2] It is perhaps worth noting here that both qualitatively and quantitatively the data obtained confirmed our belief that it would not have been worth while attempting this in the main sample, particularly bearing in mind the additional time that would have been involved.

[3] The research workers made no check on this information from the administrative case notes kept in the general office.

the number to 33,971 in 1976 (0·65 places per 1,000) these figures again mask great inequalities between different areas. Eighteen authorities' plans show a ratio in 1976 no higher than the national average for 1965, and the national average for 1976 is lower than the provision made for 1965 by 20 authorities. *Health and Welfare, the Development of Community Care*, HMSO, Command 3022 (June 1966). These statistics are followed by the comment '. . . while showing substantial improvement over the present provision, (plans) fall short of meeting the full need, particularly for training centres for adults'.

the age of 16, were known to have a combination of parents, siblings *and* other relatives; another third of the children had parents and siblings, but there was nothing known about other relatives.

Just over 13 per cent of patients were not known by nursing staff to have any relatives; as might be expected this was directly related to age, and those without relatives were mainly to be found amongst those aged 50 or more. Only 12 children under the age of 16 had no parents alive, and seven of these had no known relatives at all.

Intelligence

The literature is full of criticisms of the use of intelligence tests for assessing degrees of subnormality[1] (though not much of the criticism is directed at their *mis*use) and no useful service would be performed by repeating such views. The position is well stated by Stott[2] who writes:

> to summarize this criticism of the present procedures of ascertainment, on the one hand they are based on a static view of the level of 'intelligence' and of the ability to predict a child's future mental development; on the other hand they rely on vaguely phrased impressionistic information which does not lend itself to objective summary or validation.

So far as our own sample is concerned, we have thought it worth while to set out the data, if only to illustrate the paucity of information, and we advise the greatest caution in its interpretation. Although tests were known to have been carried out on 57 per cent of sampled patients (see Table 4.3 below) actual test *results* were only available in 47·3 per cent of cases (see Table 4.4, page 67) and in only 37·5 per cent of cases do we know which test was used; where this information is available, the majority (23 per cent) were tested on Binet scales.[3] In 5·8 per cent of cases Wechsler scales were known to have been used, and the remaining 8·7 per cent included Cattell, Goodenough, Progressive Matrices, Kohs Blocks, etc.; a further 17·2 per cent of patients were known to have been tested, but there was no information about the test used, many such cases were recorded as 'untestable'. From the manner of recording, i.e. 'M.A. approx . . .' there was also evidence to suggest that many results entered in the case notes were likely to be no more than informed guesses.

We also asked nurses to look at the case notes in order to find out when the test was carried out and this information is set out below:

[1] See for example Gunzberg, H. C.: 'Psychological Assessment in Mental Deficiency' and 'Educational Problems in Mental Deficiency' in Clarke and Clarke, *op. cit.*, O'Connor and Tizard, *op. cit.*, p. 13 ff., Castell and Mittler, *op. cit.*
[2] Stott, D. H., writing in the *Medical. Officer*, 11 October, 1963.
[3] These include forms L and M of the 1937 Revision as well as the 1960 Revision.

Table 4.3

DATE OF LAST KNOWN TEST (PERCENTAGES)

When tested*	Patients
Within preceding 12 months	4·6
Within 1 – 2 years	5·3
Within 2 – 5 years	12·4
More than 5 years ago	25·6
Tested, but date unknown	13·0
Not tested	39·1
TOTAL	100·0
No information	177
No. of patients	3,038

* In some cases a date was given but the result was recorded as 'untestable'.

Thus it will be noted that only 4·6 per cent had been tested within the preceding twelve months, and approximately 22 per cent within the past five years: a great many tests dated back to the 1930s. In the vast majority of cases the nurses who were asked to supply the information had no idea what the patient's IQ might be and many had considerable difficulty in finding any reference to it in the case record.[1]

It might be thought that the presence of a full-time psychologist on the staff would result in a higher percentage of patients being tested and/or that tests would be more up-to-date.[2] This did not always prove to be the case: the only hospital where all tests appeared to be up-to-date employed a 'psychological tester' who could not be graded by the hospital authorities as a psychologist because she lacked the proper academic qualifications. In some hospitals the Medical Superintendent claimed that regular assessments were made by medical staff, but if this were the case, they certainly did not normally record them on the case notes kept on the wards.

The fact that almost 49 per cent of cases were recorded as either 'not tested' or 'untestable' may be thought to indicate that our method of obtaining this data was unsatisfactory. Certainly we did not ask that tests be carried out specially, since in part our objective

[1] In one large hospital case records were not kept on the wards on the female side, but the records of the patients in the sample were passed to the wards by the doctor when we gave him a list of names. This was the first time that the nurses had seen them.

[2] It is possible that psychologists kept separate records and did not record test results on case papers. However, we think we should have been told had this been the case, since we always interviewed the psychologist in charge (for further information about these interviews see Chapter 7).

Table 4.4

AGE BY IQ (PERCENTAGES)

	Age							
IQ	0–15	16–19	20–29	30–39	40–49	50–59	60 and over	Total
Under 50	20·1	17·4	34·3	40·3	38·9	38·0	35·7	33·7
50 – 59	2·3	3·2	8·2	7·6	9·6	10·9	12·4	8·2
60 – 69	0·3	6·8	4·9	4·8	4·8	7·3	4·3	4·8
70 and over	1·7	4·1	5·3	4·3	3·9	5·4	5·1	4·4
Not tested	44·6	33·3	23·1	23·8	24·5	23·0	28·9	27·6
Untestable	30·9	35·2	24·3	19·2	18·3	15·5	13·5	21·3
TOTAL	100·0	100·0	100·0	100·0	100·0	100·0	100·0	100·0
No information	19	13	43	28	47	31	44	229
No. of patients*	362	232	533	465	505	497	414	3008

* Excluding 30 patients about whose age we have no information.

was to discover how much was actually known about patients at ward level. Furthermore to have requested that tests be carried out on such a large number of patients would certainly have put an intolerable burden on psychologists and medical staff. It is interesting to note that the figure of 21·3 per cent of sampled patients actually *in* hospital and deemed untestable approximates very closely to the percentage of untestable *admissions* to all subnormality hospitals in 1960 (20 per cent).[1] On the other hand our figure of 27·6 per cent 'not tested' is considerably lower than the number of *admissions* described as 'no result stated' (41·7 per cent). This may be accounted for by the fact that undoubtedly some of this group will have been tested after admission.

We were particularly surprised to find such a high proportion of children under 16 who had apparently not been tested (33 per cent), and we can only assume that in many cases the tests were carried out before admission to the hospital but the results were not recorded on the ward case notes. Furthermore in this same age group are to be found an equally large number of patients described as 'untestable' (35 per cent) and it would, of course, be unwise to assume that they all had IQs of below 50. It may be that their physical handicap or disturbed behaviour prevented their being tested on any available test.

Our results are not comparable with those of the Working Party

[1] See Registrar General's *Statistical Review for 1960, Supplement on Mental Health*, HMSO (1964).

of the British Psychological Society,[1] since the latter were concerned only with children admitted to specific hospitals (a non-representative sample) in a particular year (1962), whereas our own information relates to the total population *in a representative sample of hospitals* at the time of the research, and includes all ages. The Working Party found that of children admitted in 1962 to 17 hospitals where a psychologist was employed, 155 out of 403 were tested and of these 98 (24 per cent of all child admissions) had IQs of over 50. However, as the authors of the pamphlet say '. . . the sample cannot be considered representative of the country's subnormality hospitals as a whole, since it excludes all hospitals without psychology departments, most of the smaller hospitals, and many of the larger hospitals in the south west and north of England . . .'. They point out that the 17 hospitals were far from uniform in relation to the kind of patients admitted, and that they appeared to be well above the national average in respect of the proportion of teaching staff with formal qualifications. The findings of the Working Party demonstrate a need for more specialized educational facilities for children in certain hospitals, in view of the number of children admitted to these hospitals with IQs over 50. But such findings tend to be obscured when a representative sample of patients in all hospitals is taken, since it seems that the overall proportion of children actually in hospitals with IQs above 50 is quite small.[2]

Whilst recognizing the danger of assuming that incomplete information is directly comparable with more specific and complete data, it is perhaps worth noting that if one *were* to redistribute the group of 'untested' patients shown in Table 4.4 above in the same proportions as those for whom we have test information, the total number of patients of *all* ages with an IQ under 50 would be approximately 47 per cent, those with an IQ of 50 or over would be approximately 24 per cent, and there would be approximately 30 per cent in the category of 'untestable'.

Physical disabilities

There have been many suggestions in recent years that a hospital is not the right place to care for the subnormal, since relatively few of them are believed to be in need of regular medical and nursing care. One medical superintendent commented: 'Half of them could live without doctors and nurses buzzing around annoying them. We had to turn them into medical cases in order to justify social care'. This particular psychiatrist considered that half the accommodation in all subnormality hospitals should be staffed by non-medical and non-

---

[1] *op. cit.*

[2] This is not, however, an argument against the need for more specialized educational facilities. Our discussion in Chapter 7 makes clear the inadequacy of present arrangements.

nursing staff, but that when patients became sick or if they deteriorated, they could be moved, probably temporarily, to the medical side of the hospital.[1]

In an attempt to obtain some idea of the type and extent of physical handicap amongst the hospital population, we asked a number of questions relating to mobility, epilepsy, spasticity, incontinence, patients' ability to dress and feed themselves, and special handicaps such as blindness, deformity, etc., as well as information about those suffering from the more severe psychiatric disorders such as psychosis.[2]

Our findings certainly lend support to the view of those who feel that professional medical and nursing skills are not required in a high proportion of cases. Most of the patients in our sample (83·4 per cent) were fully ambulant, 8·8 per cent were bedfast or confined to a wheelchair all day, and the remaining 7·7 per cent walked only with difficulty and required assistance in moving around.

With regard to incontinence our data suggests that except on children's wards the problem is likely to be less severe than would appear from discussion with the nursing staff. Whilst 50·5 per cent of the 362 children are severely incontinent[3] and 23·7 per cent moderately so, amongst adults only 12·4 per cent of the 2,676 patients are severe cases, and 13·2 per cent moderate.[4]

Yet incontinence is said by the staff to be a major problem since it involves them in a great deal of work of a somewhat unpleasant nature and puts very real pressure on the laundry service. It is also frequently mentioned as one reason why patients cannot wear their own clothing all the time, nor have the same clothes back from the laundry; the argument in the former case being that there would be insufficient clothing if all had to keep their own individual supply.[5] Furthermore, in some wards (and seemingly more so in some hospitals), nurses experienced considerable difficulty in getting rid of the smell of incontinence, nor was this confined to the older buildings; in one hospital largely composed of 'modern' villas, the

---

[1] Professor T. McKeown also believes that subnormal persons should be clearly divided into those who need basic nursing and medical attention (to be cared for by the NHS) and those who require only minor personal services or intermittent medical supervision (to be cared for by Local Health Authorities). See *The Heart of the Matter*, Report of the Annual Conference of the NAMH, 1966.

[2] All the above information was obtained from the nurse in charge of the ward who, in some instances checked the case record. Time was not available to verify the information from doctors, teachers, psychologists, etc.

[3] 'Severely' is defined as daily, and in addition most of these patients were also doubly incontinent. 'Moderate' is defined as wetting or soiling occasionally.

[4] Our total of 74·2 per cent on children's wards exceeds that obtained by Cross in his Birmingham survey; he gives a figure of 61 per cent. His figures for adults were 18 per cent for males and 12 per cent for females. The discrepancies may be due to the use of different definitions; Cross refers to 'habitual incontinence' but gives no more precise definition.

[5] This will be discussed in more detail in Chapters 5 and 10.

sanitary annexes all smelt appalling, irrespective of the time of day.

The majority of the 3,038 patients, 65·6 per cent, could both feed and dress themselves; 16·8 per cent could feed but not dress themselves; 0·5 could dress but not feed themselves and 16·9 per cent were unable to do either, but this group includes the 1·1 per cent of under fives in the population who might be unable to do this irrespective of their subnormality or physical handicap.

Table 4.5 sets out the number of sampled patients suffering from various physical handicaps and from severe mental illness (separate figures are given for epilepsy and spasticity later in the chapter).

The information contained in this table was obtained from the nurse in charge of the ward. We do not consider that it presents an entirely accurate picture, and in particular we believe it to be an underestimate of the true incidence of physical handicap and serious mental illness – particularly the latter.[1] This may have arisen for a number of reasons: firstly because nurses seemed often ill-informed about physical symptoms, partly because so few appear to have had a general nurse training, and partly because the older staff who tended to be in charge of wards had no up to date training in subnormality or psychiatric nursing.[2]

A second factor which may have resulted in an underestimate of reported symptoms arose from a tendency on the part of nursing staff to assume that physical disabilities were an intrinsic symptom of subnormality and they did not, therefore, consider the two factors independently. Thirdly, where patients had been looked after for many years by the same nurse (and those in charge of wards from whom we sought information tended to stay on the same ward indefinitely, as did the patients) they seemed no longer to notice the patient's disability, they become adapted to it. Thus we sometimes saw patients who were clearly deformed, or partially crippled, yet the nurse would say that they had no disability and when this fact was drawn to their attention they seemed quite surprised and commented, for example: 'Oh, but he can get around and do things for himself all right'. Sometimes nurses would ask what we meant by physical disability and when it was suggested that this was intended to include any symptom which would require special apparatus or treatment outside the hospital, or which might result in problems of

[1] In a study of 1,652 Birmingham residents in local hospitals for the subnormal, Leck, Gordon and McKeown report 37 per cent as considered to have 'significant associated psychiatric disorders'. *Brit. J. Prev. Soc. Med.*, Vol. 21, No. 3, July 1967.

[2] We did not, in the national survey, inquire about the qualifications of nursing staff, but we did so in the intensive study where we found that amongst *registered* nurses, only 14 per cent in one hospital and 7 per cent in the other had a general nursing training. The figures for qualifications in psychiatric nursing were 42 per cent and 10 per cent respectively. Although we are not qualified to comment upon the training of psychiatric nurses or mental subnormality nurses, we think it likely that their training is somewhat limited in relation to physical disabilities.

Table 4.5
PHYSICAL HANDICAPS (PERCENTAGES)

Type of handicap	Number of patients*		
	Under 16	16 and over	All ages
Physical deformity symptomatic of subnormality	9·7	3·5	4·2
Total paralysis (including severely or completely crippled)	12·4	4·6	5·6
Partial paralysis (including moderately crippled)	10·2	4·2	4·9
Motor handicap (difficulty in movement, walking, etc.)	6·9	5·6	5·8
Infectious illness (including tuberculosis)	0·6	0·6	0·6
Other deformities (e.g., curvature of spine)	1·9	2·8	2·7
Cardio-vascular disorders	1·1	0·9	0·9
Mutism	11·3	2·8	3·8
Severe speech defect	6·1	3·5	3·8
Severe deafness	0·8	1·2	1·2
Blindness	2·2	2·1	2·1
Severe ocular condition (including blind in one eye)	3·6	1·2	1·5
Deaf/mute	1·7	0·7	0·8
Metabolic disorder (e.g., diabetes, phenylketonuria, etc.)	0·8	0·4	0·5
Other (including mental illness)	0·8	0·4	0·4
None of the above handicaps	41·7	67·5	64·4
No. of patients	362	2,676	3,038

* 8·9 per cent of all patients suffered from two or more of the handicaps listed.

adjustment in the community, they were again surprised that we should use such criteria. We feel that this illustrated to some extent their expectation that physical handicap must, almost of necessity, accompany mental subnormality and in this respect nurses appear to reflect the attitudes of a large proportion of the general public.

Fourthly and probably most importantly, we think that interviewers did not probe sufficiently, particularly in relation to mental illness, and case-notes made virtually no reference to mental symptoms.

Even bearing in mind that the information set out in Table 4.5 may be unreliable (and it is likely to be so only in terms of underestimation) it is clear that generally speaking the proportion of children suffering from the particular forms of physical handicap listed is greater than in the case of adults. As we shall show later in this chapter, the same situation applies in relation to spasticity and epilepsy.

Knowledge about mental illness appeared also to be somewhat limited amongst nursing staff. The fact that so few patients were described as suffering from serious mental illness may, we believe, be due to the fact that as in the case of physical disabilities nurses expect the mentally subnormal to show symptoms of mental illness, and they cannot easily distinguish between the two. This view is supported by the fact that although we did not obtain information regarding the presence or absence of disturbed behaviour amongst our sample of patients, we did ask the nurse in charge of each ward to give the total number of severely disturbed patients in her care. Again this caused considerable difficulty, since the interpretation of 'severely disturbed' was likely to vary from one nurse to another. In general terms we explained that this category should include those patients whose mental condition (as distinct from the problem of subnormality or physical handicap) would make them a problematical group requiring treatment outside the subnormality hospital setting. We suggested that those who showed symptoms of exceptional aggression or bizarre behaviour, as well as those who were unduly withdrawn or depressive should be included. Nurses also found difficulty in answering this question because so many patients are emotionally labile and may 'blow up' at any time. Clearly our findings must be regarded as highly tentative and we suggest that the figure they gave of 9·2[1] per cent severely disturbed patients in the total population of the hospitals sampled includes mainly those patients who *frequently* show symptoms of serious disturbance.[2] It seems legitimate to postulate that many of these patients could be genuinely described as

---

[1] In this and any other references to the total population of patients in the sampled hospitals, the results have been weighted to take into account the varying probabilities of selection of the hospitals.

[2] These patients were almost always receiving drug therapy for their mental state.

mentally ill, and the fact that only 0·4 per cent were included in our sample is likely to be an underestimate of true prevalence, due possibly to the fact that when completing our questionnaires, nurses did not always record (or possibly did not recognize) mental illness as a separate handicap.

Information was also obtained from the nurse in charge of each ward with regard to epilepsy and spasticity amongst the sampled patients. It will be noted that the proportions are particularly large, especially in relation to epilepsy (see Table 4.6 below).

Table 4.6

SAMPLED PATIENTS DIAGNOSED AS SPASTIC OR
EPILEPTIC ACCORDING TO AGE AND SEVERITY OF SYMPTOMS
(PERCENTAGES)

	Severe		Moderate		Severe and Moderate
	Under 16	16 and over	Under 16	16 and over	Total all ages
Spastic	14·0	3·4	12·1	5·7	11·6
Epileptic*	8·3	4·1	24·0	14·5	20·6
No. of patients	362	2,676	362	2,676	3,038

* Severe is defined as having attacks more than once weekly.

From this table it is clear that amongst those suffering from epilepsy, and more particularly in its severe form, the proportion of children to adults is approximately double. With regard to spasticity, whilst only 5 per cent of the total population sampled (adults and children) were diagnosed as *severely* spastic, the proportion of children in this group was far higher than in the case of adults (the ratio being about 4:1 in the case of *severe* spasticity, and 2:1 in the case of moderate spasticity.[1])

If we include both spasticity and epilepsy with those other forms of disability set out in Table 4.5 *supra*, we find that 38 per cent of the children in the sample and 14 per cent of the adults, suffer from some form of multiple handicap involving two or more different disabilities.[2] No clear pattern of combination exists, a large number of

[1] It has been suggested to us that ideally the Spastics' Society would like to remove spastics from subnormality hospitals and to care for them in a spastic society home. This appears impracticable at present, not only because there is still a shortage of places in such homes, but also because it is said to cost approximately £150 more per annum to keep a patient in such a home, as compared with an NHS hospital, and Local Health Authorities may be reluctant to consider transferring a patient from hospital care where he is the financial responsibility of the NHS. (View expressed by member of Spastics' Society Staff.)

[2] In view of our earlier comments regarding the likelihood of nurses' underestimation of physical handicaps, this may also be reflected in this figure.

spastics are also epileptic, and many spastics are either totally or partially paralysed, but apart from this, only one or two patients suffer from any one particular grouping of disabilities. Whilst acknowledging the unreliability of the data, we feel that it may be useful to give detailed information about the combinations we found, since such data are not apparently available in published form elsewhere. A table setting out the data is therefore to be found in Appendix E.

From the foregoing discussion it seems likely that it is on the children's wards that most of the secondary features requiring nursing care are to be found, particularly paralysis, severe cases of spasticity, epilepsy and incontinence, and the proportion of children having multiple handicaps is considerably higher than in the case of adults. The reason for this situation is not clear, but it seems probable that subnormal children who do not also suffer from physical handicaps can be cared for in the community until they reach adulthood. It may also be related to the fact that amongst the lowest grades (idiots) the death rate for children is particularly high. Of the 930 persons who died in mental subnormality hospitals during 1960, 22 per cent were idiots, and amongst males half of these deaths occurred at ages under sixteen years eight months, and amongst females at ages under thirteen years five months.[1] Furthermore reference was made earlier[2] to the fact that although there has been no *overall* change in average IQ and mental age of admissions, more of the children coming in now are severely subnormal than in the past. These facts suggest that different staffing ratios will be required on children's wards. The question of the most satisfactory allocation of medical, nursing and ancillary staff within subnormality hospitals, may at least equal in importance the discussion of *where* patients should be treated: in the community, in the district general hospital, or in a specialist hospital; this we shall refer to again later.[3]

Legal status

Approximately 7 per cent[4] of the 3,038 sampled patients were compulsorily detained; only three such patients were under the age of 16, the great majority being between the ages of 20 and 49. It is however,

[1] The Registrar General's *Statistical Review of England and Wales for the Year 1960: Supplement on Mental Health*, HMSO (1964). See Table MD 8.

[2] See Chapter 3, p. 49.

[3] In their survey of Birmingham residents, Leck, Gordon and McKeown (*op. cit.*) found that only about half the patients needed nursing care because of their mental and/or physical condition.

[4] In 1965, 55 subnormal persons and 6 severely subnormal patients were made the subject of Hospital Orders with Restriction by the Courts. A further 14 subnormal patients were transferred from penal institutions to hospitals for the subnormal with a Restriction Order and 9 subnormal patients without such an Order. *Criminal Statistics for England and Wales* (Command 3037, HMSO, July 1966).

interesting to note that by no means all patients who were compulsorily detained were prevented from leaving the hospital unaccompanied. Approximately one-third were confined to the ward, a further third were allowed out either alone or with other patients, and almost as many again were allowed to wander freely in the grounds of the hospital. Since at most hospitals there existed virtually no effective check on comings and goings at the entrance, this latter group of patients could quite easily walk outside the grounds, and seemingly did so, accompanied by other patients, if there was a village nearby to make the trip worthwhile. This raises important questions of principle regarding the compulsory detention of patients: are they detained allegedly for their own protection, or for that of the community? The fact that rather less than one-third of them are confined to the hospital ward suggests that if they are detained for the protection of the community, such an intention is being disregarded. On the other hand, if they are not considered by the hospital authorities to be a security risk, then it seems legitimate to ask why it is necessary that they remain as compulsory patients. One answer may be that in some hospitals patients who were recorded as compulsorily detained were in many instances detained prior to the 1959 Mental Health Act. Such persons could have been made informal patients but the necessary administrative steps were never taken. We think that this may be particularly true in the case of those compulsorily detained patients who were over the age of 50.

Summary

We have attempted in this chapter to give a picture of the type of patient at present in our subnormality hospitals; in subsequent chapters we shall try to describe the various services available for them, but first we shall discuss the physical conditions under which the patients live.

Chapter 5

THE PHYSICAL ENVIRONMENT
AND FACILITIES

IT is not easy to present a generalized picture of the hospitals studied in terms of bricks and mortar, firstly because unlike the majority of institutional buildings that house individuals who, for one reason or another, are segregated from the community, the hospitals for the subnormal tend, as we have already suggested, to consist of highly variegated complexes of buildings, rarely purpose-built, and often scattered between several sites. Only in the case of four of the thirty-four hospitals in the sample were all the units to be found on a single site, and a further nine were divided between two sites. The remainder comprised institutions scattered over between three and fifteen sites, many as much as thirty miles apart, and in two instances as far as ninety miles from the main administrative centre. The sense of isolation felt by the staff in some units is not difficult to understand. More detailed descriptions of the buildings, and the number of patients living in each unit, as well as the distance between the units and the main administrative centre are set out in tabular form in Appendix F. For purposes of simplification a summary of this information is set out in Table 5.1 below:[1]

Table 5.1

Total no. of pts. in hosp. complex	No. of hospital complexes	Average no. of sites	Mean distance of units from main hospital (miles)
1,800 and over	4	4·0	30·4
1,000 – 1,799	15	5·0	19·0
300 – 999	12	4·7	23·8
Under 300	3	1·7	9·0

A second difficulty in classifying information of this kind arises because although the majority of patients are administratively and medically the responsibility of large hospital units, the fact that so many are housed in ancillary units means that the 'real' administra-

---

[1] The information given here is not weighted since variation in weights within size strata is small.

tive and social unit is smaller than is often assumed. Thus of a total of 38,097 patients in the thirty-four hospitals visited, almost one-third lived in relatively small units away from the main administrative centre, a situation which has an important bearing on the nature of social life in the institution.[1]

The buildings

This discrepancy between the apparent total size of the hospital from an administrative point of view[2] and the 'real' size of the unit in which the patient is living is further illustrated in Table 5.2 by reference to our sample of 3,038 patients:[3]

Table 5.2

Size of hospital complex	Percentage of sampled patients in hospital complex	Percentage of sampled patients in a living unit of this size
1,800 and over	27·5	12·8
1,000 – 1,799	33·9	17·6
300 – 999	34·3	37·6
100 – 299	4·4	24·2
50 – 99	—	4·9
Under 50	—	3·0
TOTALS	100·0	100·0
No. of patients	3,038	3,038

By 'living unit' we do not simply mean a separate ward or villa, but a unit at some distance from the main hospital. Twenty-two per cent of our visits were to main units; of the remainder, 51·6 were to subsidiary units which had a very high degree of autonomy and the remaining 26·1 per cent were to non-autonomous units which were dependent upon the main hospital for most services.

Many of the buildings are very old and not suited to modern purposes; of the thirty-four hospitals studied, almost two-thirds were based upon a building or nucleus of buildings constructed before 1900.[4] Certain of these had been purpose-built for other requirements;

[1] See also comments in Chapter 3, p. 43 ff. *supra.*
[2] As has been pointed out earlier, in some instances the Hospital Management Committee is different.
[3] No information was obtained about the number of patients living away from the hospitals on licence, but attached to them for administrative purposes.
[4] It is not possible to say from the data collected exactly how many patients live in the different types of building. This is because of the extreme heterogeneity of the buildings even on a single site. It must also be remembered that patients do not necessarily spend their entire day in one particular building.

thus among the buildings in use were former workhouses built in 1830, 1838, 1840, 1848, 1856 and 1860; in other cases the precise date was unknown. The Victorian workhouse, the Victorian prison and the Victorian hospital were in certain respects remarkably similar, in that they were designed to hold populations under varying degrees of containment or control. Like most nineteenth-century public buildings they tended to be large, sometimes with internal proportions excessively out of human scale, draughty and poorly heated. Designed to be maintained by an unlimited supply of patient or inmate labour, the difficulties of keeping them clean in the mid-twentieth century scarcely need elaboration.

Perhaps even more unsatisfactory than the former workhouses are the innumerable former mansions currently used as hospitals. Apart from a tower reputedly dating from the eleventh century and currently used as a ward, the oldest mansion appears to have been built in 1660. Five mansions were of eighteenth-century construction, but the remainder, and majority, were of Victorian date. At least the workhouse was built around the 'ward' or 'dormitory' and was so constructed as to allow the staff to observe the inmates with relative ease. Furthermore it is possible to modernize and sub-divide these units, as has been demonstrated by the efforts in this direction that have been made by some Regional Hospital Boards. The mansion, on the other hand, was built to allow perhaps a dozen members of a wealthy household to enjoy a large amount of personal space which was nevertheless compartmentalized so as to provide privacy and isolation when required. The vast army of domestics were accommodated essentially out of view; children were produced by their nannies when required, but had to remain largely out of sight and sound, and master and mistress required separate, as well as joint, facilities. Functionally these great houses were appallingly inefficient in the plumbing, the location of their kitchens, and their reliance on coal fires; they were designed around the concept of the conspicuous consumption of cheap labour. As houses their scale was appropriate to the social status of their owners, as hospitals the dimensions of their rooms and corridors are quite inappropriate and their physical inconveniences legion.

Such mansions have one other major disadvantage in that whereas in their pristine state of good repair and decoration they were places of dignity and even beauty, the sheer cost of maintaining their often elaborate fabric has been such that they are in most cases run down and dilapidated to the point where they are, if anything, more depressing than the gloomy old workhouses.

Among the institutions visited, only one of those constructed before 1900 and holding around a thousand patients was purpose-built for the mentally subnormal. This was opened in 1868 on the basis of public subscription. The period 1900–14 saw the building of a number of special institutions for inebriates, and one of these forms the nucleus of a hospital on a single site accommodating around two thousand patients. In the period after World War I however, there were a number of purpose-built units constructed, generally of the two-storey 'villa' type. These buildings were provided to meet the expanding population of patients recognized to be mentally subnormal and requiring hospitalization;[1] this 'villa' type construction was resumed after 1945 and has continued to the present day. Such accommodation is human in scale and is far less institutionally oppressive, though often by no means ideal for nursing this particular type of patient. There are very few hospitals where the buildings are exclusively 'modern' and the common pattern is for a site to contain a number of buildings of widely ranging age and type.

Although comparatively little new building has taken place since 1950, in many of the hospitals visited a great deal of renovation and 'upgrading' was in progress. Desirable as this may be, if patients are not to be housed in buildings that are falling into decay, one could not but feel that in some cases the authorities were engaged in a vain (and expensive) struggle against damp, dry rot, and dilapidation. In at least one hospital an old mansion is due for demolition, so hopeless has the task become.

It must on the other hand be emphasized that by no means all the hospitals studied, and specifically not all the units of any one particular hospital, were in a state of deterioration; indeed the range of conditions was very wide indeed. Where physical conditions were poor they tended to have a negative effect on staff morale, not simply in terms of the overall atmosphere, but in consequence of the very considerable additional burdens placed upon nursing staff by having to cope with difficult stairs, a lack of lifts, unsatisfactory dining and sleeping arrangements, and outside sanitary annexes. The matron of one subsidiary unit housing approximately 180 patients complained that when patients died (they generally had only one death each year) they had to be carried down the fire-escape, past the dining room windows, because there were no lifts. The fire-escape stairs were steep iron ones, very awkward to manoeuvre.

Although the general overall condition of the physical plant was a *serious* problem in a minority of the hospitals visited, overcrowding was far more widespread; indeed it was overcrowding and the consequential effects on staff and patients, rather than decrepitude of buildings, that was the most striking single feature observed by the research team. But again, it is necessary to stress that, whilst not underestimating the undesirability of these conditions, the nursing staff in the majority of hospitals, however overcrowded, were fundamentally concerned about their patients as individuals, though their working conditions were such that their care and concern could often

---

[1] Whether for medical or social reasons.

only be expressed in ways more limited than they might otherwise desire.[1]

The old and overcrowded buildings were not the only ones with serious limitations; some of the most recently built villas failed to provide nursing staff with the facilities they needed. For example, in one hospital a children's ward had been built as recently as 1964 where the day room had also to serve as a dining room. As a consequence staff had to choose between returning the children to their dormitories after meals, or clearing away, stacking the furniture and wiping the floor while other staff 'potted' and cleaned up the children and attempted to keep them away from the debris of the meal. In other buildings of recent date, the staff often complained of sanitary annexes built too near the day rooms and with inadequate ventilation; alternatively they were built too far from the day rooms so that incontinent patients could not reach the lavatory in time, or had to be carried through a series of rooms, past many other patients and possibly upstairs in order to be cleaned up. Very few of the new villas were of the bungalow type and lifts were almost totally absent, although one would consider them an essential feature for the easy movement of patients with physical handicaps, or those confined to wheelchairs. Where lifts have been installed in old buildings, there are instances where the dimensions of the lift are such as to preclude their being used to transfer wheelchair patients. Due to overcrowding it was rarely possible to locate all such patients at ground floor level, a situation which resulted in a good deal of hardship for the nursing staff. Sometimes these arrangements meant that patients were confined to verandahs (or external covered corridors converted for the purpose) rather than being able to wheel themselves about in the grounds.[2]

Inside the hospitals

Our discussion so far has centred essentially upon the physical setting and fabric of the buildings and we shall now look more closely at the prevailing physical conditions inside the hospitals visited.

The research workers visited all wards (totalling 761) in the thirty-four hospitals sampled. Before describing the conditions we found, it might be useful to describe the way in which patients are allocated to them since it could be argued that different conditions may be needed for different types of patient. However the situation is fairly summed up by the Superintendent of a large, and for the most part

---

[1] For discussion of nurses' attitudes to their work see Chapter 6.

[2] Hospital grounds were almost always attractively laid out and well maintained, usually by groups of patients under the supervision of at least one professional gardener. At one hospital in particular, gardening is regarded as a form of therapy for a special group of patients who have built an ornamental garden.

modern, hospital who said: 'Ideally, like in most hospitals there is classification by age, grade of defect and physical handicap; but in practice it is a question very largely of where there is a space. Some regard is paid to age in the case of children, and of course to sex.' In another, much smaller hospital, the Medical Superintendent told us that age was only important in relation to keeping adults and children separate, and he specifically considered it advisable to have an adolescent ward. However in the 'adolescent' ward of the hospital concerned, we found a mixture of adolescents, adult psychopaths and geriatric patients. A third Superintendent told us that all patients were 'swapped round' as necessary in order to put a new admission in the right place. In general there is little doubt that apart from young children's wards, where the sexes are often mixed, the only factor which receives *effective* consideration is that of sex.

Almost 25 per cent of patients were in wards where the Medical Superintendent concerned admitted that they had to go wherever there was a space, and in a further 10 per cent of cases the Superintendent said the decision was based upon such vague criteria as 'where they will be happiest' or 'it depends upon their behaviour pattern'. About 9 per cent of patients are in hospitals having only one ward available for all subnormal patients. For the others, some 56 per cent, once segregated by sex, the formal policy of allocation is said by superintendents to be based upon a combination of factors namely grade of defect, age and physical handicap, usually in that order of priority.

The comments by Superintendents were confirmed by our research observations. With certain obvious exceptions, any administrative attempt to classify patients in terms of ward allocation was thwarted by overcrowding and the need to counterbalance such disparate factors as sex, age, and physical handicap with grade of defect. Nurses in charge of wards were asked about the type and/or grade of patients on the ward, but in fact the degree of overlap was so great as to make the question virtually meaningless, except as a means of illustrating the point we have made above, and to stress the difficulties of nursing patients with such a wide variety of differing abilities and needs. Table 5.3 shows our findings in relation to the sampled patients.

Two categories of patient were most likely to be in wards exclusively reserved for a particular type of patient, namely high grade patients and children.[1] With regard to the former category, we know that at least 9·2 per cent of patients in our sample had an IQ of 60 or more[2] and the fact that 6·4 per cent of such patients lived in wards

[1] Cross, K. W.: 'A Survey of Mental Deficiency Institutions in the Birmingham Region', *Brit. J. Prev. Soc. Med.* (1954) 8, 162–71, found that wards containing high grade patients and those containing mainly imbeciles were relatively homogeneous; although we would in general agree about the high grade patients, we found very little evidence of homogeneity on most other wards in our national sample.

[2] See Chapter 4, Table 4·4, p. 67.

Table 5.3

DISTRIBUTION OF PATIENT POPULATION BY MAIN
WARD CLASSIFICATION (PERCENTAGES)

General classification of ward by main category of patients*	Sampled patients on the ward†
High grade exclusively	6·4
Subnormal (high to medium grades)	15·5
Severely subnormal (medium to low grades)	41·9
Mixed (all categories)	25·1
Cot and chair	5·8
Children/babies	11·1
Hospital/Admissions/TB	4·8
Geriatric	5·3
Refractory	2·2
No. of patients	3,038

* As described by nurse in charge of ward.

† Totals do not add up to 100 per cent as these classifications are not mutually exclusive. Thus some wards housed geriatric *and* cot and chair patients, or some wards for severely subnormal patients were also geriatric wards, etc.

specifically designated as 'high grade' suggests that many patients classified in this way do live in the better conditions usually made available for them. Nevertheless in our experience, many mixed wards contained a proportion (usually quite small) of high grade patients. The danger here is that they may get overlooked when consideration is given to plans for rehabilitation, particularly if they are useful in caring for children or physically disabled patients.

In the case of children, the total number of patients in the sample under the age of 16 was 12·1 per cent[1] and we found that 11·1 per cent of patients lived in wards designated for babies and children under that age. This suggests that relatively few children are housed on wards with adults. Even where they are, it is sometimes a deliberate policy decision; in one hospital children slept in a separate dormitory but shared the day room with adults and were cared for by the same staff, since it was felt that this replicated the more normal situation to be found in the community.[2]

Most hospitals had some wards which were described primarily as 'cot and chair' wards, but although 8·8 per cent of the sampled patients were either bedfast or totally confined to a wheelchair, only

[1] See Chapter 4, Table 4·1, p. 62.

[2] Compare this with the view expressed by the Superintendent mentioned earlier (see p. 81, *supra*) who felt it was important to keep adults and children quite separate.

6·4 per cent were in wards designated for such purposes. Furthermore, we observed that a proportion of patients on these wards, although usually crippled to some extent, were by no means totally immobilized, so that a considerable number of genuine 'cot and chair' cases were being nursed in mixed wards.[1]

The total number of patients in the sample aged 60 and over amounted to 13·8 per cent, but only 5·3 per cent were in wards described as being mainly for geriatric patients, and from our observation it was apparent that many patients in 'geriatric' wards were well under the age of 50.[2] These figures confirm our view that so far as adults are concerned, apart from the higher grades, there appears to be very little classification according to age, nor according to grade. Some 60 per cent of adult patients were in wards which the nurse in charge described as 'mixed', or alternatively 'medium to low grade'.

At the time of our visits, 2·2 per cent of sampled patients were living in refractory wards; restrictive conditions in such wards varied greatly, as is suggested by the fact that rather more than two-thirds of these patients were in locked wards, and the rest in wards which remained unlocked at all times.

In addition most wards had 'side rooms' which were officially reserved for disturbed patients both during the day and night, but in fact they were put to a wide variety of uses, and again it should be noted that wide discrepancies existed between units of the same hospital. For example, in the main unit of one very large hospital, on the female side all side rooms were referred to as 'correction rooms'; they contained no furniture at all, even on those wards housing mainly high grade patients. However these conditions did not prevail on the male side where attitudes were much more liberal in every way. Another large hospital reserved many of its side rooms on the male side for homosexuals.[3]

According to staff, most patients were allocated side rooms as a privilege, or at their own request, and such rooms were usually better equipped than the main wards. The patients were normally those considered by nurses to be relatively stable and capable of looking after their own belongings. Sometimes they were elderly and/or suffered from some physical handicap. In wards where overcrowding was most acute, privileged occupants of the rooms were moved out at night if another patient became disturbed and had to be removed from the main ward.

[1] This should not necessarily be taken to imply criticism of the arrangement; the fact is recorded here merely to illustrate the unreliability of existing classificatory methods, particularly in relation to the assessment of staffing requirements.

[2] It should be noted that it is often extremely difficult to assess the age of a mentally subnormal patient solely by appearance, and our information is based on case records rather than relying solely on observation.

[3] One charge nurse described the side rooms as being for 'sexy types who like getting into bed with others'.

Internal arrangements and conditions

Over a third of the sampled patients were living in large wards containing 60 or more occupied beds, but again some qualification is necessary since we defined a 'ward' as any unit of patients administered and cared for by one or more senior nurse (usually a sister or charge nurse), with an allocation of nursing staff and orderlies working under his or her direction. Tables 5.4 and 5.5 attempt to give an impression of the layout of accommodation for the patients in our sample:

Table 5.4

SIZE OF WARD BY NUMBER OF PATIENTS (PERCENTAGES)

Size of ward	Number of patients
60 beds or more	38·2
40 – 59 beds	39·9
20 – 39 beds	18·4
Under 20 beds	3·5
TOTAL	100·0
No information	8
No. of patients	3,038

It should be noted that Table 5.5 oversimplifies the situation and a quarter of all patients do not live on wards with a single layout; the most frequent combinations are column (a) with column (c) or (d). The single rooms are usually attached to large wards for administrative purposes, alternatively a series of single rooms may be treated as one ward (e.g. in hostels). From this table it is clear that over 40 per cent of patients were living in a single dormitory with 20 or more beds, whereas 1 per cent had single rooms and approximately 25 per cent were in small rooms with fewer than seven beds.

Conditions of overcrowding in many wards comprising a single dormitory with 40 or more beds are undoubtedly extremely unsatisfactory, and we saw many wards where the beds were head to tail and there was barely room for the patients to stand between them. However in our opinion the situation which often resulted in the worst overall conditions was that prevailing in categories (c) and (d) in Table 5.5, where a series of rooms on different floors may lead off one another, or off snake-like corridors. There are usually at least two staircases,[1] and steps between rooms are not uncommon. Such conditions are particularly inconvenient and at times dangerous for those patients who may be physically handicapped. Nor are such

[1] One is often the 'maids' staircase' and may be exceptionally steep or narrow and dilapidated.

Table 5.5

LAYOUT OF WARD BY NUMBER OF PATIENTS (PERCENTAGES)

Layout	Number of patients				
	60 or more;	40–59	20–39	Under 20	Total
(a) 1 large dormitory, beds in rows	33·3	39·4	40·2	35·2	37·2
(b) 1 large dormitory, beds grouped or partitioned	4·3	6·6	9·4	3·8	6·2
(c) 2 or more rooms each containing 7 or more beds (no partitions)	28·6	25·0	14·9	8·6	23·9
(d) 2 or more rooms each containing 7 or more beds (with partitions)	3·8	4·2	0·1	3·8	3·3
(e) 2 or more rooms each containing 2–6 beds	29·5	23·9	32·9	45·7	28·5
(f) Single rooms	0·5	0·8	2·3	2·8	1·0
TOTAL	100·0	100·0	100·0	100·0	100·0
No. of patients*	1,158	1208	559	105	3030

* Excluding 8 patients for whom there was no information on size of ward.

rooms necessarily small, a few contained more than 20 beds, but the average was nearer 15.

In expressing the view that these conditions are often the most unsatisfactory and dangerous, we are less concerned with the bricks and mortar or the state of decorative repair (although physically handicapped and low grade patients are often housed in these very old multi-storey buildings), than with the impossibility of supervising, let alone nursing patients under these conditions, especially at night. There are no central observation points from which a night nurse may hear or observe patients who have fits, become disturbed, are incontinent, or who require any special attention, and we feel that this puts an intolerable burden of responsibility on the night staff. Because of the heterogeneity of the type of patient on these large wards, it is usually necessary for all such wards to be checked at intervals during the night. One night nurse who covered a series of rooms on different levels commented that she had fifty doors to open and shut on a ward round.

The degree of overcrowding in wards is indicated by the fact that 69 per cent of patients sleep in rooms with only two feet or less between the beds. There is only slightly more evidence of overcrowding amongst patients housed in one large dormitory as compared with those housed in a series of large rooms, though patients in the former type of accommodation are more often found to have one foot or less between beds. For all other types of layout of accommodation the usual space between beds was approximately two feet.

We tried to devise some method of measuring the physical conditions and provisions on the ward, as well as the degree of comfort and homeliness. As was discussed in Chapter 2 (see p. 40 ff. *supra*) we do not claim that our procedure was a wholly satisfactory one, and the most that can be said is firstly that it was used in a consistent manner (that is to say that every ward in the hospital was scored by the same criteria) and secondly that these criteria were set out in such a way as to eliminate, as far as possible, the element of subjective judgment by different interviewers.

Each ward was scored separately for dormitories, day rooms, and sanitary annexes. In both the dormitory and the day room two scales were used: the first an 'environment' index aimed at quantifying the basic provisions and in the dormitories comprised such items as the state of decorative repair, the adequacy of beds and bed linen, the presence or absence of unpleasant smells,[1] the heating arrangements and the provision of curtains or blinds. In the day rooms the comparable 'environment' index covered the same items but also included the presence or absence of carpeting, an adequate supply of armchairs or settees, and the provision of separate dining facilities. Items on these scales, although they could in some circumstances be considered amenities for individual patients, if taken together make up the rather indefinable atmosphere of the ward which is responsible for the overall impression it creates. For example the carpeted area of the day room belongs to everyone, just as the smell, if any, will be obnoxious to all concerned.

The second index could be termed an 'amenity' index since it was intended to cover items which either provide amenities for individual patients, or alternatively those 'extras' which make the ward homely without necessarily being essential to the basic comfort of the patient. Thus pictures, flowers, ornaments, and personal possessions have been included in the amenity index, whereas armchairs and settees have not, since we consider the provision of the latter to be a basic essential in any residential community. Other items included in the dormitory 'amenity' index are the availability of lockers, bedside chairs and bedside mats and in the day room 'amenity' index, consideration has been given to the general availability of ornaments, books, toys, etc. bearing in mind the type of patient on the ward.

[1] As noted at time of visit. 'Unpleasant' refers specifically to incontinence, body odours and undissipated cooking or laundry smells.

Thus we would not necessarily expect to find toys on a high grade ward, whereas we would expect books and personal possessions to be in evidence.

An additional point was also given in both scales in those cases which seemed to warrant special merit; for example where particular efforts had been made to avoid an institutional atmosphere, a situation which usually involved the staff helping patients to decorate rooms or sew cushion covers, bedspreads, etc. In one ward the cripples each had special chairs made for them individually, in striking contrast to other wards of the same hospital where there was a noticeable lack of chairs of any kind. Similarly a score of zero was given if conditions were really unpleasant, despite the existence of a few items which otherwise might have been scored. For example, if a day room were completely bare except for a few benches round the walls, if it smelled of incontinence and contained no toys, games, flowers, etc., even though it was warm, we would score zero. The information set out in Table 5.6 relates to conditions in the dormitories and day rooms.

It will be noted from the table that while in the dormitories 'environment' scores are generally higher than 'amenity' scores (average environment score 8, average amenity score 2), the discrepancy between the two is not nearly so great in the day rooms (average for both scores is 4). Further analysis shows that a high score for 'environment' in dormitories is usually accompanied by a similarly high score in the day room, but this is not true in terms of 'amenities' where low scores in dormitories are often accompanied by higher scores in day rooms.

Although it is important to note that comparisons which are too direct are not really justifiable, since not all the items scored were identical, we feel these findings reinforce our previous emphasis on the danger of rating hospitals, or even different units within the same hospital complex, for comparative purposes. As we have shown earlier in this chapter,[1] subnormality hospitals are rarely, if ever, homogeneous; within the same unit one may find buildings put up before 1860 and others built after 1950. The specific environment of the patients may vary widely from ward to ward, so that any attempt to rate the hospital as a whole in terms of one criterion is likely to bear no more relationship to reality than the 2·4 child family of demographic calculations. For this reason we have concentrated on the ward and not the hospital as the unit of our analysis in this context.

As far as dormitories are concerned, what emerges is that whereas the vast majority of patients live in an 'environment' that meets their essential needs, a substantial proportion, some 59 per cent, were in dormitories having an 'amenity' score of two or less. In other words the *milieu* in which their lives are spent tends to be characterized by

[1] See also Appendix F.

Table 5.6
ENVIRONMENT AND AMENITY SCORES IN SAMPLED PATIENTS'
DORMITORIES AND DAY ROOMS (PERCENTAGES)

Score	Dormitory		Day Room	
	Environment	Amenities	Environment	Amenities
	(Maximum score – 9		(Maximum score – 8)	
0	2·7	19·6	4·6	2·9
1	0·1	15·1	1·3	0·9
2	—	24·8	7·8	9·5
3	0·2	14·0	22·7	17·9
4	2·9	15·3	24·6	23·5
5	6·9	6·4	23·7	29·1
6	12·8	1·5	12·2	10·7
7	15·0	1·5	2·2	4·7
8	25·5	1·1	1·0	0·8
9	33·9	0·7	—	—
TOTAL	100·0	100·0	100·0	100·0
No information* or no day room	7	7	29	35
No. of patients	3,038	3,038	3,038	3,038

* Usually because ward was in process of redecoration and no assessment was possible.

spartan adequacy rather than the kind of civilized comforts which might be thought desirable, particularly for patients for whom a general atmosphere of homeliness and security may be important. Furthermore, it must be remembered that for a substantial number of patients this will be their only home for a large part of their lives.

There is a positive correlation between the worst physical conditions and the size of ward. Thus of those patients (2·7 per cent) living in dormitories scoring '0' on 'environment' almost two-thirds were in wards of 60 patients or more, and approximately a quarter were in wards of between 40 and 59 occupied beds. However by no means all large dormitories scored badly and of the 33·9 per cent of patients in dormitories scoring nine for 'environment' a third were in wards of 60 or more occupied beds and rather more in wards of between 40 and 59 occupied beds.

So far as 'amenities' and ward size are concerned, of the 19·6 per cent of patients in dormitories scoring '0', the great majority were in wards with 40 or more occupied beds, and at the other end of the scale, of the small number scoring eight or nine in dormitories or day rooms, two-thirds were in wards with under 20 beds.

Dormitories

If we look in more detail at the items from which these total scores were derived, we find that in the majority of cases beds and bedding were satisfactory in so far as the mattresses were soft, the number, thickness, and general condition of the blankets adequate, the bed linen of reasonable quality and unstained, and two pillows provided. Most rooms smelled fresh, had full curtains and were warm. The item which consistently scored lowest was the actual state of decorative repair, which was 'good' in only 61·1 per cent of cases; in 24·8 per cent there was some dirt or wear and as was mentioned earlier, in 2·7 per cent conditions were so bad as to warrant a zero rating. This leaves 11·4 per cent of patients living in conditions which were 'bad' but not dreadful.

In relation to comforts there were much greater differences between items comprising this scale. Far more patients had lockers and chests than any other item: even so, only 43·4 per cent had exclusive use and 24·7 per cent shared them. Toys were clearly available for use and ornaments displayed in 28·5 per cent of cases; the presence of flowers and/or pictures was noted rather less frequently. More patients shared chairs and bedside mats (23·8 per cent) than had exclusive use of these items (10·6 per cent), but the majority had none.

Almost 60 per cent of patients were in dormitories where no personal possessions were displayed on beds, tables, window sills, etc., and 27·6 per cent were in dormitories where they were visually evident, but belonged to less than half the patients in the ward. Sometimes nurses have to combat the views of matrons on this matter; in one 70-bedded female ward where personal possessions *were* in evidence, and all patients had exclusive use of a locker, the sister commented: 'Matron nearly shoots through the roof when she comes in here, but they haven't got nearly enough space to put their little personal things'. All the patients were in a room with only one foot between the beds, but despite these cramped conditions, all patients had their slippers under their beds and dressing gowns hanging on a hook. Many little personal possessions were scattered round the ward, and sister had made it look as homely as possible. This contrasts with a smaller ward for 40 male patients where *no* personal possessions were in evidence, and the charge nurse commented that there were no lockers because this would mean reducing the number of beds, and he added: 'If these patients had lockers, most of them would only fill them up with rubbish.' Nor is this merely a matter of difference between male and female wards; in another male ward, a verbose, but efficient and knowledgeable charge nurse commented: 'I'd like carpets in the day room and corridor, and to get some of those murals . . . I think the addition of carpets would have a wonderful effect on the patients . . . I'd like to make the day room more homely with more money. And I want some more chairs.

You've got to make things comfortable for these patients. But I'm going to keep on for my carpets, apparently all the money has been spent, but I'll keep on and on.' It should be noted, however, that it is by no means always the nurses who complain about the matrons' rigidity; matrons too say that they find it difficult to persuade some nurses to allow individuality and a degree of untidiness.

Day rooms

With regard to conditions in day rooms: 64·4 per cent of the patients in our sample lived in wards which had only one day room, 21·8 per cent had two day rooms, and almost 12 per cent had more than this number; about 2 per cent had none and the dormitory was used as a day room. In most of these latter instances, however, the dormitory was the hospital unit[1] and patients were mainly short-term cases awaiting transfer back to their own ward, or too sick to get up much.

The larger the ward the more likely it was to include more than one day room. There were as many as five day rooms in some wards with 60 beds, but this was exceptional and most of the largest wards had either three or four day rooms. However not all patients in large wards were so well provided for, and 31·8 per cent had only one day room. If there were two or more day rooms, their use was usually divided by type of patient and there was a marked tendency for patients of lower intelligence to have much less satisfactory living conditions. In one large mansion where there were a number of different day rooms shared by all the patients, one of the rooms was particularly well decorated and extremely comfortable, but no patients appeared to use it. The research worker asked the nurse about this and was told that the patients preferred the more austere conditions of the other rooms, a view which was confirmed by matron. Possibly patients were put off by the 'Ideal Home' like appearance of the room which contrasted markedly with the other rooms where they could scatter their belongings without it being too obvious. So far as size was concerned, almost all patients had plenty of space in the day room, in fact the rooms tended to be rather too large for comfort. Over half the patients lived in rooms where the ratio of floor space to patients exceeded twenty square feet.

In terms of the individual items comprising the two scores for day rooms, two items predominate in the 'environment' index: the presence of curtains and warmth.[2] About half the day rooms had

[1] All large subnormality hospitals have a special building or ward set aside for nursing patients who are temporarily sick or who may suffer from a disease such as tuberculosis. Patients may be sent to the main hospital unit for nursing if suitable facilities are not available in the ancillary units where they normally live.

[2] We could, of course, only assess wards at the time of year when visited, and this item is not really a reliable guide in so far as some of the visits were paid on warm days and no heating was necessary. Where available, temperature was recorded from thermometers.

separate dining rooms, and 43 per cent of patients lived in rooms that were in a very good state of decorative repair. For 33 per cent of patients conditions were described as 'fair', a term indicating either that walls or paintwork would have benefited from washing, or that certain parts of the room required repair or repainting, though not with any real degree of urgency. Approximately 20 per cent of patients lived in rooms requiring early decoration, that is to say in a poor, but not dilapidated state, and the remaining 4·5 per cent had day rooms in such a bad condition that we gave a zero score.

The most obvious lack in day rooms was of armchairs; only 11·6 per cent of patients were in rooms containing sufficient comfortable chairs or settees for even 80 to 85 per cent of patients to be able to sit down at any one time.[1] Again we must stress the wide discrepancies existing within a particular hospital.

So far as 'amenities' were concerned, the most striking fact was probably that almost all wards were equipped with items which entertained the patients with the minimum of supervision, i.e. television and radio, often supplied through the League of Friends. It is interesting to note that in many hospitals the League of Friends have provided television sets and record players, and their main function (as will be discussed in a subsequent chapter) appears to be collecting money for 'comforts', but we did not find that any such monies had been used to provide comfortable chairs, this despite an acute shortage. Over 89 per cent of patients were in wards where both television and radio were available as well as record players, this compared with 70 per cent of patients in wards with toys or games and books. Where the latter had been given by outside organizations, these particular items were usually kept under lock and key, or allowed to be used only by certain patients. Nursing staff appeared to feel that the donors would be upset if their gifts were damaged or broken. The same fear may explain the reluctance of nursing staff to encourage relatives to send or bring in personal gifts. The nurses feel responsible for damage done to such belongings by other patients (and they are usually unable to avoid this happening), and some also feel that it is a reflection on the hospital (and at one remove on themselves) for failing to provide adequately for patients' recreation.

By virtue of their mental age, most adults in such hospitals (with the exception of patients of higher intelligence) play with toys and games in much the same way as children. Soft toys, beads, jig-saws, cards, bricks, etc., were to be found on most wards. This was not always the case, however, in one ward 'toys' consisted of one huge stuffed animal in a completely bare room.

Almost three per cent of patients were in day rooms with no 'amenities' whatsoever, while 5·6 per cent were in day rooms scoring an additional mark for exceptionally good facilities or provisions. There was some difficulty in assessing the extent to which patients

[1] We were careful here to take account of bed patients and those in wheelchairs.

had their own personal possessions other than clothes; so far as we could tell almost half the patients obviously had at least a few items, but this figure may be an underestimate since they often had small suitcases which they either carried around with them or which were kept in an annexe near the day room to which they had access, but we did not necessarily see the contents. Furthermore it is often difficult to define personal possessions; amongst the lower grades in particular, a ball of wool, an old postcard or a scrap of material may be treasured personal possessions, to be carried everywhere and the suitcases we saw were often filled with such items. Nurses frequently commented that to give such patients lockers would only encourage squalid and unhygienic conditions, since they often stuffed food in them amongst other bits and pieces. No doubt the ideal solution would be for nurses to help patients look after their own belongings in an orderly way, but under present staffing conditions they apparently have no time to do this. Generally speaking female patients tend to have more private possessions than do males, but probably as few as 15 per cent in all had more than six recognizable items that could be legitimately claimed as their own. It is, of course, not always easy to establish whether a patient actually 'owns' a particular book or toy, or whether they have 'appropriated' it for as long as their interest is held.

Toilet facilities

Finally, when considering the physical structure and facilities of the ward, we obtained information about the sanitary annexes. The index covered the state of decorative repair, temperature, presence or absence of smell, availability of showers as well as baths, number and size of mirrors, and facilities for individual patients as opposed to communal provisions. The maximum score was again nine, and again the intention in establishing a maximum was to suggest what would be represented by civilized provision. In addition to this rating scale we noted the ratio of lavatories, baths and washbasins to patients, the degree of privacy afforded, and whether special adaptations were available for physically handicapped patients.

Probably the most striking feature of Table 5.7 is that 5·6 per cent of patients were in wards where conditions in the sanitary annexes were so bad as to warrant a zero score, almost all of them wards of over 40 beds. In one hospital visited where the annexes were in the basement and necessitated a long walk down stairs, through corridors open on both sides to the weather, a completely new sanitary annexe had been built, but the charge nurse said it could not be used as they were waiting for the 'official opening' by the Chairman of the Management Committee!

If we consider the state of decorative repair in dormitories, day rooms and sanitary annexes, and compare the number of patients

Table 5.7
SANITARY ANNEXES:
TOTAL SCORE BY PERCENTAGE OF PATIENTS

Score (Maximum 9)	Patients
0	5·6
1	0·8
2	6·1
3	19·4
4	28·1
5	24·9
6	10·4
7	2·2
8	2·3
9	0·2
TOTAL	100·0
No information	7
No. of patients	3,038

living in 'good', 'fair' or 'bad' conditions, the following table shows clearly that least attention is paid to the sanitary annexes:

Table 5.8
STATE OF DECORATIVE REPAIR (PERCENTAGES)

State of decorative repair	Patients		
	Dormitory	Day room	Sanitary annexe
Good	61·1	43·2	33·4
Fair	24·8	33·2	41·3
Poor	11·4	19·0	19·6
Very poor	2·7	4·5	5·7
TOTAL	100·0	100·0	100·0
No. of patients	3,038	3,038	3,038

The majority of annexes were warm and fresh-smelling (over 83 per cent of patients lived in such conditions), but few provided full-length mirrors as well as horizontal ones. Twenty-one per cent of patients had individual facilities and equipment for cleaning teeth, shaving or brushing hair, but in most cases the provisions were communal and had to be shared by a number of patients. In a number of high grade wards there were excellent arrangements and facilities for personal laundry, hairdressing, etc. Very few annexes had showers or hand sprays in addition to baths, and this seemed particularly unsatisfactory when so many patients are incontinent, particularly on children's wards.

Over 50 per cent of patients lived in wards where the ratio of w.c.s or urinals was 1:7 or more; for 19 per cent of patients the ratio was 1:10 or more. Similarly with baths, 64·2 per cent of patients shared a bath with at least 15 others and a further 1·2 per cent had no baths available at all;[1] in one instance a ward of 77 patients had no bath and the research worker reported 'a terrible stench and numerous flies'. In another ward there were four baths, but three of them were used for storing clothes, since no special provisions for clean clothes and linen were available. The position regarding washbasins was rather more satisfactory, these being shared mainly between four, five or six patients.

Most lavatories had doors which could be closed but not locked, but baths rarely had screens or partitions. About a quarter of the patients were in wards where the sanitary annexes contained special adaptations for disabled or handicapped patients, such as handles or rails, lifting equipment, etc. Baths were often very old in design and far too large and too low for the nurses to help bath patients comfortably. Very few had taps that could be used by the patients themselves. Despite the shortage of adaptations and the lack of suitable equipment, nurses generally expressed satisfaction and thought no additional facilities were required. If one looks at the distribution of special adaptations in terms of the type of patient on the ward, one is left with a strong feeling that nurses were either unwilling to be critical of the lack of equipment (though this seems unlikely since they were prepared to be far more critical of other, more sensitive areas, such as staff relations and communications), or alternatively that, having never had any opportunity to use such equipment, they were unaware of the extent to which it could be useful. For example only just over half the cot and chair patients were living on wards where provisions of this kind were made,[2] yet only about ten nurses expressed dissatisfaction either at having none, or at the nature of the provision made. Where any dissatisfaction *was* expressed, it was usually in wards housing the lower grades of patients. Even then not all the criticisms related specifically to special adaptations, for example a deputy charge nurse in one of the largest hospitals com-

---

[1] The Ministry of Housing and Local Government recommend one w.c. to 5 beds and one bath to 10 beds: *Housing for Special Purposes*, HMSO (1951).

[2] Such provisions were usually *very* rudimentary. For example only 1 bath-lift was seen in all the hospitals visited.

plained that on his ward, which was intended to be a medical ward, there was no clinical room, nor were there any sterilizers.[1]

Linen and clothing

Closely linked to the physical conditions and material comforts on the wards are the physical appearance (clothing) of the patients, and the food they eat. On every tenth ward visited questions were asked about the supply of clothing and linen.[2] Almost all nurses interviewed expressed satisfaction with the quantity of *clean*, as opposed to new linen and clothing provided. The exceptions were three large hospitals: at one of these, three out of five ward nurses complained of shortages, at another two nurses out of four complained, and at the third, slightly smaller, hospital, two out of three complained. There appeared to be some relationship between size of hospital and degree of satisfaction with supplies, in so far as there was very little complaint of this nature in the smaller hospitals and more likelihood of dissatisfaction in the larger ones. So far as *new* clothing was concerned, all but one ward nurse expressed satisfaction, though in a further two instances there appeared to be sufficient new clothing, but not bed linen.

However, it seems that satisfaction with supplies may simply be a function of the fact that patients do not normally keep the same item of clothing when it is returned from the laundry, the stock being 'communal'.[3] Thus availability of clothing was often unrelated to fit, and the appearance of some patients led one to feel that whilst total supplies may have been adequate, the right size was not so readily available. Only in one-third of the wards visited did patients retain the same clothing (apart from 'best clothes' whether provided by relatives or by the hospital). Again the question of hospital size appears to be a relevant variable, and whereas in most (though not all) smaller hospitals clothing was kept for individual patients, this was less likely to be the case in the larger hospitals. There were no hospitals where patients did not wear at least some private clothing for special occasions, even though this did not usually include underclothes.

Finally we enquired about the type of clothes *not* provided by the hospital. The items most frequently mentioned were dressing gowns and slippers, the former being supplied in only very few instances. Brassières and corsets were not by any means generally supplied, and

[1] According to a private communication from a member of the staff of the Ministry of Health sterilization is no longer considered safe, and ward sterilizers are not being provided in new planning. Autoclaving in central supply departments is preferred.

[2] 761 wards were visited and information on laundry facilities, supplies of clothing and linen, etc., was obtained on 78 wards.

[3] For a more detailed discussion of this matter, see Chapter 10 on the intensive study.

I

this may account for the fact that clothing on female patients often appeared to be more drab and ill-fitting than would have been the case had they had better foundation garments. Occasionally gloves were not provided, though this deficiency was sometimes covered by supplies through the League of Friends.

In addition to these formal questions, interviewers were instructed to record in note form general impressions of clothing in all hospitals visited. Most of the clothing worn was provided by the hospital and was, on the whole, dull, unimaginative and often ill-fitting, mainly one felt, due to the inadequacies of the laundries. It is doubtful whether the 'remodelling' of clothes that went on in the laundry was worse than much bulk work carried on outside, and certainly it was no worse than that found in other types of institution. Nevertheless, since there is no 'uniform' as in prisons (which at least gives a semblance of cleanliness and smartness), nor are the patients mainly in bed as in general hospitals, the extent of the devastation was only too obvious in many cases.[1]

As in all other matters, it is again important to remember the wide discrepancies existing within the different units of the same hospital. In one large hospital a lot of personal clothing was worn, but the staff were under considerable pressure from the Hospital Management Committee to explain why the laundry bills *per capita* were higher than in other hospitals. Particularly in the small hospitals the clothing was described by research workers as 'good' and mention was often made of individual styles. One hospital in particular provided very good clothing bought and fitted individually, although other aspects of the same hospital were much less satisfactory (i.e. physical conditions and provisions). Sometimes clothes were incongruously matched, for example ankle socks worn with best clothing, or clumsy boots worn with best suits. Only in one small unit of a hospital was reference made by the research worker to inadequate clothing in terms of temperature. In one 1,200 bedded hospital patients wore generally dirty and ill-fitting clothing, particularly on the male side where battledress was worn. The Medical Superintendent commented that he knew the clothes were awful but what could you do when the supplies officer said there were surplus forces uniforms going cheap, and it would save the country £100. This, in his view, was the sort of thing the Management Committee liked. In this hospital, the women's dresses were said to be better in quality than they had been in the past, and the shoes had recently been changed. They looked generally better cared for than the male patients.

In one very large hospital the research worker described the clothes as 'nondescript and baggy' (though a special hairdressing salon in the hospital resulted in their hair always looking neat).

[1] See also discussion of laundries in Chapter 10 concerning the two hospitals studied more intensively.

With certain notable exceptions, females were cleaner and neater than males; the exceptions tended to be in the larger units. By its very nature female clothing, particularly outer clothing, is much easier to launder, an important point with incontinent patients. So far as male patients are concerned there might be advantages to experimenting with more unconventional clothing such as denims, rather than relying so heavily on flannel. Similarly pre-shrunk cotton for underwear and nylon socks might prove more economical in the long run.[1] However it should not be thought that poor clothing necessarily reflected lack of interest by senior nursing staff, and the writer was present during many unprompted discussions amongst staff on the subject of how clothing could be improved and made more suitable for the type of patient concerned.

Food

No formal questions were asked about food, but again research workers were asked to comment on meals served, and in many cases kitchens were visited and copies of menus obtained. In general comments made by interviewers were reasonably favourable, though there were frequent references to food being adequate in quantity, but rather stodgy and dull. The quality of the catering service appeared to bear no relationship to the size of the unit: in many very large hospitals the food was described as ample, appetizing and nicely served, whereas in others, equally large, the reports were less glowing. In one hospital which employed a specialist catering officer, careful consideration was given to the needs of different kinds of patient, for example those who could not chew easily, young children, or the physically handicapped. Unfortunately this did not appear to be general, and too often all patients in the same hospital tended to be given the same kind of food, and had to eat it as best they could with the help of higher grade patients or staff. Interviewers often ate with the nursing staff and in general the comments were much the same: ample, but dull and stodgy.

It is worth noting that despite differences between hospitals in different regions, the total national average amount spent on food in subnormality hospitals for the year ending 31 March, 1967 was £1 4s. 5d. per person fed per week. This amount is lower than that spent in any other type of hospital, the average for mental illness hospitals being £1 8s. 3d. and for all other hospitals £1 13s. 4d.[2]

Summary

The importance of the physical structure of any institution lies in the fact that not only does it help to create a 'psychological' atmosphere –

---

[1] See also Chapter 8, p. 167.
[2] Ministry of Health, Hospital Costing Returns year ending 31 March, 1967.

which is as important for the staff as it is for the patients – but that it determines the ease or difficulty with which everyday tasks are performed. For the patients this is their world, within whose circumscribed limits their lives are lived out twenty-four hours a day, seven days a week. Inmates in institutions of all kinds tend to set great store by material objects some of which, to the outsider with his more varied experience, may seem trivial. It is constantly said, particularly by those nursing the mentally subnormal, that what they need is warmth and affection in human relationships, 'we are their family', 'we are all they have got' are remarks which are frequently heard. But such relationships when they exist in the setting of the normal family tend to take place in an environment which is warm and secure. At the most fundamental level, most human beings make their shelter as comfortable as possible, warmth and comfort being a component in physical contentment and psychological well-being. Barrack-like institutions with spartan provisions are a negation of what is normal in human experience, and it is within the context of human experience that subnormal patients seem most likely to respond to care and training.

Similarly with clothing and food; choice and adequacy are normal for ordinary persons. Food presents special problems in all institutions, if only because of the difficulties inherent in mass catering; but as far as clothing is concerned, there can, in an age where mass production has produced a 'quality revolution', be little excuse for allowing patients to be drably dressed. For convicted offenders, institutional clothing might still be justified by some as part of the punitive sanctions, but for hospitalized patients there can be no such rationalization. A patient whose clothes are ill-fitting can scarcely be rationally encouraged to take care of them, and pride in personal appearance is fundamentally related to the individual's expression of his self-concept as a person.

The importance of the fact that until new methods of treating and training the subnormal are developed, the hospital remains the patients' world for a very long time, cannot be overstressed. He is already handicapped by his mental subnormality; by what justification then may his additional material deprivations be maintained? The answer lies partly in history and partly in our current social philosophy. In the past, the handicapped, like the destitute, were provided for by charity that had one eye continually cocked on the size of the public or private purse. The recipient (or his relatives) was obliged to be grateful, and was in no position to be critical. At the present time, public policy dictates along different lines, along those of harsh priorities which may be altered more readily by pressure on the part of interested groups than by an initial stirring of the public conscience. Mental subnormality comes low on the list of public concerns and therefore a long way back in the queue for public money. In a materially prosperous society, the conditions of overcrowding and dilapidation which we have described in this chapter bear testimony to the harsh paradox of private affluence and public squalor.

Chapter 6

THE PROBLEMS OF STAFFING

THIS chapter discusses the numbers, quality and morale of medical and nursing staff. It starts by furnishing basic information about staff and staffing ratios, and goes on to describe the work of the hospital as senior staff see it, how these staff are recruited and what qualifications they have. The principal themes of the chapter are then developed, namely the physical and organizational problems with which staff have to cope, and the crucial relationship between morale and patterns of communication within the hospital.

Staffing structure

Each main hospital is formally organized into three autonomous hierarchies. The medical administration, headed by the medical superintendent, includes all medical staff, although Consultants are directly responsible to the Regional Hospital Board in matters concerning the treatment of their patients and are subordinate to the superintendent only on matters of administration.

The nursing administration is subdivided into two independent departments, male and female, although their formal organization is similar. The Chief Male Nurse and Matron are the respective nursing heads and normally have a deputy and a number of assistants working under them, depending upon the size of the hospital. In some hospitals Matron is the sole supervisor of the nurse training school, but this function is sometimes shared with the Chief Male Nurse. Charge nurses and sisters are each responsible for running their own ward, usually on a shift basis with a deputy to take over when they are off-duty.

The third hierarchy is that of the lay administration, headed by the Group secretary who, in some instances, is also the hospital secretary. The hospital secretary is in charge of all the hospitals' business administration, although much of the work is often delegated to the finance officer, the supplies and records officer and the maintenance or engineering superintendents.

Most of the subsidiary units have either a Matron or Chief Male Nurse in residence, supported by nursing staff at all levels. Medical staff visit from the main hospital and many such units receive regular calls from local GPs, but this depends upon the size of the subsidiary unit and its distance from the main hospital. The administration is normally carried out from the main unit. A few ancillary units are run by Lay Administrators who are directly responsible to the Hospital Management Committee; in such cases medical responsibility rests with a consultant from the main hospital and appointed by the Regional Hospital Board. Such units also have either a Matron or Chief Male Nurse in charge of the nursing hierarchy. As we have indicated[1] the structural relationship between ancillary units and the main hospital varied widely, and some lay superintendents resented the idea that they had any connection with the parent mental subnormality hospital and its superintendent; his involvement was seen as interference by those working in the subsidiary unit.[2]

Sources of information

So far as the medical staff are concerned, the data used in this chapter are drawn from formal interviews with the superintendents of the 34 hospitals visited, as well as with two deputy superintendents and three lay superintendents. Both the deputies interviewed were in charge of a sizeable unit at some distance from the main hospital, though in one case the incumbent complained that he was in a very difficult position since he did not conceive of himself as being 'in charge' of the patients as they were admitted and discharged through the main unit. Other deputy superintendents were not interviewed formally since they were based on the main unit and were, to all intents and purposes in the same position as other consultants, except that officially they became the senior doctor when the superintendent was absent.

Whether lay superintendents were interviewed or not depended largely upon their own perception of their role. Thus, if they saw their function as resembling the role of an administrative secretary, they themselves declined to be formally interviewed, since the questions asked were primarily directed towards medical or nursing matters which they felt could best be answered by the matron or chief male nurse. In such units the matron was sometimes married to the lay superintendent, a situation which could, on occasion, present a very resistant face to examination by the outside world.

The data on nursing staff are drawn from formal interviews with 141 matrons and chief male nurses in main hospitals and subsidiary units;[3] in hostels it was usually the warden who was interviewed. It was sometimes necessary to see deputies if the incumbent of the post

[1] See Chapter 2, p. 32.

[2] One lay superintendent who had been requested by the medical superintendent of the main hospital to co-operate in our research claimed that he had been told by his Management Committee (which differed from the Management Committee of the main hospital) to ignore the request.

[3] Although in this section we refer to matrons and chief male nurses and their deputies, since they constituted the bulk of our interviewees, our remarks also include Principal Nursing Officers and Chief Nursing Officers and their deputies, of whom a few were in post at the time the research was carried out.

was away for longer than the research workers remained in the hospital. As a result of personality difficulties one of the matrons interviewed was unable to answer the questions asked, so that we obtained as much factual information as possible from her deputy and assistants, and for the rest we simply listened to her reminiscences.[1] In a second instance, the superintendent made it difficult for the research worker to see the matron of a subsidiary unit alone, and when we attempted to do so later, she was found to be severely ill.

In addition, we interviewed the nurse in charge of every ward at the time of our visit. These were nearly always charge nurses or sisters (or their deputies) but in a few instances students, state-enrolled nurses or assistant nurses were in charge.

Medical and ancillary staff [2]

Each hospital had a medical superintendent, though in some instances these superintendents were attached to the local mental hospital and included the subnormality hospital or ancillary units in their jurisdiction. In addition the hospitals visited employed a total of 36 full-time and 21 part-time consultants, all of whom had a DPM. There were also 55 full-time and 44 part-time medical officers who had no DPM, and 25 part-time GPs. If one assumes that part-time staff work approximately half the number of sessions worked by full-time staff, this gives a weighted ratio of approximately one doctor to every 219 patients, though the ratio varied considerably even between hospitals of comparable size.[3]

In 24 of the 34 hospitals visited at least one paediatrician was employed on a regular consultant basis; seven had the services of a paediatrician readily available as required, and three had to make special arrangements for this type of service.

Eleven hospitals had a neurologist on a regular consultant basis and ten had one readily available. All but two hospitals had at least one dentist on the staff, usually part-time. Fifteen hospitals employed a chiropodist, only two of these full-time. Many hospitals employed opthalmic opticians, physicians and ENT specialists on a consultant basis and the larger hospitals also included a dermatologist, pathologist, and radiologist.

Nursing staff

As we pointed out earlier in this report,[4] any overall assessment of

[1] Various different interviewers attempted the interview, all were equally unsuccessful.

[2] The figures relating to staff have been weighted where appropriate.

[3] See Chapter 3, p. 51, *supra*, where figures obtained from Ministry of Health sources indicate a ratio of 1:250. The difference may be due to the fact that we have no details of the amount of time worked by part-time staff and we may therefore have over-estimated this, particularly in the case of GPs (see p. 121).

[4] See Chapter 3, p. 52.

staff/patient ratios does not take into account the fact that approxim. ately only one-third of the staff are available for duty at any one time (one-third being off-duty, and one-third on leave, sick, or absent for some other reason). Nor do such figures give any picture of staff distribution on the different types of ward, nor how many staff are actually on the ward at any given time. We heard constant complaints from senior ward staff that nurses are allocated to a ward but are transferred elsewhere at a moment's notice if there is a shortage- Alternatively they may be sent on errands, or to escort patients from a different ward to various departments, or even outside the hospital. We shall, therefore, first discuss the overall staffing ratios, and then look at the actual situation as we found it on the wards.

In general terms it is difficult to extract any meaningful patterns from the data; only one point emerges clearly, namely the inconsistencies between the staff/patient ratio of qualified nurses and the staff/patient ratio of *all* nursing staff. Thus a hospital in the Manchester region with a ratio of qualified nurses of 1:13·4 has a *total* nursing staff/patient ratio of 1: 4·5, whereas a hospital in the Oxford region having an almost identical ratio of qualified nurses (1:13·1) has a total staff/patient ratio of 1: 8. Similar examples can be found throughout the sample, the most striking being the fact that one of the worst off hospitals in terms of qualified staff (ratio 1:20·1) has one of the best ratios when one includes all nursing staff (1: 3·5). The average figure for all hospitals visited was 1:13·9 for qualified staff and 1: 4·7 for all nursing staff but these data should be interpreted with the greatest caution, since the variations in staffing as between regions, individual hospitals and units within hospitals are very large and cannot conceivably be accounted for by variations in the needs of patients, particularly in view of the heterogeneous nature of the patient population on most wards.[1]

Looked at in terms of *total* hospital size (though it must be borne in mind that this includes all the units in a particular hospital and in fact one is not justified in assuming that all units are equally well or badly staffed) we find that by taking *all* nursing staff into consideration, with two exceptions hospitals of between 1,000 and 1,450 beds have a worse staff/patient ratio than any of the hospitals in other groups (see Table 6.1 below). This size of unit also contains the hospital with the worst staff/patient ratio of any hospital visited (1: 8·73), though it should be noted that this is a hospital which does not admit children (as will be shown later in this chapter, children's wards are usually better staffed in terms of numbers). Neither of these remarks follows, however, if one looks at the staff/patient ratio of *qualified* nurses, when this size of hospital (1,000 to 1,450 beds) differs little from hospitals of other sizes, though there is a slight overall tendency for the larger hospitals to be generally better staffed with qualified nurses.

[1] See Chapter 4, p. 81.

Table 6.1

HOSPITAL SIZE BY OVERALL NURSING STAFF RATIOS

Total no. of beds (all units)	Hospital	Nursing ratio	Average for group
1,750 and over	1	1:5·22	1:4·26
	2	1:4·72	
	3	1:4·54	
	4	1:3·74	
1,450–1,749	1	1:5·46	1:4·74
	2	1:5·59	
	3	1:5·11	
	4	1:5·44	
	5	1:4·69	
	6	1:3·17	
1,200–1,449	1	1:4·93	1:5·97
	2	1:6·16	
	3	1:5·87	
	4	1:7·43	
1,000–1,199	1	1:6·40	1:5·89
	2	1:8·73	
	3	1:8·10	
	4	1:6·52	
	5	1:3·29	
800–999	1	1:3·26	1:3·79
	2	1:5·44	
	3	1:3·28	
600–799	1	1:4·94	1:3·89
	2	1:4·47	
	3	1:3·41	
	4	1:5·24	
	5	1:2·88	
300–599	1	1:4·64	1:4·68
	2	1:4·04	
	3	1:5·10	
	4	1:5·28	
Under 300	1	1:3·64	1:4·29
	2	1:5·71	
	3	1:4·05	
	Average for total sample (*weighted*)		1:4·70

Turning now to the question of staff allocation, Table 6.2 shows the nursing staff/patient ratio for each hospital in the sample grouped by Regional Hospital Board, the ratio of nurses to patients actually on duty at the time of our visit to the ward,[1] and the ratio of nurses to patients on childrens wards, since data presented in the previous chapter suggest that physical handicap is more prevalent and more severe on children's wards, and it could therefore be argued that a higher staff/patient ratio is needed.

It must of course be borne in mind that column (i) includes all those senior members of the nursing staff who do not normally work on wards (i.e. matrons, chief male nurses, principal nursing officers, and their deputies or assistants) whereas columns (ii) and (iii) include only ward staff actually on duty. However, on average their inclusion makes a difference of only 0·5 or less to the staffing ratio of each hospital. In calculating the ratios in these last two columns, the total number of patients on the ward has been used, but it is in fact highly likely that in many of the wards a proportion of the patients would have been out at work or at school at the time of our visit. However since they are mostly there at the busiest times of the day, for example when getting up, going to bed, and at meal times, as well as at weekends, we have thought it justifiable to include them.

Whilst it is evident that in most hospitals the childrens' wards are more generously staffed, the differences between hospitals in any one region are quite marked and suggest that the distribution of staff as between wards varies very considerably from one hospital to another. We are not of the opinion that this can be accounted for by variations in the type of patient accommodated in the different hospitals, and we believe there must be differences in staffing policies as between hospitals, though this matter was not discussed with the interviewees.

Table 6.2

RATIO OF STAFF TO PATIENTS BY HOSPITAL AND REGION

Regional Hospital Board	Hospital	(i) Total Staff/patient ratio	(ii) Actually on duty at time of visit (average all wards)	(iii) Actually on duty in children's wards (excluding adolescents)
Newcastle	A	1:3·5	1:10·4	1: 6·1
	B	1:4·0	1:10·5	1: 9·7
Leeds	A	1:3·3	1:14·5	1: 8·0
	B	1:3·3	1:12·3	1:10·0

[1] Since almost all visits (for recording purposes) were made between 9.00 a.m. and 6.00 p.m., this will tend to average out.

Sheffield	A	1:6·4	1:16·2	1: 8·3
	B	1:5·3	1:17·9	1: 9·0
	C	1:4·2	1:16·5	1: 7·9
	D	1:5·8	1:34·0	—
East Anglia	A	1:5·1	1:17·8	1: 7·2
North West Metropolitan	A	1:5·2	1:16·9	1: 6·0
	B	1:4·7	1:15·4	1:12·2
North East Metropolitan	A	1:4·6	1:13·6	1: 8·5
South East Metropolitan	A	1:4·8	1:16·3	1: 6·2
	B	1:5·4	1:23·7	1: 7·6
South West Metropolitan	A	1:5·1	1:22·9	1:14·0
	B	1:6·3	1:19·9	1: 6·3
Wessex	A	1:4·0	1:14·7	1: 7·5
	B	1:4·1	1:12·8	1: 5·0
Oxford	A	1:8·0	1:15·2	1: 5·7
South Western	A	1:5·4	1:21·7	1:13·7
	B	1:4·7	1:14·8	1: 9·6
	C	1:4·9	1:18·7	1:16·2
	D	1:5·1	1:10·9	1: 5·3
Birmingham	A	1:6·0	1:19·6	1: 7·8
	B	1:6·1	1:20·1	1:19·4
	C	1:8·4	1:19·2	—
Manchester	A	1:4·5	1:15·6	1: 6·3
	B	1:3·6	1:14·4	1: 8·4
	C	1:6·3	1:14·3	1:12·1
	D	1:3·3	1:11·5	1: 6·1
Liverpool	A	1:2·9	1:10·3	1:10·0
Wales	A	1:5·1	1:13·9	1: 7·6
West Scotland	A	1:5·3	1:18·2	—
	B	1:3·7	1:14·9	1:10·2
Average for sample (weighted)		1:4·7	1:15·8	1:11·1

Although we do not have detailed information about the situation at night, the position was generally highly variable. Most of the larger hospitals had one assistant nurse on duty on each ward, but the smaller wards tended to share one nurse between them. The night superintendent or sister normally made two rounds of the hospital each night, and for the rest was available in her office if required. In the smaller hospitals proportionately fewer staff were on duty during the night.

Recruitment

(a) *Superintendents* All the medical superintendents interviewed were asked how they came to work in the field of subnormality. By far the largest group said that they had 'drifted' into this particular field, but had become interested in the work and so had stayed; this was most frequently said by superintendents in the larger hospitals, a situation which may be accounted for by the fact that many of those in senior positions in large hospitals entered the subnormality field at about the same time, that is at the end of the Second World War, a period which coincided with the reorganization of the health services resulting from the 1948 Act. Most of these superintendents had obtained their DPM before or during the war, and having married and started families, they were looking for jobs where pay and promotion prospects were good. Thus one superintendent, typical of many, said that he might have preferred general practice, but this meant buying a practice, knowing that it would soon be nationalized. Since he had obtained his DPM during the war and practised as a psychiatrist in the army: 'the most obvious thing to do was to go back to mental deficiency'. Only a quarter of those interviewed said that they deliberately chose subnormality because they were interested in it, and these were mainly superintendents working in hospitals with under one thousand beds.[1] In a few instances the superintendents were in charge of, or attached to, a mental hospital, and the subnormal patients were already part of it, or were absorbed into its orbit at some later date.

Superintendents' views about the future recruitment of doctors to the service seemed to indicate that whilst they themselves claimed to have grown interested in subnormality as the years went by, potential recruits were as uninterested in the subject as had been common in the past. 'Subnormality is a medical backwater'; 'there is insufficient knowledge of subnormality'; or simply 'they don't like it'; were generally considered to be the most important deterrents to new entrants.[2] Other factors such as the conditions of service or pay, the

---

[1] Some replies to the question contained an element of humour, thus one superintendent told us that he became interested in the mind at the age of six when his family had a maid who cut up frogs and dangled them in front of hens: 'I became interested in the minds of the frogs and the hens'.

[2] An editorial comment in the *J. Ment. Sub.*, Vol. VI, Part II, No. 11, December 1960 refers to the fact that the field (of subnormality) is seen by doctors as 'static, sterile and frustrating'.

geographical isolation of the hospital, or the general shortage of doctors were rarely mentioned.

(b) *Administrative nursing staff* As might be expected, there were considerable differences between male and female staff as to why they came into this kind of work. The men mainly 'drifted in' and became interested, or they came in because pay and promotion prospects were considered good at a time when employment prospects outside were poor (1930s). One chief male nurse said that both his parents were mental nurses and 'in those days hospitals were staffed by the children of mental nurses. In the thirties often this was one of the few kinds of secure employment'. Another sizeable group came in after the Second World War, many having done some nursing in the forces; since opportunities for male nurses were very limited in general nursing, they had little choice and tended to gravitate towards mental or subnormality nursing. Some came for apparently irrational reasons, as illustrated by the following comment: 'I used to do a lot of hammer throwing, I was going into the police force, but had an accident with a hammer and was unfit for the force. I decided to go into mental nursing as I used to deliver milk when younger, and the mental hospital was on my rounds and I became interested in the patients'.

On the female side, although again more said they 'drifted in' than any other single category, far more females than males came in because they were always interested in the work, and this reason was even more frequent amongst acting or deputy matrons than amongst matrons. Hostel wardens, both male and female also tended to come in because of a genuine interest in the type of patient. Matrons were far less willing than chief male nurses or superintendents to admit that they chose subnormality nursing because of the better opportunities for promotion; however it is our impression that this factor was not unimportant in determining the type of hospital selected, a view which is reinforced by the fact that in the smaller units a general nursing qualification was not always a necessary pre-requisite for promotion to matron. (Further details of qualifications will be given later in this chapter.)

A minority of matrons took their present job in order to be near their family or because their husbands worked in the area, but in fact not many were married. It is conceivable that the selection of subnormality nursing, which involved the care of very dependent persons, may have presented an opportunity for the expression of maternal feelings which might otherwise have remained dormant.[1]

Where subnormal patients were in hospitals catering primarily for other types of patient (mental illness, geriatric, general, etc.) the chief male nurses and in particular the matrons, did not consider them-

[1] This view is reinforced by the differences in attitude towards nursing as between male and female staff (see p. 117 ff.).

selves as being generally concerned with subnormality; the patients were usually there when they first came to the hospital and these nursing administrators varied in the degree of interest they took in such patients.

(c) *Nursing staff* All the matrons and chief male nurses involved in recruiting staff used advertisements in the national and/or local press, nursing journals, and more particularly the Irish press.[1] One matron ensured that members of her staff going to Ireland on holiday all took brochures of the hospital with them! A chief male nurse complained that the Hospital Group would not advertise in the national press because it was too expensive; he felt that this was a mistake since such advertisements attracted a better *quality* of nurse. Another chief male nurse tried to attract policemen due for retirement, and he had also approached the county cricket ground for 'failed' staff (sic). Two matrons said they had no difficulty in recruiting staff; one of them claimed to have a waiting list for jobs in the hospital. In general talks, exhibitions, open days and the Labour Exchange, were all mentioned, and a great many relied on personal recommendation.

On a number of occasions we found that part time staff were working full time at a local mental hospital. One subsidiary unit caring for 75 patients employed six part-time staff, most of whom worked full time at the local mental hospital, and this included two staff nurses. The situation arose in reverse when regulations prevented charge nurses from being paid overtime and they therefore took part-time jobs in local mental hospitals. Although quite 'legal', this was regarded as most unsatisfactory by administrative nursing staff.

Only very few references were made by administrative nursing staff to coloured nurses: one matron did not think they were a good idea 'because they don't chat to patients' and another reference was to foreigners generally: 'they don't settle down'. The particular hospital where this matron worked was situated in a very rural area and there was only one such person on the staff. It was mostly by charge nurses that hostile opinions were expressed: the objectives were nearly always to immigrants being foreign rather than specifically coloured and the views expressed were very generalized, for example: 'foreign staff are not an asset on the ward, they are a liability. They have great difficulty in making rapport with the patients. The patients don't understand them and they get upset'. Another charge nurse referred to coloured staff as 'imported labour' and was most emphatic that they should not be used: 'they can't do enough for you for the first few days, then *they* take over and try to tell you what to do', and he went on to describe them as 'lazy and lacking initiative'. A deputy charge nurse working in a mixed occupational/industrial training department said the Spanish and Italian nurses were dirty and

---

[1] One chief male nurse specifically advertised abroad.

illiterate, and he added: 'the sheets had to be burnt after two Irishmen left – how can *they* give patients any sort of habit training?'

The number of nurses who did not have English as a native tongue, or who were coloured, was in fact very small; in the thirty-four hospitals visited, just under five per cent came into one of these categories. In one hospital the chief male nurse had five foreigners on his staff, but he commented 'no coloured people'. In the hospital where the matron claimed to have a waiting list of applicants there were no foreigners or coloured nurses, and the chief male nurse commented that he 'wouldn't have them'.

Although we have no hard facts which would explain the relatively small number of coloured nurses, data obtained in the intensive sample may give pointers: firstly the ratio of older to younger staff is high in subnormality hospitals. Secondly the turnover of staff is small – nurses tend to remain in subnormality hospitals (usually the same one) for long periods. Furthermore, it is well known that immigrants tend to settle in urban areas and to remain in closely integrated groups. This may explain the fact that most of the coloured or foreign staff found in our sample were concentrated in two hospitals in the Manchester region, and the others were mainly in hospitals near large urban areas such as London and Birmingham.[1] Another factor which may be important is that coloured students may come to this country for training and then return home: training in subnormality nursing will be of limited value to them as compared with general or even psychiatric nursing.[2]

Finally it should be borne in mind that matrons and chief male nurses in subnormality hospitals have sole responsibility for the recruitment of nurses, and it may well be that selection is influenced by the very obvious hostility often expressed by other nursing staff to which we made reference earlier.

Staff shortages and conditions of work

Most of the nurses interviewed complained of a shortage of trained staff. Certain duties, such as the distribution of drugs, could only be carried out by qualified nursing staff, although students in their third year were usually allowed to do such work. Ward sisters or charge nurses and their deputies felt anxious about leaving the ward in charge of state-enrolled nurses or assistant nurses during their off-duty periods and the recently adopted method of up-grading assistant nurses to become state-enrolled nurses was widely disapproved. A

[1] It must be stressed that this applies equally to foreign, as distinct from coloured, nurses. Although we did not check their nationality or country of origin, Italians appeared to predominate.

[2] Informal discussion with coloured persons in this country suggests that the mortality rate for subnormal children is very high in the West Indies and that few enter institutions; if this is the case there will be virtually no demand for staff trained only in this branch of nursing.

charge nurse discussing his work explained that there were no other trained staff on the ward and he was a 'jack of all trades' and he added: 'The state-enrolled nurses are the same nurses as they were before the enrolment. One day they are not allowed to inject, and the next day they are! . . . That's my biggest grumble, not enough trained staff'. Another charge nurse (who was also secretary of the nurses' union and a representative on the joint consultative committee) commented: 'State-enrolled nurses can't give injections, matron and chief male nurse won't have it. It's bloody ironical because sometimes the assistant nurses are running the ward and officially they can't give out the medicines although they're responsible for eighty-odd patients. At the same time matron and chief male nurse are sponsoring their application for enrolment as trained state-enrolled nurses; in fact, they are saying officially they can do what in effect they have not been allowed to do'. A chief male nurse explained it to the research worker in this way when referring to a particular assistant nurse: 'He's not very bright, but he's useful, he's done his job satisfactorily for six years and there's no reason for him not to be made a state-enrolled nurse. If he and others don't deserve the state enrolment then we should have sacked them. I see no reason why they shouldn't get the golden handshake'.

The normal working week was 42 hours and we found that overtime was much more likely to be worked on the male wards, since the married male nurses (and they were often married to nurses on the female side) did not normally have home domestic duties and were glad to earn the additional pay.

There was an acute shortage of domestic staff and almost all the hospitals visited had unfilled vacancies for domestics or orderlies. A few hospitals used cleaning contractors, but the views of staff were mixed about this arrangement and some expressed dissatisfaction. In view of the constant complaints made by nursing staff about having to do domestic chores, one might think that the use of contractors could usefully be extended to more hospitals.

The larger hospitals provided married quarters and single sex homes or hostels for nursing staff, but in at least one 1,000 bedded hospital, staff were living on the wards, a situation about which the matron was highly critical: 'I have been crying out for accommodation; I've got eleven nurses and eighteen domestics living on the ward and it's disgraceful . . . I think perhaps I was wrong to make over rooms on the ward to the staff because while I can manage the Regional Hospital Board won't provide any more'. Nor was this matron happy about the accommodation offered in the nurses' hostel: 'The Ministry are ridiculous, they drive us crazy. Even when I make out a watertight case I still can't get anything. We took photographs and showed them what dreadful places they were and they haven't the proper facilities there'. This matron felt that the previous superintendent was to some extent to blame since he was

K

'satisfied with so little'. Another hospital where accommodation was at a premium provided a caravan site for nursing staff, some of the caravans being privately owned, and others being the property of the Hospital Management Committee.

Almost all non-resident staff had a canteen or dining facilities available, and most had a sitting room. However the same could not be said of changing rooms and about half the non-resident staff had to change on the wards. In a few of the smaller units situated in rural districts, transport was provided to and from the hospital, but for the most part nurses lived in, and we heard little complaint about conditions, although it should be pointed out that nurses were not questioned individually on this point.

Training

In those hospitals where there was a training school, matrons and chief male nurses were asked their views about the current syllabus for training subnormality nurses. For the most part they were satisfied with the training, but there were plenty of reservations, some of them contradictory. Some thought the syllabus contained too much theory, others thought it did not contain enough. However, the overwhelming mass of criticism related to the need to link the training far more closely with general nursing, and it was thought that the General Nursing Council, as well as general hospitals, should do more to help over secondment problems. One matron said she tried to send her nurses away to a general hospital for one month, but the General Nursing Council said it must be for three months or not at all, and as this matron pointed out, they could not spare the staff for that period. She also added: 'The general hospital will not let their nurses come to us'. Another matron thought that those trained only in subnormality should have three months compulsory secondment to general nursing, and a chief male nurse in a very large hospital said the syllabus was 'over-simplified' and there was 'too little general training'. Another chief male nurse commented: 'I feel that general nursing and the mental side are two distinct things entirely. I think mental nurses are born not made'. A few thought that psychiatric and subnormality training should be combined, and some thought the academic standard of the students was insufficiently high to cope with the current syllabus.

Qualifications of administrative staff

No single member of the nursing administration had sole responsibility for the largest hospitals (1,745 beds and over); this arose partly because of the subdivision of these large hospitals into male and female 'sides', and partly because almost all were subdivided into units, many of which had autonomous nursing administration. The larger the number of patients for whom the matron or chief male nurse was responsible, the more likely were they to have qualifications in general as well as subnormality nursing. The alternative qualification was usually general nursing with mental nursing, and a very few had qualifications in all three branches. Nevertheless it is important to note that almost one-third of our sample of patients were in units where the matron or chief male nurse had no general nursing qualification, and a third were in units where they had no qualification in subnormality nursing. The matron of one geriatric hospital which had a separate block for approximately 100 subnormal patients said she had no need of any qualification in subnormality nursing as the deputy matron was trained in mental nursing. However when asked if the deputy matron was specifically concerned with the subnormal patients, we were told that this was not so, and the matron included this block in her rounds. According to the interviewer she expressed no interest in the subnormal patients whom she had 'inherited', a word she also used in referring to the fact that the subnormal block was kept locked. She said it saved the added responsibility of watching straying patients 'some of whom would make for the males in the grounds'. Some patients were in hospitals or units where the matrons or chief male nurses had no qualification in general nursing or in subnormality nursing, but they may have had a qualification in mental nursing; many of those in charge of hostels had no nursing qualifications at all.

Under regulations brought out by the Ministry of Health in 1965 a nurse appointed to a post for which he or she does not hold the appropriate qualification has his or her salary abated at all points on the scale,[1] and we were told that as a result of this subnormality hospitals had lost a considerable number of nurses who had only mental training. Previously their pay had been 'made up' but under the new regulations this had to be stopped.

The question of qualifications has some relevance to the question of whether there is a need for patients to be in a hospital, as opposed to a home or hostel, since it is assumed that a hospital provides specialized nursing skills. The data obtained on this point suggest that a substantial minority of subnormal patients are in hospitals where the most senior members of staff are trained only in a limited branch of nursing.

Staff views of hospital function[2]

Staff perceptions of the function of subnormality hospitals varied with status positions in the hierarchy and the role they performed. In general the ideas of the medical superintendents were global in

[1] This varies from £25 to £35 per annum according to seniority.
[2] A more detailed discussion of this topic will appear in Chapter 10 relating to the two hospitals studied intensively.

concept and somewhat idealistic. They are well summed up by the superintendent who said that the hospital function was:

> The investigation of all suspected cases of subnormality, where possible their treatment and training to a point where they are able to leave hospital and lead an independent existence. For those for whom this is not possible, to provide facilities for them – occupation and recreation – to enable them to live as full and happy lives as possible in spite of their disability. Both investigation, therapy and rehabilitation, it should be a village; the old idea of a 'colony' was a good one, although it has an unfortunate connotation now. In our investigations we ought to be contributing to the causes and treatment of subnormality – it must be on a wider scale than just the individual patients.

Thus for most superintendents ideally there were different goals for different groups of patients.

Virtually all superintendents considered that the provision of medical and psychiatric treatment was important, although in the smaller units this was not necessarily the case and one-third of the sampled patients were in hospitals where the superintendent did not hold this view. The same situation obtained in relation to training, and it was primarily in the larger hospitals that this was viewed as an important function. The position was reversed however with regard to the provision of a sheltered environment: here superintendents in the smaller hospitals were more likely to see this as the function of the hospital, although it was also true in those units of larger hospitals housing older patients. A few superintendents mentioned research as a desirable function,[1] and some referred to the importance of providing accommodation for psychopaths. One superintendent thought that 'long-term psychopaths' should be accommodated in subnormality hospitals rather than in mental hospitals: 'There is the problem of mixing intelligences, nevertheless the place for the psychopathic personality is in *this* type of hospital. I would divide the hospital into two halves and in one half have IQs up to 50 or 60 and in the other have IQs over 60 and have no ceiling. The division in the Act is stupid'. This view was exceptional, and others who mentioned psychopaths thought that only *subnormal* psychopaths should be accommodated in subnormality hospitals, and then only in those having a special security unit.

One or two superintendents thought the subnormality hospitals should incorporate a day hospital which would also provide an outpatient advisory service; one of these consultants firmly believed that

---

[1] In an address given to the NAMH Annual Conference (1968) Prof. A. Crisp referred to a general lack of research in the field of mental health and added that some appointment committees were reluctant to appoint doctors who had research interests.

the subnormality hospital was *not* appropriate for the long term care of those imbecile patients whom he felt did not require much nursing care. He thought they should be in hostels situated in rural areas where they could live a quiet life away from the hurly-burly and temptations of the city. Several superintendents referred to the provision of short term care to relieve relatives, though with one or two exceptions we found little evidence that this took place on any large scale basis.

Once superintendents had discussed their views of the function of the subnormality hospital they were invited to say how many patients at present *in* hospital could be satisfactorily cared for in the community were adequate hostels, sheltered workshops, etc., to be provided. As might be expected the superintendents experienced considerable difficulty in replying to this somewhat hypothetical question, since obviously the answer hinged around one's definition of 'adequate'. In asking the questions, it was hoped that careful probing would result in their clarifying their own views of adequacy, but in fact their ideas were very diffuse, and no clear pattern emerged of what was required. Thus one superintendent of a very large hospital commented that none of his patients could live outside, either because they are 'too low grade to be acceptable to local authority hostels, or too dependent and inadequate to be dealt with other than by nursing or medical staff, or those whose criminal or psychopathic tendencies make it essential for them to have a period of training in hospital . . . there are no signs that the kind of provisions at present available meet the needs of our patients'. Another said he had already discharged six or seven per cent, and that for every ten 'boys' six would return, and for every five 'girls' two would return. 'The hostels are not very attractive to them. They haven't enough outlets in work or recreation. Employers are not so sympathetic and large numbers of patients are being sent to hostels staffed by people who have very little experience, and to buildings which soon deteriorate. We can't afford to duplicate hospital services in hostels'.

A superintendent who was reasonably community oriented also pointed out that it would be no advantage if hostels merely became small hospitals run by Local Authorities. He estimated that he had at the time of interview about six male patients who would be able to live in a hostel, but because they came from other local authority regions many years ago, unless these authorities contributed to their upkeep in a hostel near the hospital, they could not be accepted there. The suggestion was that they should return to hostels in their own local authority area, but as the superintendent pointed out, this ignored completely the fact that all their contacts, work, associations, etc., were in the area of the hospital.

Another superintendent thought that about one-third of his patients could live in hostels if they were 'fully supervised'. This meant having their meals cooked, clothing looked after and outings supervised 'to prevent their getting damaged or harmed'.

Attitudes of superintendents to the question of patients being cared for in the community did not appear to vary according to size of hospital, this seemed to be purely an expression of individual points of view with, as we have suggested, very little agreement between them. However, the larger hospitals mostly had one or more hostels attached to them, and patients in such hostels were usually considered suitable to live outside in due course. The views held by superintendents regarding the possibility of patients living in the community *did* seem related to their attitude towards sexuality amongst subnormal persons; the more fearful they were the greater the tendency to consider institutional care essential.

Nurses' perception of their role[1]

The attitudes of the nursing staff regarding the functions of subnormality hospitals were very varied; they found some difficulty in expressing their views about abstract concepts such as treatment and training and were largely concerned with the day to day handling of patients on the wards. Again this tended to vary with their status in the nursing hierarchy, and, as we shall suggest, as between male and female nurses.

It was a little easier for nurses to conceptualize their own role in terms of what they aimed to achieve for the particular patients in their care, though many had considerable difficulty in doing even this, and much probing was usually necessary.

According to those nurses interviewed (and in 95 per cent of cases these were trained nurses or hostel wardens), only in wards with fewer than 20 beds did the nursing staff feel that time was generally available for helping patients with their social training, or in other ways. Once the number of beds exceeded 20, size of ward appeared to make little difference: in the majority of wards, nursing staff thought that about one-half of the patients received adequate attention to their social needs, but we have no information about their criteria of adequacy.

What did the staff feel they accomplished for patients? As might be expected, the age of the patient was an important variable in this respect: for *all* age groups, 'nursing and care' was the item most frequently mentioned, and 'custody' – in the sense of protecting either the community or the patient – was the item least often mentioned. Table 6.3 sets out the position in relation to the number of patients in each age group:

[1] For an interesting discussion of the role of the nurse in subnormality hospitals written by a nurse, see O'Hara, J. O.: 'The Role of the Nurse in Subnormality: A Re-appraisal', *J. Ment. Sub.*, Vol. XIV, Part I, No. 26 (1968).

Table 6.3

NURSES' ESTIMATE OF TYPE OF CARE BY AGE OF PATIENT
(PERCENTAGES)

Type of care	Age of patients									
	0–4	5–9	10–15	16–19	20–29	30–39	40–49	50–59	60 and over	Total*
Nursing and care	78	66	62	57	56	63	61	62	71	61
Rehabilitation	—	6	7	14	11	11	11	12	6	10
Homely atmosphere	20	32	37	25	27	32	31	30	31	30
Social and/or habit training	57	53	42	46	35	35	38	31	36	36
Custodial	—	—	1	4	5	5	6	4	4	—
Counselling‡	—	1	1	4	7	9	10	9	12	4
Very little	7	7	18	18	16	15	12	12	9	8
Other§	—	2	2	1	4	2	3	2	3	2
Total patients in age groups†	33	125	204	232	533	465	505	497	414	3,008

* Totals exceed 100 per cent since two or more types of care were usually mentioned.
† Excluding 30 about whose age we have no information.
‡ Usually giving advice to patients at an individual level and on personal matters.
§ 'Other' often included contact with parents.

Some of the nurses who said they achieved 'very little' set themselves very high standards bearing in mind the type of patient they had to care for; thus a charge nurse responsible for a group of 42 severely subnormal and very disturbed boys commented: 'I've been in charge of this ward for nine months and in that time I've taught twelve boys to use a knife and fork, that's the kind of progress you can hope for'.

However, in looking at all the answers to this question one must necessarily bear in mind not only the reliability of the responses, but also the fact that some nurses are both more intelligent and more able to express their views than others. Most nurses found the question difficult to answer and we feel that it would be dangerous to assume that those who replied 'very little' necessarily achieved less than those who expressed themselves more fluently.

Bearing this in mind, however, the difference in role perception between the male and female staff appeared quite noticeable, although it would be dangerous to generalize too widely from these findings. Parsons'[1] discussion of instrumental and expressive roles may be

[1] Parsons, T.: *The Social System*, Routledge & Kegan Paul (1951).

relevant here, since the tendency was for the male staff to stress rehabilitation, custody and social training, whereas female staff stressed nursing and care. Thus a sister in charge of 53 children of mixed grades commented: 'I see what we do as care, education and bringing out what is not there. I'm very fussy about the way food is served, little things like that help to build up a family atmosphere'. Another in charge of 52 severely subnormal females aged between 16 and 32 said: 'We keep them clean, well dressed and well fed. I try to look after them as I would my own kids. We write letters for those who have the sense of wanting to write. I like to create a homely atmosphere. I never mind about the din so long as they're not fighting. This is a ward of throw outs, so we have problems. When they've saved so much money we take them out shopping'. And in a so-called geriatric ward[1] the sister said: 'the attitude towards the patients is motherly and friendly. There have never been any complaints and the atmosphere is friendly and homely. We try to make them as happy as possible'. There is a tendency for nurses to reinforce the child-like dependency of the patients, thus an assistant nurse in charge of a ward of 60 high and medium grade females in a subsidiary unit commented: 'The patients are more like little children, you have to treat them like children. They rely on you for mostly everything. They come to you as though you're their mother'.[2]

The creation of a homely atmosphere and counselling, were mentioned with equal frequency by male and female staff, but from our own observations there was often a marked difference in the *achievement* of the former between male and female wards and we believe that whilst male staff viewed this as an aim which they hoped to achieve as often as did female staff, the male nurses had other priorities and so achieved it less often. This may also be related to the fact that male nurses more often expressed dissatisfaction with their own achievement: if in fact they more frequently aimed at rehabilitation and training, then they were bound to be faced more often with failure, or at best very slow progress indeed.

The question of priorities naturally affects the whole situation of role performance, and to some extent obscures other factors; patients who suffered from multiple handicaps, those who had difficulty in moving about, or feeding and dressing themselves, were likely to require nursing and care quite irrespective of other factors such as their IQ, the length of time they had been in the hospital, or even the size of the unit. It was interesting to note that nurses did not mention habit training (for continence) any more frequently in connection with incontinent patients than any other type of patient.

---

[1] Six patients in this ward were in our sample and although nominally a geriatric ward, two were aged 34 and two aged 46 and 47 respectively. This exemplifies our earlier discussion (see Chapter 5, p. 83) concerning the heterogeneous character of most wards.

[2] Nursing staff almost always refer to patients of all ages as 'boys' and 'girls'.

This may not be a very meaningful relationship however; if only about a quarter of all the adult patients are incontinent,[1] and these patients tend to be distributed throughout the wards, then even if nurses were to be concerned with habit training, the number involved on each ward would be relatively small and therefore might not have been mentioned. However we think it more likely that habit training is reserved for children only; once they are in adult wards, the attempt is, for the most part, given up.

There was, however, a clear relationship between the aim of rehabilitation and the IQ of the patient.[2] Amongst those for whom test results were available, rehabilitation was mentioned as a goal in respect of only 6 per cent of patients with IQs under 50, but in respect of 25 per cent of those with IQs known to be above this figure, although this latter group represented only 17·4 per cent of the total sample.

Some of the attempts at rehabilitation were quite remarkable on both male and female wards. The sister on a ward of one very large hospital said that she tried: 'to avoid allowing them to become bedridden. We had one twelve months ago from another hospital in the Group, saying she could only be nursed in bed, had no speech and was doubly incontinent. I got her up into a spastic chair, she could count up to 13 and her speech was blurred but I got her to communicate. With hard nursing we get patients up who have been allowed to become bedridden on other wards'.[3] It would only be fair to point out, however, that this was a small ward of 17 patients.

Patients living in very small units (under 25) were generally those living in hostels situated at some distance from the main hospital. As might be expected rehabilitation and social training were usually the main concern of the staff at these units, since the patients were fully ambulant and usually relatively young (i.e. under 45).

In general the length of time a patient had been in the hospital bore little relationship to the type of care given by the nursing staff. An exception to this was, however, the custodial role, which tended to apply more frequently to recently admitted adult patients. This may be explained by the fact that a high proportion of compulsory patients admitted through the Courts were young offenders or those diagnosed as psychopaths, and for them custody was an integral part of their hospitalization. One other interesting factor related to counselling: this was relatively rarely mentioned by staff as being a role they performed, but those who did mention it, did so most

---

[1] See Chapter 4, p. 69.

[2] Always bearing in mind the cautionary comments relating to IQs mentioned in Chapter 4.

[3] This example, from a ward sister, shows the danger of generalising about role perception, but we still feel that the difference between male and female nurses suggested above is worth recording.

frequently in connection with patients who had been in the hospital for twenty years or more.

In considering this discussion of staff perception of their role, it must be borne in mind that information was collected on a ward basis, and as we have already indicated in Chapter 5, apart from a fairly consistent division between adults and children, and between the sexes, wards are usually very heterogeneous. This fact would tend to obscure any relationships that might exist between various types of care and the characteristics of patients, except in relation to children and adults.

Supervising ancillary units

We referred earlier to the fact that approximately one-third of all patients do not live in the main unit of their hospital but in an ancillary unit some distance away. Table 6.4 sets out the frequency with which the medical superintendent or a consultant from the main hospital is said to visit these units.

Table 6.4

FREQUENCY OF VISITS BY SUPERINTENDENT OR
CONSULTANT TO ANCILLARY UNITS (PERCENTAGES)

Frequency of visits	*Patients affected*
Daily	5·4
Two to three times per week	3·5
Weekly	12·6
Fortnightly	0·6
Monthly	3·8
No regular visits	7·1
Does not apply (patients live in main unit)	67·0
TOTAL	100·0
No information	129
No. of patients	3,038

The infrequency of visits from senior doctors was often the cause of great dissatisfaction amongst nursing staff in ancillary units. The superintendent was said to have visited one unit of 103 patients only three times in eighteen months, and another consultant had attended twice in the same period. Even where the consultant visited three or four times monthly there was resentment that the medical superintendent did not come himself. Nor did visits usually last for more than an hour or two at the most, and this did not necessarily include a ward round. Certain patients may be selected by the person in charge for attention by the consultant, but the remaining patients usually do not even know that he is in the building. In one unit where the male subnormality patients were housed in an annexe of a general hospital, the superintendent of the local mental hospital who was responsible for their care was said never to visit. Physical conditions were extremely poor; patients appeared dirty and ill-kempt, they had no occupation, and the atmosphere was entirely negative. The nurses had no facilities for their own or the patients' comfort, and they were totally isolated from the staff working in the general hospital. This same superintendent showed slightly more interest in the women's and children's unit (which was also separate from the general hospital) but even this he visited only rarely, and the staff of both units expressed the view that he was uninterested in subnormality. In another unit, the matron told us the superintendent came twice a year, but in addition a consultant was supposed to visit weekly. According to the matron concerned he had, however, been only twice in the preceding eight months, despite the fact that the unit was only thirty miles from the main hospital.

There was also considerable variation in the ancillary units regarding their contact with the local general practitioner; in some instances he called daily whether or not patients required medical attention, and in others he called weekly or 'as required'. As the matron in one unit put it: 'the GPs don't know anything about subnormal patients, and the hospital doctors don't come unless asked'.

Some of the ancillary units were run by matron/superintendents; one medical superintendent in particular favoured this arrangement. But whether the day-to-day running of the unit was carried out by lay superintendents, matrons, chief male nurses, matron/superintendents or principal nursing officers, the infrequency, and often irregularity, of visits by medical superintendents or consultants often presented several disadvantages. It is probable that were a patient in need of urgent medical or psychiatric treatment, the person in charge would send for a consultant who would call immediately; but for the most part subnormal patients do not need this kind of emergency attention. They might, however, benefit from changes in treatment and training and these may be less likely to take place if patients are seen only infrequently. As a result of this practice, in some ancillary units much of the medical responsibility was delegated to the nursing staff and inevitably much depended both upon their knowledge and skill as well as their interest.

The situation applied equally to specialist and auxiliary medical staff. We believe that their services were by no means so readily available to patients living in ancillary units. In cases of serious illness this was unlikely to be the case, and patients were returned for treatment to the main hospital if necessary; but where chiropody, dentistry, and opthalmology are concerned (to give but a few examples), we feel sure that generally speaking patients in main hospitals had a better chance of receiving attention.

From a social point of view, the situation was also unfortunate, since patients in ancillary units had virtually no access to senior medical staff with whom they might wish to discuss personal problems. We suggested earlier in this chapter that the nurses' attitude towards patients usually includes considerable reinforcement of child-like dependency, and any attempt by patients to see or talk to the doctor, particularly when visits are less frequent than weekly, tend to be quickly discouraged. One superintendent who visited all units weekly said that patients could make appointments to see him, but he added: 'When you talk to some of the patients you get the impression that they have difficulty in getting the interview. It's the nurses' attitude I am afraid: I think we ought to have more personal contact with the nurses, but in these small units it is difficult to find more than two nurses on duty at any one time and they would feel persecuted and feel you were attacking them if you talked to them about personal relationships with patients'.[1]

From an administrative point of view, the present arrangement means that the superintendent who has overall administrative responsibility for patients (and often for other aspects of the hospital) may never visit the units for which he has such responsibility unless patients for whom he is medically responsible are housed there. Thus he will never be known to the patients, and only to those members of staff in senior administrative positions who attend meetings at the main hospital. Patients may have access to a consultant from the main hospital having responsibility for their actual treatment, but such consultants are not in the same status position as the superintendent *vis-à-vis* the Regional Hospital Board or the Hospital Management Committee, and they are certainly not perceived to have the same degree of authority by staff or by those patients who are able to distinguish between roles. It might, of course, be argued that the presence of the superintendent is unnecessary since it is a function of the Hospital Management Committee to safeguard the interests of the patients, but as we shall see later in the report, their involvement with the hospital appears to be inadequate to meet these requirements.

Finally, as we have already indicated, whilst a few of the senior nursing staff may enjoy the freedom from medical supervision, most would welcome it, if only in order to feel that someone cared about what they were doing. Apathy is very apparent in many of these units, and the more junior nursing staff have no contact whatever with medical staff, and consequently little opportunity to learn.

---

[1] This view is not necessarily shared by the nurses, but in the units of this particular hospital, it is the matrons who discourage contact between either nursing staff or patients and superintendents.

It would, however, be a mistake in this area of hospital care, as in all others, to assume that all subsidiary units suffered from a sense of isolation, or that relationships with the main unit were always either negative or non-existent. And again we must stress that this was not simply a function of differences between *hospitals* but of differences between units within the same hospital. Thus for example, in a large hospital one subsidiary unit was under the care of a very motherly matron who created a comfortable home-like atmosphere and had close and frequent ties with the medical superintendent, the hospital secretary, and the psychologist. In another unit of the same hospital the matron claimed to be very overworked and suffered from a sense of isolation. She felt out of her depth when she attended matrons' meetings, and so gave up going. Since visits from medical staff were rare, her attitude dominated the home and staff too felt resigned and apathetic.

Communication between medical and nursing staff

(a) *Social mixing* None of the doctors were interviewed formally, but members of the research team took every opportunity of listening to their views informally. This was not always easy to do, since most of them lived in married quarters in or near the grounds of the main hospital, and when not actually on duty, they returned home. Relatively few of them used the staff canteen or social club, and our contact with them usually took place either when their visit coincided with ours on a ward, or alternatively when we met them in the corridors or walking between villas.

Eighteen hospitals had a staff sports and/or social club, and in one instance this was a joint staff/patient club; 'more like a family' said the chief nursing officer. These clubs were, however, almost exclusively used by nursing staff, thus a situation existed where the reference point for the different types of staff reinforced their 'differentness': the nurses looked 'inwards' to the hospital community, the doctors, many of whom had young families, were largely 'home-centred' and their social life took place away from the hospital. Many medical superintendents were in the process of moving away from the houses provided by the hospital service, preferring to buy homes in areas of their own choice. Their social life took place well away from the hospital, and the local golf club rather than the hospital sports club appeared to play an important part in their lives.

Many of the nursing staff, even those working in the main units of hospitals felt extremely isolated.[1] This isolation was both physical

[1] An article in *The Lancet*, 16 January, 1954, by Jarrett, Wyndham Davies, Laing and Tredgold points out that in addition to isolation, mental deficiency nursing lacks the glamour of new treatments that have developed in mental nursing, and that 'its only claim to public interest has been an unfortunate association with cases of crime, or alleged wrongful detention'.

and professional; most of them lived in or near the hospital and had little contact with the community outside. Nor did they have contact with those working in a wider field of nursing – apart from senior staff few had even been to other subnormality hospitals.

(b) *Professional co-operation* Within the hospital itself, nursing staff had very little contact with medical, training or administrative staff.[1] Any concern for the rehabilitation and training of the patients was to a large extent felt to be irrelevant, since kindness was all that was expected of them. Their knowledge of the patient's background was often slight, case conferences were rare, as were opportunities for discussion with medical staff, and refresher courses were the exception rather than the rule.

Approximately three-quarters of the patients were in wards of hospitals where the senior staff said the medical staff discussed patients with them, but this was largely a function of hospital size: the larger the hospital the more likely was it that such discussion took place. However it must be borne in mind that most of the smaller units were in fact subsidiary units of larger hospitals, and as has been suggested earlier, frequency and duration of visits by medical staff was often limited and opportunities for discussion between doctors and nurses were accordingly restricted.

The number of patients in wards where the senior nurses actually felt *involved* in decision making regarding their treatment or training was, however, much smaller (approximately 40 per cent), although a further 25 per cent of patients were in wards where nursing staff said they could make suggestions, but that the decisions were taken by the doctor; the remaining 35 per cent felt uninvolved. Thus a charge nurse responsible for a ward of working men in a very large hospital commented: 'I've never been asked in the 34 years I've been here. The doctor came in this morning and two patients who had been ordered to bed for a week for misbehaving on the farm – he just ordered them up – not a word to me'. On the other hand in the subsidiary units the position was often reversed, since in view of the infrequent visiting by doctors, decisions regarding treatment and training were of necessity much more often taken by senior nursing staff.

We do not, however, think that our data are wholly reliable on these points. This may have arisen as a result of poor wording of the question; thus nurses would answer 'yes' to the question whether medical staff discussed patients with them, but then go on to indicate that such discussions were often a mere formality: 'We get the opportunity to discuss and suggest, but I know nothing is done. It's

[1] It was noticeable for example at mealtimes; even in hospitals where dining facilities were shared by all staff, nurses did not mix with other types of staff. The situation was, of course, reinforced structurally by the existence of separate common rooms.

all dictatorial here: sit up, stand up, you're told and your opinions are not considered'.[1]

Nor were formal meetings between superintendents and other medical and senior nursing staff for the purposes of discussing policy very frequent. In some of the larger hospitals they took place from time to time, but 35 per cent of patients were in hospitals where no regular meetings took place at which policy matters were discussed. In one hospital the medical superintendent said that the staff made excuses for not being kept in the picture: 'All the machinery is available but information is not disseminated. It's the usual story of the wrong people on the wrong committees and the right people uninterested in sitting on them . . .'.

Some hospitals had joint consultative committees at which all levels of staff were represented, but there was a good deal of criticism of this system, since the elected representatives were not always thought by nurses to be those best suited to this function. Generally speaking they were a relatively new innovation in the subnormality hospital and existed almost exclusively in the larger hospitals where meetings were for the most part infrequent. In one hospital where the joint consultative committee had existed for nine years (an exceptional case) the charge nurse who had been a representative throughout the whole period complained that he had never seen 'the Board'.

Almost two-thirds of the nurses interviewed said that either they were given no information about hospital policy, or alternatively that the methods used (usually cyclostyled notices sent round the wards) were quite inadequate. As one charge nurse in a very large hospital complained: 'The morale is absolutely down here, no one tells you anything. They tell you what to do, but they hardly ever come round. It's all due to bad administration'.

It is important to bear in mind that almost all these views about meetings and opportunities to be involved in discussions either about the care and treatment of patients or about hospital policy, were expressed by senior nursing staff. It is, therefore, not hard to imagine how much greater must have been the sense of isolation and apathy experienced by those lower down the hierarchy.

Nor were formal opportunities for communication between the various ranks of the nursing staff satisfactory. Although in many of the larger hospitals meetings between matrons and ward sisters (or their male counterparts) were officially held on a monthly basis, we found no hospitals which held meetings which included more junior staff members, and many even excluded deputy charge nurses or sisters.

In the smaller units (mainly those with fewer than 300 beds) it was not unusual to find that no formal meetings took place. Sometimes it

---

[1] The fact that there was apparently so little discussion of patients between doctors and nurses may to some extent account for the difficulty experienced by nurses in answering our questions regarding the mental and physical handicaps of patients (see Chapter 4, p. 70 ff.).

was said that they occurred 'as and when required'. As the chief male nurse of one 400 bedded hospital put it: 'If there's anything exciting to discuss, they all go to the local pub to discuss it'.

Furthermore there appeared to be a considerable difference of opinion between matrons or chief male nurses and nurses in charge of wards as to the frequency of formal meetings: in a subsidiary unit with over 200 patients the chief male nurse told the researcher that he held charge nurses meetings every three months; there were five wards in this unit and one charge nurse claimed that meetings were held monthly, another said there were no regular meetings and a third said they were held every two months. Such *major* differences of opinion are not typical, but it was rare for there to be any general consensus.

Furthermore even when meetings took place with some degree of regularity, there was often considerable dissatisfaction expressed. Charge nurses in one very large hospital were all agreed that they were a waste of time since the matters discussed did not result in any action being taken. At another hospital there were references to the 'secret service' and the fact that there was no opportunity to discuss views about hospital policy at such meetings, only trivialities were allowed an airing.

Finally we asked nurses whether they had any opportunity to attend refresher or training courses. Only very occasionally could they do so readily, since even where courses were available the general shortage of nurses prevented them from attending. Approximately 60 per cent of nurses interviewed said that they had never been on a course, and it was not unusual to hear a ward sister complain that she had to rely on her students to keep her in touch with current developments.

Morale

(a) *Medical staff* In some of the medium-sized hospitals the superintendents seemed very apathetic and uninterested, even depressed, and as a result they were often away sick, on leave, at conferences or meetings, and left the running of the hospital to the matron and/or chief male nurse. One superintendent commented:

> Why I feel so out of step is that in the olden days people had a duty to the patients and this involved doing something the patient or parent didn't like (sic). We are really quite helpless now. I don't really know how we can help these sorts of patients. You get bad habits and throw off much responsibility because there's nothing you can do. The time is coming when doctors will be superfluous. The coming of the lay administration is inevitable because of the new set-up.[1]

[1] The attitudes of medical superintendents will be discussed in more detail in Chapter 13 of this report.

Inevitably the attitude of the medical superintendent towards his work affected that of other doctors in the hospital. We were impressed by the interest and enthusiasm of many of those to whom we talked; they were anxious to improve the service, and were fearful lest we criticized in a wholly destructive way. They were aware of the problems resulting from shortage of money, overcrowding, poor quality staff, as well as insufficient staff, but since they felt these aspects of the situation were unlikely to change at all rapidly, they wanted to develop ways of improving the hospital service *despite* these disadvantages, and it was here that they hoped we would help. But this was a self-selecting sample; perhaps those who were less interested did nothing to seek us out, and were rarely seen by research workers on the ward. A superintendent who was very anxious that his deputy should obtain his DPM had suggested he took some time off for further training, but he declined the offer and was described by the superintendent as 'too damn lazy'.

In only nine of the hospitals visited were individual doctors reported to be engaged on some form of research, and there were no research departments. This information was, however, obtained from the medical superintendents and it is possible that other doctors were doing research work unknown to them; nevertheless in general we obtained the impression that this was an activity for which relatively little encouragement was given and little enthusiasm evinced. Such research work as *was* carried out appeared to be largely biological and there was no apparent attempt to introduce a sociological approach to the problem.[1]

(b) *Nursing staff* The nurses' overall sense of achievement was small, and morale tended, in many hospitals and units, to be very low. Thus in one main hospital on the male side the research worker reported: 'Staff restless and unhappy; many retired nurses employed, some deaf, others worn out. Many complaints from senior staff about the standard of nursing assistants'. In another hospital where staff attitudes were positive, the research worker reported: 'Job dissatisfaction amongst staff due to pressure of work and mundane tasks involved'.

As in all other spheres we must emphasize the wide differences often existing between units of the same hospital. Thus of one unit of a medium sized hospital the research worker wrote: 'A happy hospital ... overriding humanitarian attitude' and in another unit of the same hospital: 'Not a good atmosphere, very dominated by "us" and "them"; tolerance but not sympathy shown'.

It is virtually impossible to pinpoint reasons for the discrepancies; sometimes shortage of staff was an important determinant of low morale, but this was by no means a consistent factor. The most that

---

[1] A number of psychologists claimed to be carrying out research. This will be discussed in Chapter 7. See also footnote 1 on p. 116 *supra*.

L

can be said is that usually personality factors were of the utmost importance; thus in one large hospital where the matron was well liked by her staff and praised to the research worker by the medical superintendent, the atmosphere was good on the female side, whereas the chief male nurse was described as 'pathetic' and 'a muddler' and the deputy medical superintendent (who had responsibility for the male side of the hospital) was considered to be 'lazy and ineffectual', so that in consequence of this combination, morale on the male side was generally poor. In another hospital the matron was treated as 'a bit of a joke' and was usually 'missing', a situation which other senior staff felt accounted for the shortage of staff, their poor quality, and very low staff morale.

It was interesting to observe that in those hospitals where the lay administration sought to dominate the medical side, there was sometimes a particularly close relationship between medical staff and senior nursing staff. This reflected itself in a genuine concern for the patients which almost appeared as a closing of ranks in the face of a common opponent.

The fact that nurses did so much domestic work may have had a serious effect on morale, particularly that of the trained nurses, since it reduced their self-perceived status and was thought to be responsible for their feeling that other specialist staff looked down on them. Time after time we found ward sisters and charge nurses cleaning, laundering, sewing, preparing breakfasts and, mainly in the case of male nurses, barbering.[1] One sister commented: 'Nurses are not allowed to do domestic work, but no one minds if the ward sister does it'. Domestic chores included scrubbing floors, cleaning windows, ovens, paintwork, and in one case even the boiler was mentioned. In one very large hospital the female ward staff did all the linen repairs for their own wards by hand, although there was a sewing room with a machine. No one was quite sure why this was so, it seemed to be 'traditional', and although the nurses blamed the matron for retaining the system, she was a somewhat vague administrator, who probably had not even noticed the situation.

As a result of the very considerable amount of domestic work done by trained staff, a strange situation emerged: although domestic work was also done by untrained staff, they did not normally have administrative duties, nor were they usually responsible for the supervision of other staff, nor did they dispense drugs. This meant that time not spent on domestic chores could be spent with patients, in a way that trained staff claimed was not possible for them, since they had so many other duties. This they greatly resented, as most of them maintained that they would have preferred to spend more time with patients. On the other hand it seems likely that had they passed

---

[1] In one hospital a hairdresser was employed and came when asked to do so, but matron commented 'the nurses do a lot of hairdressing', and it seems that only rarely was the hairdresser invited to attend.

over *all* the domestic chores to untrained staff they might have lowered morale even further, and might even have been faced with resignations. It would seem to us that part of this difficulty could be overcome as suggested earlier, by increasing the amount of contract cleaning work done by outside firms, or alternatively by increasing the number of ward orderlies or domestic staff. Unfortunately the isolation of most of the hospitals from large centres of population makes it very difficult indeed to obtain the services of domestic staff and as a result it is the nursing assistants and state enrolled nurses who are forced to perform such tasks, assisted by more senior nurses.[1]

A general dissatisfaction with their role and status was expressed by a nurse in these terms: 'Everyone looks down on nurses, even the teachers and other people in their white coats talk down to you'. In the same hospital a charge nurse, looking after a ward of patients working out on licence said:

> Nurse is a misnomer actually, we're not nurses, we're jailers. Most of these boys are criminals nowadays. . . . Nurses don't do anything any more, all the plum jobs are for other people, teachers, social workers, etc. The only thing that's important for promotion here is cleaning and being a good yes man. . . . They're scraping the bottom of the barrel now; they've lowered the standard of exams so much that they daren't do it any more or they'll be had up for negligence.

A charge nurse in another hospital said he thought there had been a deterioration in charge nurse status due to staff shortages: 'We have to do menial tasks and there is a tendency to forget why the patients are here'.

Summary

In this chapter we have attempted to give a picture of the medical and nursing staff and their relationship both to each other and to the patients. It is widely believed that shortage of staff is a vital factor preventing the implementation of many improvements now generally recognized as being necessary if mental subnormality hospitals are to be brought into line with current medical thought.

Our data seem to suggest that staff shortage is perhaps only one factor in producing poor staff morale. Equally important are the isolation of the hospital, the debasement of the nursing role, and the failure of communication, all of which tend to stultify creative thinking. Furthermore the fact that staff turnover is so slow, parti-

---

[1] It is, of course, possible for nurses to carry out domestic chores *with* patients in a way which may have considerable therapeutic value. To be successful the nurses concerned need to be made aware of this therapeutic role, otherwise they will continue to see the performance of chores as being due solely to shortage of domestic staff and they will continue to feel resentful.

cularly at senior level, means that there is little opportunity for new ideas to penetrate the service.

The fact that so few patients are physically ill and requiring medical attention places the nursing staff in a position of power *vis-à-vis* patient care which would not be possible in a hospital where the medical staff had a more obvious and positive role to play. Under the present circumstances only those doctors in subnormality hospitals who are interested in the psychiatric treatment of patients, or in research, have any major role to play. For those who are concerned primarily with the physical care of patients, the subnormality hospital offers very little.

In this study not a great deal of attention was paid to the question of training for both medical and nursing staff working in this field, but sufficient information was forthcoming in informal discussions to lead us to believe that especially in the field of medicine, subnormality is an uncharted sea and one which receives short shrift on training courses.[1]

In the following chapter we shall introduce a third dimension into the situation, that of the specialist staff; one might expect them to play an important part in the training of patients, and not until we have examined their role in the hospitals can we really assess the situation in relation to staffing generally in subnormality hospitals.

[1] This view is confirmed by the findings of the Royal College of General Practitioners in their report No. 7, *Education in Psychology and Psychiatry*, September 1967.

Chapter 7

EDUCATION, TRAINING AND
OTHER SPECIALIST SERVICES[1]

IN this chapter we shall attempt to describe the facilities available for
the treatment and training of patients, other than those of a strictly
medical or nursing nature. The information upon which our data are
based were obtained largely through interviews with the relevant
heads of the departments and, in the case of schools, workshops, etc.,
periods of observation were spent in the relevant department, which
included talking informally to as many staff and patients as possible.

In some cases medical superintendents were asked for their views
about certain aspects of these various departments, and in addition a
considerable amount of useful, but unsystematic information concerning the specialist departments was forthcoming from members
of the nursing staff; we have also drawn on these sources for illustra-
tive purposes.

Children's schools

' "When *I* use a word", Humpty Dumpty said in a rather scornful
tone, "it means just what I choose it to mean – neither more nor
less".'[2] This may perhaps be only too true of what are termed schools
in hospitals for the subnormal; they range from imposing new
buildings, well-equipped and well-staffed, to what can best be
described in the terms used by the medical superintendent of one
hospital as 'no more than rotas of assistant nurses playing with
children'.[3]

Not that fine buildings necessarily make for good schools; one of
the schools visited had completely inadequate classrooms, both in
number and size, no regular access to a recreation hall, no proper
playground, and ill-ventilated and insufficient toilets leading off the
classrooms. The poor building did not, however, prevent the head
teacher from having good relationships with doctors, nurses, and
psychologists; experimental work was being carried out with teaching

[1] Throughout this chapter weights have been used where appropriate.
[2] *Alice Through the Looking Glass*, Chapter V.
[3] Since our fieldwork was completed at least one large hospital is known to
have opened a new school with excellent physical conditions, two others were in
the course of construction when we were at the hospital, and a further three
were at the planning stage.

machines, and nurses attended the school for a period of six weeks' training. The head teacher's only real criticism concerned working conditions which compared unfavourably with those in occupation centres and ESN schools: 'The Ministry's attitude has always been, are your conditions worse than those of nurses – well they aren't, but that's beside the point'.

In the thirty-four hospitals visited, all but four offered some kind of teaching facilities either in the main unit, or, if they had no children there, in a subsidiary unit. Of the four hospitals that had no provisions for teaching, two did not normally admit children under the age of 16, and the third was a unit of approximately 30 children aged between 2 and 15, but where there were no provisions for schooling. In the fourth case the school had been closed for two years due to lack of qualified staff, though some therapy was carried out with adolescent boys on the ward by two untrained staff. No facilities were available for girls.

Four of the main units had two schools each, and 24 subsidiary units offered some kind of teaching programme. Thus, by interpreting 'school' in its widest sense, and by including the therapy with adolescent boys referred to above, we have a total of 59 in our sample. According to the head teachers concerned, a total of 2,671 pupils received full-time schooling and a further 356 part-time,[1] but these would not all be between the ages of five and sixteen, since some schools included pupils up to the age of 19 or even older, and in occasional circumstances others took them under the age of five.

So far as our sample of patients was concerned, a total of 15·8 per cent were in hospitals which provided day-time schooling for their particular age-group;[2] of these just over one-third attended school. Within the specific age-group five to sixteen, approximately 43 per cent attended school. The criterion of measured intelligence appeared to have little bearing upon whether or not a child attended school, though thirteen of the fifteen school-age children with IQs known to be over 50 did in fact attend.

Information regarding the staffing of schools is set out in Table 7.1 below. From this table it is clear that the majority of those teaching in hospital schools for the subnormal have no formal qualifications. The British Psychological Society Working Party,[3] who obtained information relating to the year 1962 on 17 schools (not a representative sample), found that 35 per cent of their staff came into our first two categories as compared with our figure of 18·8 per cent; their

---

[1] The total number of children aged between 5 and 16 in the 34 hospitals concerned amounts to 4,249.

[2] This figure exceeds the number of school-age children shown in Chapter 4, p. 61, Table 1 (11·0 per cent) because in a number of instances hospitals provided educational facilities for patients up to the age of 19, and in general there were no very rigid age limits to school attendance.

[3] *op. cit.*

Table 7.1

QUALIFICATIONS OF TEACHING STAFF

Nature of qualifications	Percentage of total*
Teaching certificate	9·3
Teaching certificate and NAMH diploma†	9·5
Specialist subject qualifications‡	4·6
NAMH diploma§	4·2
No teaching qualification but nursing or other qualification (e.g., SRN, SEN)	4·8
None (including untrained nurses)	67·5
TOTAL	100·0
No. of staff	307

* These figures are based upon the assumption that part-time staff work half-time. Almost all those with qualifications work full-time but 13 per cent of those who are untrained work part-time.

† The information in this table is based upon replies given by head teachers; Ministry of Health officials consider that there are *fewer* teachers holding both a teaching certificate and the diploma than our data suggest.

‡ e.g., art, music, handicrafts, etc.

§ Since 1964 the name has officially been changed to the Diploma for the Teachers of the Mentally Handicapped. The training council is concerned that even amongst staff it continues to be known by its old name.

figure for those with no training was 57 per cent compared with our 67·5 per cent; however it is not known whether the working party included part-time teachers – these *are* included in our percentages.

The presence of qualified staff did not appear to be related either to total size of hospital, nor to region, though it happens that two hospitals in the Manchester region did have more qualified staff than other hospitals sampled. In one of these cases the information paints a somewhat distorted picture because of an abnormally high teacher/ child ratio in a special children's unit (1:8 – all being qualified), whereas in the main hospital employing five teaching staff the ratio was 1:10 but only one teacher had any formal qualifications.

Three of the 'schools' had no classrooms – in one case where 10 children attended part-time and two part-time specialist teachers were employed they used the day-room on one of the wards. In another 'school' attended part-time by 38 children and staffed by two unqualified teachers, we were told that there was no need for a separate building as classes could be held either in the hall or in the garden. In the third hospital where no classrooms were provided, 'school' consisted of 58 children attending part-time for sensory training given by two full-time unqualified staff in the hall. In two of these three instances the medical superintendent said the 'school' was big enough for the requirements of the hospital concerned, and in the third case we do not know his views on the subject.

Forty-two of the 59 schools had a playground, and 15 had a kitchen: in most cases children returned to their ward for lunch. Only 20 schools had sanitary annexes attached to the school, in one of these there was no running water and 'potties' had to be used. In some schools where no sanitary annexes were provided, the children had to be dressed and taken outside to lavatories attached to one of the wards. A few schools had additional facilities such as cloakrooms, one had a 'rumpus' room and a greenhouse in the garden. Another had a sick bay and a music room, and a number of schools had additional playrooms, sometimes equipped with television. Very few had any storage space and the head teacher's office was usually no more than a box-like partition which had often to be shared by all the teaching staff. Nevertheless almost half of those in charge of educational facilities expressed themselves as satisfied with the accommodation provided.

A number of schools excluded children, most frequently because their behaviour was said to be too disturbed. They were also excluded on medical grounds, but only very occasionally as a result of being too physically handicapped. Eight hospitals ran 'play-groups',[1] either in a special room set aside for the purpose, or more frequently teachers (usually assistant nurses acting in that capacity), were sent to the wards to play with special groups of children. Sometimes they were too young to attend school: in one such case the group comprised brain-damaged children. In another hospital two classes were held on the ward for those considered too noisy or emotionally disturbed to attend school, and in a few hospitals the school staff were concerned with habit and sensory training on the wards.

Only seven of the fifty-nine teachers in charge said they were dissatisfied with the equipment provided; most said they received whatever they asked for.

Twenty-eight schools were in hospitals where no psychologist was employed on the staff. Of the remaining 31, 18 head teachers said they had contact with the psychologist about individual patients and two of these also discussed teaching methods with him/her. But the other 13 had no such contact, and in one case expressed surprise that there *was* a psychologist, and in another, confused him with the medical superintendent. Nine teachers had some contact with the Local Education Authority psychologist or school inspector, but in four of these cases it was only on isolated occasions.

A few teachers said they used formal teaching methods, but most claimed to use a mixture of directed and undirected play. Too little

[1] It is possible that more did so unofficially, but they were not drawn to the attention of the research workers.

time was spent in the schools to make any assessment of curricula, or of the efficacy of their teaching and training methods, nor were the interviewers qualified to comment on these matters.

Any proper assessment of schools would require a much more rigorous and specialized examination than we were able to carry out. However, on the criteria we were able to apply during our visits, that is taking into consideration only such items as the facilities available, the use made of the equipment, the size of the class and the general atmosphere, we would estimate that seven schools appeared to meet the kind of requirements we looked for,[1] 10 failed totally to do so, and the remaining 42 fell somewhere in between.

Finally we asked head teachers about any special problems they experienced, and these are set out in Table 7.2:[2]

Table 7.2
SPECIAL PROBLEMS IDENTIFIED BY HEAD TEACHERS

Nature of problem	*No. of times mentioned*
Too little contact with relatives	33
Lack of accommodation and/or space	20
Unsatisfactory communications/relations with other disciplines	11
Unfavourable conditions of service	10
Insufficient staff	7
Lack of equipment, materials, poor maintenance facilities	6
Unfavourable attitudes of other staff towards education	5
Other*	5
Difficulties due to grade/handicap/behaviour of patient	4
Sense of isolation from general field of education	4
Transportation difficulties to and from ward	2
Insufficient contact with LEA	2
None	7
Number of head teachers	59

* e.g., dissatisfaction with NAMH training course, need for smaller groups, insufficient clean clothing for children, etc.

The number of teachers mentioning insufficient contact with relatives is interesting; of the 33, nine referred to it as a *major* problem. One

[1] This is not to say that all the children who could have benefited from attendance did so, our assessment refers simply to the service provided for those who *did* attend. Nor are we implying that the staff were themselves satisfied with the school provisions, and in particular some would have preferred to come under the Department of Education and Science.

[2] This was an open-ended question, coded subsequently.

teacher, typical of many, said that she had only seen two parents in the 18 months she had worked there. Most said the situation arose because parents visited at weekends when they were not on duty; there was a general feeling that more parents would visit the school on weekdays if they knew that this would be allowed. Most head teachers said they saw parents in the grounds once a year at Open Day, but it seems that they were unsuccessful in using this occasion as an opportunity to encourage parents to visit the school during the rest of the year.

Lack of contact with relatives is only one aspect of the almost complete isolation of the schools from general involvement in treatment, and from the field of education generally. This same sense of isolation lies behind many of the comments under such headings as 'unfavourable attitudes towards education',[1] 'unsatisfactory relationships with other disciplines', etc. The fact that in some cases 'schooling' is carried out on the wards does not appear to result in closer integration with other aspects of training, since children who are taught on the wards, as compared with those attending in a building set aside for the purpose, receive only very limited educational training. We have already noted that this work is usually carried out by nursing assistants seconded to work under the head teacher, rather than by educators, and the normal amount of time spent on the ward rarely exceeds an hour each day during term time.

Throughout this report we have frequently referred to the differences which exist between units of the same hospital. This situation is equally true in relation to schools: in the main unit of one hospital the school was extremely well-equipped, the teaching was imaginative and included many outings to places of interest, news discussions, training in citizenship, as well as more formal education and play. The school staff did 'dinner duty' on the children's wards, a situation which not only helped counteract the shortage of nurses, but also gave nursing and teaching staff an opportunity to understand each other's work and problems.

In a large subsidiary unit of the same hospital (approximately 400 patients) conditions were very different: only a very small proportion of children attended school, the accommodation was poor, there was no contact with the school staff or the psychologist at the main unit, nor with the Local Education Authority psychologist or inspectors. The two teachers in the subsidiary unit worked in total isolation and when questioned about this the senior of them said she was not worried by it, her only concern was lack of running water. The research worker commented: 'There is very little activity in this school, the teachers are kind but lack enthusiasm or interest, a situation which contrasts markedly with the school at the main unit'.

---

[1] The isolation of hospital schools and training centres from the main stream of education is also referred to by the British Psychological Society Working Party, *op. cit.*

So far as conditions of service are concerned, teachers compared their own position unfavourably with those working for the Local Authority. The administrative responsibility for almost all the schools lay with the Hospital Management Committee,[1] and in order to attract new staff or to keep teachers already in post, some committees appeared to have modified hours of work and periods of leave, a situation which had sometimes achieved the attempted aim only at the cost of considerable resentment amongst the staff themselves. In one school, three of the teachers were each entitled to three weeks holiday, five had an entitlement of nine weeks and the head teacher had an entitlement of four. This school was also used as a training centre for teachers of subnormal children, and of the twelve staff seconded for training, eight had left after the two years' compulsory work and had taken jobs with higher pay and longer holidays.

In another unit of the same hospital all teachers had nine weeks holiday, but new entrants were only to have three. At the time of the research only one new entrant was affected by this ruling, but the head teacher visualized that it would cause considerable ill-feeling as the number of new teachers increased. In one school the teachers had taken matters into their own hands: three of the staff were entitled to twelve weeks leave and two of them to only three weeks. As a result, two of those with longer holidays voluntarily gave up three weeks of their leave in order to allow the others to have six weeks, but, we were told, 'the Group Secretary is not happy with this, because some are getting more than they are entitled to and others less'.

Some teachers thought schools in subnormality hospitals should come under the auspices of the education authority: 'It's not good for professional relationships to have educationalists under the control of medical staff. No one is sure where to place teachers. School staff work different hours from other staff, and this leads to rivalry. There is no reason for the school to be under the Health Service'. But on the whole very few mentioned such professional susceptibilities possibly because very few are trained teachers.[2]

Adults' schools

In addition to the children's schools, 13 of the 34 hospitals provided day-time schools or evening classes for adults. One of these had no provisions for adults in the main unit, but had adult schools in two subsidiary units. Altogether approximately one-third of the patients in the hospitals sampled were in units where some facilities for adult education were available.

[1] One hospital school was run by the Local Education Authority and a few others, although run by the hospital, had children attending from outside and therefore had close links with the LEA.

[2] At the time of writing (March 1968) discussions are proceeding at Ministerial level regarding the transfer of responsibility for the education of subnormal children in hospital to the local education authorities.

The total number of adults attending classes is difficult to ascertain since numbers tend to fluctuate; so far as we could tell, approximately 1,350 patients attended for between one and six hours per week,[1] 38 attended for ten hours, and 111 attended for approximately 30 hours. In addition 36 patients in one hospital were being trained full-time in domestic science, and some attended children's schools full-time. It seems that approximately 12·3 per cent of those for whom the facilities are available actually attended classes.

The smallest adult school (approximately 20 patients) was in one of the largest hospitals. This may be related to the fact that this particular hospital sought predominantly to train patients in their industrial workshops. In the past they had catered largely for high grade patients only, but like all other National Health Service hospitals they now took all grades of patient and seemingly had some difficulty in adjusting to the presence of the lower grades.

The three evening schools which took between them the vast majority of patients were run and staffed by the Local Education Authority and the hospitals provided only the accommodation and some of the equipment. In general, provision for adults tended to fall into two groups – those aiming to provide education or training, and those aiming primarily to provide a social club. Occasionally the two functions ran side by side as in the three major evening schools mentioned above. The wide variety of provisions, the enthusiasm of the staff, and the interest of patients, were obvious to the research workers, who also were impressed by the high level of achievement. At one of these hospitals a 'social' was regularly held after the classes when patients, teaching and nursing staff all went to the hall for refreshments. The atmosphere was described by the research workers as 'informal and friendly, staff and patients mixed, chatted, and danced together'. They also watched the annual pantomime and were impressed by the performance of allegedly severely subnormal patients. One of these evening schools provided a library, and whereas on the wards books were torn, destroyed or scribbled upon, in the evening school they were properly handled. The head teacher commented: 'It is so essential that they feel needed and wanted and this is what we try to provide'. Typical of the type of provisions made in these three schools are classes in reading and number work, tape recordings used to train patients in job applications, speech training, arts and crafts, dressmaking, domestic science, woodwork, educational films, special lectures, drama, and PE. Since the type of patients in these three large hospitals[2] did not differ in degree of subnormality or physical handicap from those in other similar sized hospitals, we feel it would be possible and helpful for Local Education Authorities to extend this work to hospitals throughout the country.

[1] 1,055 of these were in three large hospitals.
[2] All over 1,400 beds.

Psychological services

Seventeen hospitals in our sample provided some kind of psychological service, but as in the case of schools, the range covered by this term was wide indeed, as is indicated by the staffing situation: ten main units and one subsidiary unit employed one or more full-time professionally trained psychologists, making a total of 25 in all.[1] There were a further seven part-time psychologists, one of whom was the only member of the department and visited the hospital monthly. One of the other part-time psychologists was employed full-time at the local mental hospital, but was said by the matron to carry out psychological tests for the subnormality unit and so is included in our figures.

Six university students were employed, one being attached to a hospital which does not officially have a psychology department: she visited only during the vacations in order to carry out psychological tests. Finally, there were five persons with other qualifications working full- or part-time in the psychology departments (this does not include clerical workers); one was a psychological tester, one a teacher, two were nursing assistants, and one a laboratory technician.

Only in one hospital was there a different psychologist working in an ancillary unit, in addition to those working in the main unit; this situation arose because the ancillary unit concerned was highly autonomous, was medically but not administratively responsible to the main hospital, and had a different Hospital Management Committee. In one hospital where a psychologist had, in the past, been employed in a subsidiary unit but not in the main unit, he had since left and not been replaced.

Approximately 34 per cent of sampled patients were in hospitals which provided a psychological service; for a further 12 per cent the services existed in the hospital, but not in the particular unit in which they were living. For the remaining 54 per cent no service was available. This information was obtained from the medical superintendents, and we think that where it was said that a psychological service was also available to patients in subsidiary units (using staff from the main unit), this usually covered no more than an initial test on admission or, if a case was to be reviewed, a special IQ test may have been requested. It should be noted that the non-availability of a psychological service did not necessarily mean that no patients were tested.[2] On the other hand, 'availability' meant anything from the services of one or more full-time psychologists, to a monthly visit.

Where there was no psychologist we asked superintendents whether they would have preferred to have one; 62 per cent of patients were in hospitals where the superintendent would have liked one but said he could not get one, and 38 per cent were in hospitals

---

[1] Nine of these were employed in one hospital.
[2] See Chapter 4, p. 66, which refers to IQ tests carried out by medical staff.

where he did not want one. In one of the largest hospitals the super-intendent expressed his ambivalence in terms of the *nurses'* hostility to them: 'All these extraneous people are viewed with great suspicion by the nursing staff and it is particularly difficult if these people gang together and don't mix with nursing staff. The nurses have in the past done everything and they are very conservative indeed'.

The most senior psychologist on the staff was interviewed in each unit.[1] Almost all cases were referred by medical staff: five interviewees said they also came through nursing staff and four through other specialist staff, such as school or training department. Five said they found patients upon their own initiative.

We asked psychologists about the type of work they carried out.[2] All but two said that the department carried out routine tests and assessments on admission. Certainly the IQs of patients were a little more readily available in hospitals employing a psychologist, but unless psychologists kept their own records and did not enter the test information on the case records, it seems likely that a considerable number of patients slip through the net, or alternatively that the time lag between admission and testing may, in some instances, be quite considerable.

Eight psychologists said that regular follow-up tests and assess-ments were carried out: it is noteworthy that they were all in reason-ably well-staffed departments[3] with a tradition of psychological services, or alternatively the psychologist was regarded by colleagues as forward-looking in ideas and attitudes. Nevertheless it is our strong impression that even in these departments the process was a selective one, and the majority of patients were not followed up.[4] Most of the departments did reassessments only at the request of the medical staff.

Ten departments claimed to carry out research: five of these were concerned with training and rehabilitation, two with intelligence and learning processes, two departments were involved in research in three different areas: hearing, motor reflexes and the effect of drugs in one case, and in the other cognitive processes, stress in psychopaths and neurological factors. One psychologist was not prepared to co-operate fully with our research and merely said she was working with a well-known professor.

[1] The information given in the remainder of this section is derived from interviews with him/her. We were not able to interview the part-time student, nor the psychologist who visited only monthly, leaving a total of fifteen inter-viewed.

[2] For an interesting discussion of the role of the psychologist in the sub-normality hospital, see Gunzberg, H. C., in *Inter. J. Soc. Psychiatry*, Vol. 1, No. 4, Spring 1966.

[3] An exception to this was the hospital referred to in Chapter 4, p. 66.

[4] Again the situation may have appeared worse than it actually was due to poor recording of information, though one might think it would be important to make this kind of information available on case records for the benefit of medical and nursing staff.

Ten departments said they were involved in teaching, through the nurse training school, and one psychologist said the department was concerned in interviewing prospective students. Four departments did post-graduate staff counselling.

The staffs of nine departments were also involved in work at out-patient clinics run by the hospital (sometimes in conjunction with the Local Authority) and seven of the more senior psychologists also spent time on committee work.

Eight departments claimed to be doing counselling or therapy with patients, but we have no information as to the number of patients involved, other than that it was a very small case load. One psychologist said she organized outings for patients and one claimed to have 'unofficial' contact with patients after discharge.

Undoubtedly the greater part of the psychologists' time in sub-normality hospitals is devoted to IQ testing; their presence in the hospitals is viewed with suspicion by other staff, particularly if they attempt to move outside the role of psychological tester. With few exceptions an air of apathy pervades the departments and one would require exceptional pioneering qualities to persuade medical and nursing staff to accept a wider definition of their role.

Psychologists were asked about the adequacy of opportunities for discussion with medical and nursing staff: eight out of fifteen said they were satisfied with the situation in relation to medical staff, ten out of fifteen were satisfied in relation to nursing staff. We consider that the extent of their isolation from other staff may have been underestimated. The question was poorly phrased: by asking if they had 'adequate' opportunity we may have missed the fact that some did not *want* such an opportunity and therefore 'no contact' was considered 'adequate'. Again, one psychologist who replied 'Yes' to the question, later modified this in relation to medical staff saying: '. . . I meant the younger MOs. The medical director I do not see. . . . He is not as accessible as he should be. If I do ask to see him he is not here, if he is here he is too busy'.[1]

We think that the true state of affairs was much more accurately depicted when we asked psychologists to discuss their problems.[2] This showed that unsatisfactory communications and/or relation-ships with other staff (medical, nursing, training or school), was mentioned eight times and that in addition unfavourable attitudes towards psychology by other staff was mentioned six times. One psychologist referred to lack of status, closely connected with a poor relationship with medical staff. Gunzberg refers to the need for the psychologist to be given 'full clinical responsibility to the same extent as his medical colleagues of equal seniority, so far as non-medical

---

[1] The superintendent in question appeared to spend a considerable time away from the hospital (research observation).

[2] In addition to the two psychologists not interviewed, two declined to answer this particular question.

matters are concerned', as well as to the need for the relationship between the psychologist and the medical superintendent to rest on 'complete mutual confidence and respect'.[1] From our research observations it would seem that both these situations are rare to the point of non-existence.

For the most part psychologists tend to be housed in accommodation far from the main administrative block where the medical and administrative nursing staff have their offices, and this physical isolation symbolizes a more general attitudinal isolation. This is no doubt partly the fault of the psychologists themselves – most are uncertain of their function and status in the subnormality hospital and are content to isolate themselves from the general run of treatment and training. One psychologist referring to this isolation commented: 'It is partly our fault (that the nursing staff see them as unapproachable), we tend to be seen as specialists accessible only to other specialists'.

Shortage of staff was mentioned as a problem only five times (in one case this was lack of secretarial help) and conditions of service twice. But there was a great deal of criticism of other departments such as schools, social work, occupation and training departments, for their use of untrained staff. There was also much criticism of the quality of the nursing staff, and of their rigidity of attitude: 'They are glorified domestics in sisters' uniforms' expressed succinctly the views of many.

Occupational therapy and industrial training[2]

All the main units visited and 62 of the 119 ancillary units provided facilities for occupational therapy or industrial training, in a total of 130 departments. As in all other aspects of hospital life, the provisions varied markedly not only as between hospitals, but between units of the same hospital. Although training departments often provided one of the few opportunities for male and female patients to mix, fewer than one-quarter of the departments were integrated; industrial training was generally (though not exclusively) reserved for male patients and females most usually did occupational therapy. In practice there was often no clear distinction between the work undertaken by these two types of department, and to the extent that differences did exist, we believe that they reflect the differences in the attitudes of male and female nursing staff referred to earlier,[3] since nurses are usually the real arbiters of where patients work.[4]

The proportion of patients in each hospital unit attending either occupational therapy or industrial training varied widely. In some

[1] *op. cit.*
[2] For a useful discussion of vocational and industrial training in institutions see Gunzberg, H. C., in Clarke and Clarke, *op. cit.*, p. 390 ff.
[3] See Chapter 6, p. 117.
[4] This will be discussed in some detail in Chapter 8.

hospital units the figure was between 60 and 75 per cent, in others it was as few as 3 per cent, an average figure would therefore be misleading.[1] Moreover, as Table 7.3 illustrates, the availability of departments did not mean that patients attended – thus a further 35 per cent and 25 per cent respectively did not attend departments which existed in the hospitals in which they were housed, nor were they engaged on other occupations.

Table 7.3

PATIENTS ATTENDING OCCUPATIONAL THERAPY AND
INDUSTRIAL TRAINING DEPARTMENTS* (PERCENTAGES)

Availability of department and attendance	*Occupational therapy*	*Industrial training*
Department available, patients attend	21·2	13·5
Department available, patients do not attend (no occupation)	35·0	24·6
Department not available	43·8	61·9
TOTAL	100·0	100·0
Does not apply (patient too young or otherwise occupied)	1127	1079
No information	13	11
No. of patients	3,038	3,038

* Where the department is a joint one, the patient is included under industrial training.

Generally speaking, patients working full-time in occupational therapy or industrial training departments worked about 30–35 hours per week and those working part-time about 15 hours. With certain notable exceptions (in hospitals recognized as having particularly good opportunities for training), it would be true to say that whilst most of the large hospitals had a smaller percentage of patients attending, the facilities, the supervision, and the type of work undertaken were in general superior to that found in the small units. Often the proportion of patients in small units attending occupational therapy was high, simply because there was little alternative occupation, but the scope of the work was in many cases extremely limited.

The type of activity undertaken in the various departments is set out in Table 7.4. As a generalization it could probably be said that all occupational therapy departments did handicrafts and all industrial departments did industrial contract work; this was, generally

---

[1] See also Chapter 8, p. 177 ff. which discusses patients at work. This section indicates that 12·5 per cent of sampled patients attended occupational therapy departments and 9·4 per cent attended industrial training.

speaking, the factor which determined what the department was called. One charge nurse who ran a mixed unit deplored the policy of the medical superintendent, which was to run down the occupational therapy side and develop only industrial contract work: 'A lot of this industrial work is nothing but a modern gimmick – if you're not doing it, you're not a modern hospital, there's just as important part to play in a hospital this size from craft work as from industrial work'.

Table 7.4

TYPE OF WORK UNDERTAKEN BY DEPARTMENT

Type of work	No. of occupational therapy departments	Type of work	No. of industrial training departments
Handicrafts	82	Industrial contract work	48
Art/pottery	23	Carpentry	24
Musical activities	11	Printing	8
Physical activities	11	Building/decorating	10
Sedentary games, (jig-saws, beads, etc.)	17	Gardening/farming	12*
Industrial contract work	5	Domestic science	6*
Other	8	Brush making, tailoring, boot repairs, upholstery, etc.	21
		Other	3
Total number of OT departments	82†	Total number of IT departments	48†

* This does not include hospitals where this type of work is undertaken but not under the auspices of the industrial training department.

† These totals include nine joint departments.

In one hospital a 'launderette' was attached to the occupational therapy department and we were told that if they were able to do so, patients came from the whole hospital to use it. There was no washing machine – simply a spin drier and three irons. No one was taught how to use the 'launderette' and we did not ever see it in use.[1]

Table 7.5 sets out the qualifications and experience of the staff working in these training departments.

[1] In some hospitals certain high-grade wards have launderette facilities attached to the ward and these are in frequent use.

Table 7.5

QUALIFICATIONS AND EXPERIENCE OF STAFF IN OCCUPATIONAL
THERAPY AND INDUSTRIAL TRAINING DEPARTMENTS
(PERCENTAGES)

Qualifications	*Number of staff* *
Qualified occupational therapist (MAOT)	8·5
Specialist qualifications, i.e., industrial, arts and crafts, etc.	9·4
Nursing staff (trained and untrained)	25·6†
Journeymen	10·8‡
Other	3·2§
None	42·5
TOTAL	100·0
Total number of staff	502

   * Part-time are included here as working half-time.
   † Four of these nurses are shared with the school.
   ‡ Two are also trained nurses.
   § Mainly with industrial experience.

Almost all those with occupational therapy training, as well as those with industrial experience, worked full-time. Approximately one-third of the nursing staff worked part-time as did just under one-fifth of those with no qualifications.

As in all other departments, the head of each unit was interviewed,[1] and asked, amongst other matters, about problems. Again poor relationships with other staff was an important factor as will be seen from Table 7.6.

Far and away the most frequent complaint was the lack of suitable accommodation, and although in some cases the shortage of space referred to working room, for the most part the shortage was one of storage space. Large, light and airy workrooms had in some cases been built with nowhere to store materials, equipment or finished goods. This was not always the case, however, and a trained occupational therapist on the female side of one of the biggest hospitals expressed well the feelings of many colleagues in other hospitals:

> Our A1 problem is limited space. I believe a new occupational therapy centre is being given priority but I doubt whether it will be ready for another five or ten years. I had 80 patients here, but the pressure was just too much (she had three full-time and one part-time assistant, all untrained), with this type of patient one can deal

[1] In two units where the therapist only comes from time to time we were not able to see him/her and basic information was obtained from the matron or chief male nurse. Another unit was closed because the therapist was on leave.

Table 7.6

SPECIAL PROBLEMS AS IDENTIFIED BY
PERSON IN CHARGE OF TRAINING DEPARTMENTS

Nature of problem	*No. of times mentioned*
Lack of suitable accommodation/space	50
Unsatisfactory relationships/communications with other staff	32
Insufficient staff	29
Problems relating to grade/handicap/behaviour of patient	16
Difficulties in obtaining suitable work	14
Unfavourable conditions of service	12
Insufficient equipment/materials, etc.	7
Generally unfavourable attitudes towards department	6
Unsatisfactory system of payment to patients	4
Sense of isolation in profession	2
Difficulties in selling goods	2
Transport difficulties to and from wards	2
Other	2
No problems	8
No. of persons interviewed	127

with fewer because they need more intensive instruction. The grade of patient I get has gone down over the past few years as the cream is skimmed off to the industrial training unit or the sheltered workshop. All the patients should be having occupational therapy from a psychological point of view. It's obvious to the nurses who come up here to see what patients do. They cause very little trouble when they're occupied. A terrific lot of nurses don't agree with this, and there *is* a shortage of staff so they don't all get up here, but I found, not only in this hospital, that they are very impressed when they do. But when they go back (to the ward) it's a question of out of sight, out of mind.

Questioned about the possibility of expanding work on the wards, the interviewee said:

It's a touchy point. It has been tried – the Hospital Management Committee have given their approval. I had a part-time therapist working on the ward, but she left and hasn't been replaced. I found that I sent an occupational therapist to the ward where the doctor wanted her, but the sister didn't. *It's not that she didn't want her patients occupied, but it was perhaps an over-zealous doctor and a sister suspicious of new ideas.*[1] It hasn't been going now for nine months and nobody has questioned it. We started with the sick wards, this was the doctor's idea and I agree with it, because I

[1] Author's italics.

think if a patient can get up, they should be able to go out to work, even if they do nothing when they get there – that's why you see some of them doing nothing here. From the ward point of view, you may get the impression that they want it (occupational therapy) and that we won't co-operate, but the doctors put pressure on the sisters from time to time and for a short while they keep ringing up for me to send materials down and I do. But this dies down after a week or two until the doctor starts it all up again. There is a crying need for more activity for patients, but I can't have more staff till I have more patients, but I can't have more patients till I have bigger premises, so here we stick.

We feel that this illustrates a matter which is crucial to all our findings, namely that whether a patient has access to the facilities available or not seems to be determined not only by a breakdown in communications between the staff concerned, but by the presence – or absence – of ignorance or prejudice about what is 'right' for the patient.

The male occupational therapist in the same hospital also complained of a lack of co-operation from the nursing staff, but he felt even more strongly about failure of liaison with doctors. This view was supported by the research workers who observed that in this particular hospital the medical staff working on the female side were far more active than those working on the male side. The therapist would have liked a monthly group meeting to discuss patients, but none were held. In his previous hospital, he had always kept case notes, but was told that they would not be necessary here since no one wanted to see them. He nevertheless kept an account of each patient's progress, and felt annoyed because no one consulted him: 'They even move them to the industrial therapy unit without asking me if I think they are capable, and then they (patients) come back to us, and I could have told them (doctors) in the first place'.

In the industrial training unit of this hospital, they too complained about the way referrals were made, and in particular referred to the unsuitable people sent over by doctors. Apart from this problem the supervisor mentioned conflict with the hospital psychologist over the aims of the unit – he regarded the psychologist's view as being 'too inflexible'.

Information about these three units within the same hospital is written up at some length because it well illustrates the interdepartmental conflicts which we found to exist in one form or another almost universally, and because of an almost complete lack of communication, these conflicts are never discussed, let alone resolved. In one large hospital where meetings are rarely held, the occupational therapist commented:

Communication with the medical staff is practically non-existent. If you have a meeting with the medical superintendent he is only wanting to get it over as soon as possible. One meeting on eight patients took only 16 minutes. We feel they're not really interested in the patients. . . . All the other departments are good and it's a friendly place, only the medical staff are the weak link, they lack good leadership. Under the new system the superintendent is not really head of the female side. . . . The nurses could come in here as part of their training but they don't send them enough. . . . They could be doing so much with the patients on the wards; they don't really like coming here because it's not *sick* nursing.

In one of the few hospitals visited where relationships with the rest of the hospital were said to be very good, occupational therapists attended weekly case conferences, a situation which we were told made for much better relationships. In this hospital the occupational therapy department *collected* patients from the wards, which avoided the problem of nurses not being available to take them. The patients in two blocks (villas) were allowed to go unaccompanied, but the therapist commented that this was not popular with the nursing staff.

Four hospitals had industrial workshops where a certain number of patients worked in conditions described by the hospital authorities as being comparable with outside light industry. However in one of these units patients were not paid in cash, they went to the canteen where they could draw whatever they wanted up to a certain sum, and they were taken on day trips, given holidays, outings, etc., from the profits. Most of the work done in this unit was for the benefit of the hospital, e.g. shoe repairs, making brooms, repairing furniture, etc., and the supervisor complained that they 'don't enjoy much co-operation from local industries, because they don't know what we can do, partly because they don't want to know'. These matters tend to be glossed over in the publicity afforded to the unit outside the hospital, although it would be unfair not to point out that in these four units the workshops approximate more closely to normal working conditions than do most hospital units, in so far as patients attend during normal working hours and are expected to achieve a reasonable level of efficiency.

Some of the industrial training units made considerable sums of money. The head of one department with 41 patients and two untrained staff, claimed to earn thirty-eight pounds per week clear on industrial contract work, and said they could earn more if supplies were more regular. The money was paid into a general fund, although the staff had repeatedly asked for it to be paid into a special account, since patients working in the department received an average of only 4s. 1d. per week. The supervisor felt that patients wanted more money and would work better if they earned more, but the suggestion was turned down by the Group finance officer. This was not always the case and in some of the hospitals all the money earned was distributed amongst the patients in the department, either individually or more usually by means of outings to the seaside, pantomimes, or on shopping expeditions. In one hospital on the male side, the money was shared out at the end of the month and paid into the patient's personal account. With this they bought clothes, paintings, transistor radios, etc. The amount was graded by the supervisor according to their ability: 'It's fairly elastic'. He claimed to plough back £2,000 per annum into the department.

As in all other areas discussed in this report, the departments varied widely within the same hospital. Perhaps the most unfortunate aspect of this is that no one in a position of authority seems aware of it, or if they are, they are not prepared or able to do anything about it. Thus, in one very large hospital the female occupational therapy department was described by the research worker as 'dull and unimaginative', and the untrained occupational therapist in charge was seen to adopt very authoritarian and punitive attitudes towards patients; yet the male side of the same hospital had, in the writer's estimation, one of the most satisfactory units observed in the research, with plenty of planned activity and a real interest shown by both staff and patients. That such situations can develop must, we feel, be regarded as a reflection on the administrative competence of those concerned with running the hospital. It is clearly undesirable that there should be wide variations in the quality of a service which should be uniformly satisfactory for all patients; it is not the task of administrators to run the units; it is, however, their task to see that they operate efficiently and imaginatively with every patient being equally able to benefit within the limitations imposed by the degree of his or her handicap.

We mentioned earlier that in many of the hospitals it is only relatively few departments that cater jointly for both male and female patients; in one hospital which offered a wide range of occupational and training facilities, and which was generally recognized by the profession to have progressive ideas, the female occupational therapy building was quite new and was shared by some of the male patients. Nevertheless it had been built with separate entrances and with no way through from the male to the female part of the building. Even the paths from the two entrances went in opposite directions, so that the sexes never met. We were told that this was planned many years ago, and when it came to be built, 'they' (unspecified) refused to replan it, although it was said that it would not have been so segregated had it been a more recent plan! Even the nurses were strictly segregated and female nurses in this hospital were not allowed to go to the male workshops, even in order to buy something from the occupational therapy shop, without first ringing matron and asking for permission (sic).

In one large hospital where the industrial training department was integrated, the male nursing staff expressed considerable hostility to the arrangement saying, *inter alia*, that 'subnormals are oversexed'.[1]

[1] Further discussion of attitudes to sexuality will be discussed in Chapter 8.

Not all shared this view and we also visited departments where the supervisor admitted that initially he had been very opposed to the idea, but experience had made him change his mind, and he found that patients were happier, and therefore worked better, in a joint department.

It was suggested to us in informal discussion with staff that in the 'old days' training departments were staffed almost exclusively by nurses, and that many of the problems now existing result from the fact that professionally trained therapists and workshop instructors have been brought in from outside. This is said to account for the frequency of poor relationships between nursing and training staff, and for much of the hostility towards training departments generally, as well as for some of the low morale amongst nursing staff; not only is their traditional nursing role often irrelevant in the subnormality hospital,[1] but their training role is also rapidly decreasing.

If these comments are justified, one might expect departments staffed exclusively by nurses to have better relationships with the rest of the hospital and to have higher staff morale, even if the type of work offered to patients were less professional. The only way of assessing this at all reliably is by comparing departments within the same unit of the same hospital, where one is run by nursing staff and the other by trained therapists. Even this procedure is not entirely satisfactory since it is impossible to control other factors such as the personality of those involved, staffing ratios, facilities available, etc. Bearing in mind these warnings we found that on the whole there was no apparent difference – that is, if the training staff felt that other staff were co-operative and helpful, this view applied equally whether they were nurses or specialist staff. There was a slight indication that less generalized hostility was expressed by other sections of the hospital towards departments staffed by nurses, but whether there was a direct causal connection it is impossible to say, and it was certainly not true of all hospitals. One nurse in charge of an integrated department commented that certain of the nursing staff did not think that lay people (trainers or unqualified people) should work in subnormality hospitals, but he thought that this view was now gradually changing.

Because of the wide variety of conditions existing in these training units, it is impossible to do justice to the better ones, nor to depict the dullness of others. We were left with four overriding impressions:

1. the poor relationships with medical and nursing staff, and the lack of integration of medical and nursing care with occupational and industrial therapy;
2. the relatively large number of patients who *could* attend, and whom the therapist felt would benefit, but who were prevented either by

[1] This will be discussed further in Chapter 12 with reference to treatment ideology.

the size of the department, or by lack of interest on the part of those who might refer them;
3. the fact that relatively little attempt is made to take occupational therapy to those wards such as cot and chair, where it is difficult to transport patients to the department;[1] to very low grade wards, and even to children's wards. Occasionally nurses are provided with the equipment by the occupational therapy department, but in general they receive little encouragement to develop such work;
4. the limited scope and financial independence of existing arrangements.

Physiotherapy

Sixteen of the thirty-four hospitals employed between them ten full-time and twelve part-time qualified physiotherapists. In addition there were four full-time and eight part-time untrained assistants. They were all attached to the main unit of the hospital concerned and only occasionally included in their case loads patients from subsidiary units.

The number of patients currently receiving treatment was difficult to gauge since some patients were seen regularly and others only at very infrequent intervals. An approximate figure based on replies given by the physiotherapist in charge of each department[2] is 2·5 per cent of the total population of the hospitals visited. This figure obscures not only frequency of treatment but also duration of treatment, though the period most frequently mentioned was one hour per week. In one hospital with a special spastics unit, patients were said to receive treatment five hours per week, and in another hospital children received ten minutes each per day, and adults ten minutes twice weekly.

In terms of availability to patients, 41 per cent of our sample were in hospitals where the services of a physiotherapist were available and 59 per cent where no such provisions were made. We did not ask whether each patient in the sample was receiving treatment from a physiotherapist[3] but we did consider whether those patients suffering from total or partial paralysis (including cripples) were living in hospitals where physiotherapy was available: 40 per cent of such

---

[1] We should, however, point out that in a number of units such patients *do* attend, having been transported in their wheelchairs, and it is often simply a question of staff motivation rather than patients' incapacity.

[2] Four were not interviewed, either because they attended only part-time and did not visit the hospital during the period of the research, or because of illness. As much factual information about their work as possible was obtained from other sources.

[3] We recognize that this would have been helpful, but it was necessary to limit the amount of data collected in order to keep within the financial resources of the budget, and in particular we did not want to involve too much of the nurses' time.

patients fell into this category, leaving a high proportion for whom the service was not available even if it had been considered helpful.

So far as spastics are concerned, information obtained from charge nurses and sisters suggests that approximately eight per cent of the total population of the hospitals visited suffered from moderate or severe spasticity.[1] On the assumption that not all of the 2·5 per cent of patients receiving physiotherapy are *necessarily* spastic, it seems likely that many of this group – who might well be expected to benefit from such treatment – are not in fact receiving it. One physiotherapist commented: 'With the medical staff injuries take precedence over spastics – if I had more staff I could keep one specially for spastics'.

As was the case with other specialist services, we again asked interviewees about their problems. Table 7.7 sets out the information derived from the 12 physiotherapists we were able to interview.

Table 7.7

SPECIAL PROBLEMS AS IDENTIFIED BY PHYSIOTHERAPISTS

Nature of problem	No. of times mentioned
Lack of suitable accommodation	10
Insufficient staff	7
Unsatisfactory communications and/or relationships with other staff	7
Unfavourable attitudes towards physiotherapy by other staff	7
Transport difficulties to and from ward	4
Lack of equipment	3
Difficulty with grade/handicap/behaviour of patient	3
Other	3
Unfavourable conditions of service	2
No problems	2
Total number of physiotherapists	12

Once again it is our impression that a number of these different headings reflect two basic problems: those of relationships between staff of different types, and a degree of isolation from other aspects of treatment and training. For example the question of transport to and from the ward tended to reflect negative attitudes on the part of nursing staff more than real difficulties of transportation, though staff shortages did contribute to this situation. This view is supported by

[1] This figure is likely to be an underestimate since in one small hospital and four subsidiary units we were unable to obtain complete information on this point.

the fact that the problem did not necessarily occur on wards which were particularly poorly staffed.

Both nursing and medical staff came in for almost unanimous criticism. One of the mildest critics commented:

> I think the greatest (problem) is getting a higher percentage of the nursing staff interested in something therapeutic. The majority think of themselves as custodians rather than nurses carrying out treatment. . . . Because the staff are not generally co-operative, I tend to select patients from wards where they *are* co-operative.[1] I don't mean that they won't send patients, but if I send a patient back with certain instructions, very seldom are these carried out (exercises, re-education in walking, etc.)[2] . . . I don't very often meet the medical staff. Some years ago we met each week and we saw the superintendent once a month. I think theoretically we could still meet them, but none of the therapists do. [Why?] I don't think I'd like to answer that.

Two physiotherapists complained about the difficulty of getting calipers, surgical boots, etc. for patients. In both cases the senior nursing staff were said to be obstructive, or at best, uninterested.

Lack of accommodation and equipment is, we think, also associated with these negative or neutral attitudes, since without sufficient pressure by the superintendent, improved conditions for the physiotherapist were likely to be relegated to the end of the queue.

The shortage of staff and lack of accommodation forces the physiotherapist to choose between concentrating on the treatment of a few patients and visiting the wards 'to do a little for many'. Most choose the former, but are fully aware of the mass for whom they do nothing: 'I'm sure something could be done about the cripples here, but being long-term patients it would need years'.

It is perhaps unfortunate that so few hospitals employ physiotherapists and that the number of patients in treatment is so small, because the therapists themselves are full of enthusiasm for their work and really believe that if its nature and usefulness were more widely appreciated by hospital staff generally, it would be to their benefit as well as that of the patients. Perhaps one solution to the problem might be for the existing physiotherapists to spend more time working on the wards, enlisting the co-operation of nursing staff and attempt-

---

[1] This again illustrates, with reference to physiotherapists, the question referred to earlier in relation to occupational and industrial therapists, namely failure of communication between therapists and nursing and medical staff, and a degree of ignorance and prejudice amongst the latter groups regarding non-medical forms of treatment.

[2] Unfortunately due to insufficient probing by the interviewer we do not know whether the instructions were given to nurses escorting patients or direct to patients. If the latter it is, of course, not surprising that no action was taken since no sister or nurse would take instructions sent in this way.

ing thereby to break down some of the hostility by a sense of personal involvement:

> We need to enthuse the nurses with proper methods of handling; this could be applied to the whole field of low grade defectives, we are adding insult to injury if we are not doing something to maintain their interest and potentiality. In these hospitals there are many facilities for the ambulant patients . . . whereas the physically handicapped have *nothing* . . . they suffer from deprivation and fall back further and further. The real problem in any hospital is the re-orientation of the nursing staff; I have always found it easier to work with male nurses, they are mostly married and have outside interests.

Even if many additional physiotherapists were to be recruited, it might still be advantageous to nursing staff if they worked on the wards so that nurses could both learn to handle patients correctly, and ensure that those patients who are given prescribed exercises carry them out regularly.

Speech therapy

Eight of the thirty-four hospitals employed a speech therapist (one of these employed two), of whom four worked only part-time. In addition one of these hospitals had four part-time students working under the supervision of the speech therapist.

Their estimate of the total number of patients receiving treatment amounted to 269, which implies that for all hospitals only about four in a thousand receive treatment, mostly those in large hospitals. In one hospital where two therapists were employed, no patients were actually in treatment at the time of the research as they had only been employed there for one week and were busy carrying out a survey of needs.[1]

Of the 269 in treatment, 100 were in one hospital, 50 of them being seen monthly and most of the remainder weekly. In another hospital 30 patients received individual treatment for up to 20 minutes a week, and in addition four weekly classes were held for 20–30 minutes, each taking between 12 and 18 patients.

Whilst we do not know the number of sampled patients actually receiving speech therapy, we do know[2] that a total of 8·4 per cent of sampled patients suffered from mutism, severe speech defects, or were deaf/mutes. Of these approximately one in six were in hospitals where speech therapy was available.

In one hospital employing a part-time therapist (one and a half hours per week) we were told that she would be leaving soon and there had been no other applicants for the job. In this ancillary unit

[1] No speech therapist had been employed previously.
[2] See Chapter 4, p. 71.

of a main hospital (where there was no speech therapist) nine children out of a total of 65 were receiving treatment at the time of the research.

In five hospitals patients were selected on the initiative of the therapist; where they work only part-time (sessions varying from half to three sessions per week), much valuable time which might have been spent treating patients was in fact spent seeking out those who might be suitable for treatment.

The fact that so few hospitals employ speech therapists undoubtedly reflects a shortage in the country generally. Nevertheless we believe that it again reflects the attitudes of the hospital staff towards specialist staff from outside. We have given countless examples of this in relation to other disciplines; probably educationalists suffer least from it because it is generally recognized that education (at any rate for children), is a legitimate activity and a part of normal life which even severely subnormal persons are entitled to share. Physiotherapists, whilst being less acceptable than teachers, receive a certain degree of acceptance because the nature of their treatment is physical and therefore readily understandable. Psychologists and speech therapists, probably for different reasons, come well down on the scale of acceptability. We think that the psychologists are seen by many of the staff as a threat, their role in the hospital is not understood, and if they step beyond the boundaries of IQ testing they are felt to impinge upon the functions of others. Speech therapists are too few in number to have made any impact at all – only in one hospital did we find a therapist who, despite the antagonism or lack of interest of other staff, had sufficient confidence and interest in his job to persist with real enthusiasm.

In discussing their problems, five of the eight therapists interviewed made reference to unsatisfactory relationships with other staff, four of these relating to doctors. One therapist who worked one day a week and divided his time between the main unit and one subsidiary unit commented: 'It may be my own fault, but being one day a week I get segregated. I am out on a limb and I could sit and read a book. There should be case conferences. I haven't seen the medical superintendent in seven years. The staff don't really believe in speech therapy'. In fact occasional case conferences were held in this hospital, but the speech therapist was not invited to attend. This therapist treated 19 patients regularly and a further 15 attended occasionally.

In another hospital the therapist referred particularly to difficulties with the *female* nursing staff: 'We don't get co-operation from the female staff, the male staff can't do enough for us, but the females seem much more rigid, they don't think this is important'.[1]

---

[1] See comments in Chapter 6, p. 117, regarding differences in attitude between male and female nursing staff.

One full-time therapist mentioned too little contact with parents and expressed views which will be quoted in some detail since they seemed widely shared by other, less articulate, interviewees:

The point is that in a hospital like this you've no parents backing the child, and the adult has developed a don't care attitude anyway. It's very different from general hospital work. All our training is based on the fact that you've got *motivation*. . . . The whole attitude to speech therapy hinges on motivation and most of the people working in this kind of institution think they're all hopeless . . . it's all a big joke. The superintendent is an administrator – he doesn't get around much. . . . It's difficult to get patients here, there aren't enough staff. The nursing staff don't have any alternative to the hopeless attitude, they don't see any results, and it develops in them a very cynical attitude. They are very kind to them physically. (Doctors) are very fond of referring little mongols to me, and they will develop speech anyway, so it's a waste of time. They don't often refer deaf patients, they can't really cope with deaf patients here, they think they are emotionally disturbed and don't refer them. There are quite a few deaf mutes and it never occurs to anyone to refer them to me. I don't think medical people know what a speech therapist is for. As I've got complete freedom (to select patients) it works very well. I don't have any problems and they don't!

This therapist worked in a hospital having approximately 2,000 patients; he spent about half his time on research and half on treatment. But because patients received about two and a half hours treatment per week, only approximately 10 were in treatment at any one time. There was an establishment for another two speech therapists, but they could not get staff.

Social work

Seventeen, or half of the hospitals, employed a total of twenty-two 'social workers', though this term covers a wide range of personnel and includes many duties which one might not expect to come under the heading of social work. Three of them had a social science certificate or diploma, a further 3 had social work experience but no formal training, 6 were trained nurses, and one was a sociology student. The remaining 9 had no specialist qualifications nor experience in social work. All but two worked full-time.

Where hospitals employed more than one social worker they were usually of different sex and divided the work according to this factor.[1] In such cases both social workers were interviewed (usually jointly), and their replies amalgamated, since their experience of the hospital and their attitudes coincided – or so it appeared. Despite their lack of

[1] This appears to be yet another example of the extent to which segregation according to sex is regarded as a *sine qua non*.

formal training or qualifications, many of the social workers were referred to as 'psychiatric social workers' by the superintendent and by the staff generally.

Almost 50 per cent of patients in our sample were in hospitals employing a social worker, though many of these patients lived in subsidiary units which were rarely visited by him/her. In hospitals employing no social worker the superintendent was asked whether he would prefer to have one, and the replies are set out in Table 7.8:

Table 7.8

DISTRIBUTION OF PATIENTS ACCORDING TO ATTITUDES OF
MEDICAL SUPERINTENDENTS TOWARDS AVAILABILITY OF
SOCIAL WORKERS (PERCENTAGES)

Superintendent's attitude towards employment of social worker	*Patients affected*
Approve, cannot fill post	7·8
Disapprove, local authority responsible	11·4
Disapprove, social work unnecessary	16·7
Disapprove (no comment)	14·4
Does not apply (social worker already employed)	49·7
TOTAL	100·0
No information	8
No. of patients	3,038

Under the 1959 Mental Health Act (section 8), Local Authorities are charged with the welfare of 'mentally disordered persons of any description' and it appeared to be generally recognized by medical superintendents even in those hospitals employing a social worker, that Mental Welfare Officers are legally responsible for the social work function relating to subnormal patients *in* hospital as well as those living in the community. However, as indicated by the replies set out in Table 7.8, only 11·4 per cent of sampled patients were in hospitals where no social worker was employed *because it was considered to be the function of the Local Authority*. In the majority of cases the superintendent disapproved of the idea generally, or considered their services to be unnecessary.

Superintendents were asked about their relationship – or that of the hospital staff generally – with the local authority social workers. About 15 per cent of patients were in hospitals where the superintendent said relationships were either poor, or insufficient, or both. Our own observations suggest that even in the remaining 85 per cent of cases where relationships were said to be satisfactory or good, this was largely a superficial assessment. In one hospital, for example, where no social workers were employed, the medical superintendent was glowing in his description of the local authority mental welfare workers who, he claimed, visited the hospital for two hours each day. The research team remained at the hospital for two weeks but did not see a mental welfare officer, although the office allocated to the research was said to be the one normally used by the welfare officer. At a nearby subsidiary unit the matron said that the original intention had been that the mental welfare officer should visit regularly and that there should be case conferences. Children under 16 were visited, 'but the others come about once every two years'. In three hospitals where the *superintendent* said relationships with the local authority mental welfare officers were good, the hospital social workers said they were unsatisfactory. We formed the impression, in informal discussions with social workers, that the local authority officers had sufficient work with those mentally disturbed and subnormal patients living in the community, and in attending outpatient clinics, so that for the most part they had little time available for hospital patients, particularly those who were subnormal as opposed to mentally ill.[1] Where their services were used, it was generally in order to contact a family at the request of a doctor or social worker at the hospital, or to supervise a patient who was living outside on licence. There was no indication that local authority social workers had personal contact with patients in hospital (with the exception of the children referred to above), though we are relying here upon the views of those working in the hospital and we did not check with the local authority workers. On no occasion did any of the research workers report meeting a mental welfare officer in the hospital, and it would seem that if any contact does take place it is mainly by telephone, or at outpatient clinics which are not held at the hospital.

Social workers were asked to describe the work of their department: three said they saw patients on admission (a further one saw them a month after); fifteen said they worked intensively with some patients, four worked intensively with some families, and four said they found jobs for patients. However, when we asked the fifteen for details of the type of work they did with patients, nine said it was mostly job finding for higher grade patients. Two arranged holidays for patients, and one said much of her time was taken up in writing to patients' relatives, and visiting patients who had to attend outside hospitals.

We then further analysed the six interviews with social workers who said that intensive work with patients and/or their families took

[1] In an article entitled 'An Integrated Mental-Health Service: Nottingham's Experience' (the *Lancet*, 24 November, 1956), MacMillan describes the responsibility of the Local Authority in respect of both mentally ill and subnormal patients. However, in his discussion of the social worker's place in the scheme, references are exclusively to their role in relation to mentally *ill* patients as opposed to the subnormal. See also Rehin and Martin: *Psychiatric Services in 1975*, PEP Planning, Vol. XXIX, No. 468, 4 February, 1963.

up most of their time, but where this did not include job finding. One, with social science qualifications, said she worked with all the patients and their families – she did not specify the precise nature of her duties, but said she was out of the hospital a great deal. She had no secretarial help, but could use the typing pool if necessary. Her only complaint was that the hospital had no hostel. If she had too much work, the local authority mental welfare officers 'took over' the cases.

Another social worker, with no training, had only been in the job for four months. She said she worked intensively with patients 'the families come under the local authority'. Asked for details of her work, she said she spent most of her time checking up on children who did not get visited, but she did not herself get in touch with the relatives, that being the work of the local authority: 'They admitted the patient, and they like to do all the case notes to follow up the patient. They are very touchy and we must not tread on their corns'. She did however, transport patients' relatives to and from the hospital, or take patients to visit them if they were infirm.

A third (a trained nurse and health visitor), spent much of her time 'keeping the contact going between patient and family'. She said she would do casework if she had more staff. She also found jobs for patients and made visits for the doctors engaged on clinical research.

One social worker (untrained) who said she thought casework and counselling were unnecessary, in fact spent many evenings at the hospital counselling and listening to the problems of the high-grade patients for whom she found jobs. Another took patients to visit relatives and *vice versa*, but most of her time was spent either job finding or on clerical work, the latter being largely letters to relatives, asking them to write or visit.

The last of the six who claimed to work with patients spent much of his time with them in his capacity as entertainments organizer, and he also acted as hospital 'postman'. All patients' mail at the hospital went through him, but for the past three years it had only been opened by him if it was for a compulsory patient or if the superintendent thought it should be: 'If a patient receives money, I can then send a receipt. I record mail as it arrives and take it round. The charge nurse or sister generally hand money to me, the female side is more strict and I generally get about 90 per cent of the money and pay it into their savings'. The same social worker ran a library for the patients and there was a staff library 'available whenever I'm around'. The secretarial work was done by clerks on the administrative staff.

From this short resume of activities, it is apparent that whilst the work being done by all these people is undoubtedly valuable and necessary (with the possible exception of the 'postman/censor'), for the most part it is relatively peripheral to social work and much of it might be more legitimately carried out by the Ministry of Labour's

Disablement Resettlement Officer, if such officers could be suitably trained.[1]

All but two of the social workers felt they had sufficient opportunity to discuss cases with the medical and nursing staff, but seven complained of unsatisfactory relationships with other staff in the hospital, and three of unsatisfactory relationships with the local authority.

Although only one complained of lack of accommodation, a number had no room specifically allocated to them (e.g. they had a desk in the general office) and where there were two social workers, they almost always shared a room. One worker complained that she had no outside telephone and another complained of insufficient payment for the use of a car and expenses.

Since some of the social workers claimed to have contact with the families and to try to persuade them to visit, it might be thought that there would be a connection between the amount of visiting and the presence of a social worker in the hospital.[2] There is clearly no indication that this is the case, as is set out in Tables 7.9 (a) and (b).

Whether it is desirable, given an ideal situation, for the local authority mental welfare officers to include the patients of subnormality hospitals in their caseload, or whether such hospitals should employ their own social workers falls outside the scope of this report.[3] Nevertheless two facts clearly emerge from this discussion: firstly local authority social workers already have large caseloads comprising patients living in the community.[4] Secondly most of the subnormality hospitals are situated in very isolated surroundings so that local authority social workers find it extremely difficult to visit them sufficiently often to establish and maintain contact with patients. At present lip-service is paid to the role of the local authority social worker, and in those hospitals which employ their own, the greater part of their time is taken up in finding jobs for high-grade patients. The fact that so few social workers in subnormality hospitals are professionally trained is doubtless one factor in the very poor

---

[1] In at least one hospital known to the research the social worker does collaborate closely with the Disablement Resettlement Officer.

[2] Further discussion of visits will appear in Chapter 8.

[3] For a discussion of these matters, and for the need for social caseworkers see, for example, Grad, J. C.: 'Social Work with the Families of the Mentally Subnormal', paper read before the Health Congress of the Royal Society of Health, 1964, also Adams, M.: *The Mentally Subnormal: The Social Casework Approach*, Heinemann (1960), also Savoca, R.: 'Family Counselling for the Retarded' in *In Service Casework Training*, Nicholds, Columbia University Press, 1966.

[4] For a disturbing account of the work of Mental Welfare Officers with subnormal patients in the London area, see PEP report, *Mental Subnormality in London; a Survey of Community Care*. Lack of flexibility, the use of untrained workers, low morale, constant staff changes and infrequent visiting, all contribute to provide a very inadequate service to meet existing needs outside the hospital. Under present conditions to expect these workers to undertake the social work of the subnormality hospitals in addition, would be unrealistic, even if desirable.

Table 7.9

PATIENTS' CONTACT WITH RELATIVES WITH REFERENCE TO
PRESENCE OR ABSENCE OF SOCIAL WORKER (PERCENTAGES)

A

Time of relatives' last visit	*Patients*		
	Hosp. with social worker	*Hosp. with no social worker*	*Total*
Within past four weeks	34·1	41·7	38·4
Between 1 and 12 months ago	20·8	19·6	20·1
Not visited in past year	45·1	38·7	41·5
TOTAL	100·0	100·0	100·0
No information	36	22	58
No. of patients	1,315	1,723	3,038

B

Time of patient's last visit home	*Patients*		
	Hosp. with social worker	*Hosp. with no social worker*	*Total*
Within past four weeks	7·5	10·3	9·1
Between 1 and 3 months ago	6·8	5·6	6·1
Between 3 and 6 months ago	3·2	4·3	3·9
Between 6 and 12 months ago	3·3	3·1	3·2
Over one year ago	2·5	1·4	1·8
Never goes home	74·7	75·3	75·9
TOTAL	100·0	100·0	100·0
No information	35	21	56
No. of patients	1,315	1,723	3,038

status position in which they find themselves: most of them are
content to remain job finders: one expressed very great surprise
when she visited a hospital employing a social worker (not a subnormality hospital) and found that the social work department did a
wide variety of other work, including counselling, giving advice on
sources of practical help, and social casework with patients.

Experimental treatment and training

In a few hospitals we found that small specialist treatment and/or training departments had been established, often involving research by medical or psychological staff. Thus, one hospital set up an experimental workshop in order to see how far low grade patients could be trained to do industrial work. The unit was run by two members of the nursing staff and both male and female patients worked there. Although several of the doctors were said to evince an interest because of the experimental nature of the department, and male nurses co-operated with the unit, this was not the case amongst female nurses. The psychologists were also involved in collecting data from this department, but again they experienced more difficulty in obtaining information from female nursing staff.

In another hospital a charge nurse organized a unit specially for 14 disturbed patients who were difficult to handle on the ward: 'We cannot leave them alone, or lock them up, so we have to try and find something beyond enemas and four square meals a day'. This same charge nurse was largely responsible for setting up a special play group 'to keep low-grades out of trouble'. They were given suitable and varied games and occupations, and a considerable amount of individual attention.

Another hospital provided special 'recreational therapy'. The person in charge had been there eight years and for the first twelve months struggled against heavy opposition. The nursing staff were slow to co-operate, they thought the games were rather childish. Almost 1,500 patients were now involved in this training, divided into seven groups, and they included spastics, blind patients, heart cases and asthmatics. Activities ranged from complicated folk and country dancing, to simple clapping and stamping in rhythm. One matter to which the therapist drew our attention was that patients were *never* incontinent in the hall, and they were said to improve in this respect and to be less restless on the wards. She also claimed that the drug bill had gone down.

Four hospitals had industrial workshops where a certain number of patients worked in conditions comparable with outside light industry.[1]

Other hospitals provided units for special groups such as psychopaths, epileptics, spastics, autistic and psychotic children. One had a special baby unit with housemothers in charge; here an attempt was made to create a really home-like situation. The medical superintendent of another hospital was anxious to try and have mixed wards under a principal nursing officer, but there had been objections from the nurses' union on the male side. Meanwhile it was being tried experimentally on some wards.

---

[1] See previous reference on p. 148 *supra*.

Summary

In this chapter we have attempted to describe the wide variety of non-medical treatment and training facilities which are available in our subnormality hospitals. Two themes have run through our discussion – firstly the very small number of patients who receive any benefit from the departments, and secondly the dissatisfaction and frustration experienced by most of the staff working in them, this last factor being closely associated with poor communication between specialist staff and members of the medical and nursing profession; also the seeming complacency and pessimism of senior staff in terms of the interpretation of their responsibilities *vis-à-vis* the condition and prospects of patients.

Chapter 8

LIFE AND RELATIONSHIPS
IN HOSPITAL

WE have, in the preceding chapters, described the hospitals and those who live and work in them; we have also outlined the services available for the treatment and training of patients. In this chapter we shall concentrate our attention on the experience of hospitalization; we shall start by a discussion of the ways in which patients are admitted, and then give an account of the freedoms they experience and the constraints to which they are subject in the course of their daily lives.

Admission procedures

Much has been written about the mortification or 'rôle stripping' process of patients entering institutions,[1] but it is questionable whether the situation is entirely comparable for the mentally subnormal. We noted earlier[2] that a high proportion of patients come into hospital in late childhood or early adulthood and we believe that at home they have played essentially 'dependency' roles. The process of role-stripping may be attenuated for the simple reason that they have been almost entirely precluded from playing significantly autonomous roles in the community, and their incapacity to do so has often been an important factor in the recognition of the need for hospitalization. This is particularly the case when hospitalization arises not as the result of any immediate deterioration in the patients' condition, but, as is more likely to be the case, as a result of environmental changes such as the illness or death of a parent, housing problems, or even the strain and emotional stress engendered in the family as a result of caring for a subnormal person.

It may be that some subnormal patients, particularly those in working-class families, are accepted without discrimination, and when they are located by doctors, social workers or others and sent to hospital, they then tend to be explicitly defined by the community as 'mental' or as beyond recovery. The extent to which their self-image is affected by such 'labelling' deserves further consideration. Moreover it could be argued that they lose the opportunity for potentially loving treatment by parents, and with it the opportunity

[1] See for example, Goffman, E.: *op. cit.*
[2] See Chapter 4, p. 62.

to display selfish and assertive emotions. This, when denied in the hospital context, may well represent a form of emotional deprivation and 'role-stripping'. However, it cannot always be assumed that parents fully appreciate the implications of their children's retardation and treat them correspondingly with affectionate indulgence, particularly if they themselves are of limited intelligence.

We suggest therefore that the translation from familial to institutional status may be even more meaningful (and possibly more traumatic) for the relatives than for the patient. Undoubtedly patients are unsettled by a change in the environment,[1] but this may not necessarily, we think, arise as a result of any role change, either real or perceived. If this is correct the admission procedures adopted, and the attitude of staff towards relatives will be of the utmost importance and one which the research findings suggest is certainly overlooked.

The data used in this section were obtained solely from interviews with medical superintendents, matrons and chief male nurses. We were not able to observe patients being admitted, partly because this is not a frequent occurrence and partly because we believe that the presence of a research worker would undoubtedly have affected the situation and rendered it atypical.

Most patients entering the larger hospitals will have been seen by the medical superintendent at an out-patient clinic before admission; an important exception may be cases sent direct from the Courts. In one or two instances the diagnostic clinic takes place at the hospital itself, a situation which enables relatives of prospective patients to look round the wards of the hospital at the same time, but most clinics are held elsewhere and in addition to the superintendent or consultant from the subnormality hospital, staff from other hospitals and from the local health authority may share the facilities.

In the smaller hospitals there may be no out-patient clinic; the superintendent of a 450 bedded hospital said that if anyone needed to be seen, he visited them at home. The Regional Hospital Board kept a priority list and allocated patients to the appropriate hospital; he had no part in the decision.

We asked superintendents whether relatives were invited to visit the hospital before the patient was admitted and if so how this was done; the replies are set out in Table 8.1.

In practice extremely few relatives came; superintendents were vague about the precise number, but only one suggested that it exceeded five or ten families a year. Generally speaking visits by relatives before admission were not considered important, though few medical superintendents were as outspoken in their disapproval of them as the one who commented: 'It's very rare that they come.

[1] Even within the hospital this can be upsetting and nurses often told us of the distress caused by moving a patient who had been a long time on one ward, to another.

Table 8.1
METHOD OF INVITING RELATIVES TO VISIT
BEFORE PATIENT'S ADMISSION (PERCENTAGES)

Method used	*Patients**
By personal contact or letter	38·2
Through other agency (GP, social worker, etc.)	30·1
Cyclostyled letter or form	17·7
Not invited	22·3
No direct admissions	3·0
No information	23
No. of patients	3,038

* Totals exceed 100 per cent since some may be invited both by the hospital and by another agency.

We laugh when they do; we have so many clamouring to get in here – who are they to be particular?' Another superintendent said he did not invite relatives as this might increase the numbers seeking admission.

The possible advantages for the *hospital* (in terms of information and parental co-operation) were apparently unrecognized, a situation which was repeated by the tendency to ignore relatives even at the time of the patient's actual admission.

If hospital staff were well informed about the patient's background, medical history and home circumstances at the time of admission, the lack of contact with relatives might be understandable – at least from the hospital's point of view. But this was not in fact the case: only thirteen medical superintendents said that patients' notes were adequate at the time of admission, a further ten per cent were very dissatisfied with the information provided and the remainder said the situation varied, depending upon the doctor and the local authority concerned. Despite this only approximately ten per cent of patients' relatives were seen by a doctor or senior nurse *at the time of admission*, and in the majority of such cases, this was at the instigation of another, outside agency. Many matrons and chief male nurses expressed quite hostile attitudes towards relatives: in at least four hospitals they were completely excluded at the time of the patient's admission other than in the most exceptional circumstances (e.g. if the patient was admitted to a sick ward). Many other hospitals discouraged relatives from visiting for the first few weeks on the grounds that this was too upsetting for the patient.

Methods of assessment on admission to hospital were not universal. Table 8.2 sets out the procedures as indicated by superintendents, as well as by matrons and chief male nurses:

Table 8.2

ADMISSION PROCEDURES (PERCENTAGES)

Procedure adopted	Patients affected	
	According to Superintendents	According to Matrons/CMNs
Placed in admission ward	17·0	24·9
Routine medical examination	91·0	48·2
Routine psychological assessment	65·8	not asked
Case conference	36·9	not asked
Programme of treatment planned	61·4	not asked
Relatives interviewed	9·5	11·6
No special procedures	8·8	23·2
Settling down period in which relatives are excluded	not asked	20·9
Clothes sent home	not asked	43·7
No. of patients	3,038	3,038

Not all questions asked of these two groups were strictly comparable, but since in many cases they were, we have shown both sets of figures side by side. The discrepancy in the figure for those being medically examined might be explained by the fact that whereas superintendents were asked how many patients were medically examined, it was thought that only the matrons or chief male nurses would know whether patients were automatically put to bed on admission (whether handicapped or not) in order to await such examination. Thus the figure of 48 per cent represents only this latter group and undoubtedly almost all patients were in fact medically examined. We do not have information about the degree of thoroughness employed, for example whether dental or ophthalmic examinations were included under the heading 'medical'.

The fact that clothes were sent home in almost 44 per cent of cases may seem surprising in view of the current policy to encourage patients to wear their own clothes and for hospital clothing to be issued on an individual basis.[1] The chief explanations for the practice were: 'because the hospital doesn't want the responsibility' or 'because of laundry difficulties'. In one hospital the matron said clothes were sent home 'in case patients do not stay – this has led to complaints by relatives'. However, although these views predominated, there were a few hospitals where attitudes were quite different. Thus one matron of a very large hospital commented:

It depends entirely on the patient. If they're very distressed we don't do anything about bathing, etc., we welcome them and try to introduce them to someone of their own age. Then, when they've

[1] For further discussion of this see Chapter 10.

settled they have a bath and medical examination. Their mental age is assessed when the patient is reasonably settled in the hospital. We like them to retain their own clothes – we have a good marking system and very few articles get lost.

Similar views were expressed by the chief male nurse in the same hospital. In another medium sized hospital the matron encouraged parents to bring the children's own toys, discussed the child's diet with them, and generally went out of her way to make the admission procedure as gentle as possible.

But such attitudes appeared to be quite exceptional. Furthermore it was our impression that this is an area of activity about which the medical superintendent and other medical staff have no real information. We think it unlikely that actual admission procedures are checked or investigated by medical staff. It could be argued that a similar situation exists in general hospitals where medical staff would not normally be expected to be involved in the social aspects of admission procedures, but we feel that the circumstances surrounding admission to mental subnormality hospitals are somewhat different, and since admissions do not occur frequently, it might be thought that doctors and social workers should make a point of seeing relatives and ensuring that the patient is received with kindness. To some extent differences in procedure and in attitude reflect differences in the size of the unit. The most rigid admission procedures were found in the larger hospitals, and the greatest flexibility in those with 300–999 beds. The larger hospitals were more likely to have a special admissions ward, though hospitals with between 1,000–1,799 beds were even more likely to have one than the very largest group. The relationship between patients being put to bed automatically and size of unit was also clear; it affected 83 per cent of sampled patients in the largest hospitals and dropped to about 15 per cent as the unit size declined. However regulations about a settling down period[1] did not appear to be affected by size (between a quarter and a fifth of sampled patients were affected by this) though in units of less than 100 beds the practice was not used at all, possibly because these were not new admissions but transfers from the main unit.

The sending home of patients' clothes tended to be more common in the smaller units (under 1,000 beds) and although we have little evidence for this, we believe it to relate to the poorer laundry facilities which often existed in such hospitals. Staff were concerned about complaints from relatives regarding the way 'private' clothes were laundered and cared for, and rather than risk such complaints, they preferred patients to wear hospital clothing except for 'best' (e.g. visits, socials and outings, etc.). To what extent they were rationaliz-

---

[1] This term usually meant that relatives were discouraged from visiting until the patient was considered to have 'settled down'. The period varied widely, the minimum usually being a week.

ing or legitimizing the widespread use of hospital clothing is, of course, debatable.

Life on the ward

How did patients spend their time on the ward when not occupied elsewhere? Without any shadow of doubt, and with the exception of the exclusively high grade wards and hostel patients, the great majority spent their day sitting, interspersed with eating. Only in very few wards (fewer than 12 out of 761 visited)[1] did we find nurses helping patients with individual or group *leisure* activities; nurses were usually cleaning either the wards or the patients, helping to prepare meals, cutting and washing hair, dressing or undressing patients and feeding them. When they were not so occupied nurses tended to sit or stand around talking to each other rather than to the patients. On one or two occasions this was queried by the research worker with the sister or charge nurse. They felt that there was little they could do to change the situation, staff are hard to get and they feared that any exertion of discipline would result in resignations, and incur the displeasure of the administrative nursing staff.

Research workers made a note of the time each ward was observed and what was happening at that time. The result makes depressing reading: 'wandering around'; 'listening to radio'; 'sitting'; 'rocking and making noises'; 'waiting for a meal'; 'eating'. In one ward of 65 patients visited at 12.30 p.m. most of the patients were wandering around in the sanitary annexe waiting for dinner. A single nurse was on duty who commented: 'They can't be put in the dining room[2] or they would eat the bread'. In another hospital a student nurse was observed throwing crusts of bread at patients at tea time. Whilst the research worker was interviewing the chief male nurse in one large hospital a patient threw himself from the window of a ward and broke his leg. We were told that this was a locked ward mainly for psychotic patients, but that the charge nurse had 'little inclination, time, or facilities to act in any but a custodial role'. When this ward was later visited (at 11 a.m.), it was found to have only one nurse on duty for 41 very disturbed patients, a few of whom were doing simple assembly work but the majority were 'wandering about aimlessly'. Countless examples of inactivity could be given, but they would merely sound repetitive.

On approximately six wards a few patients were engaged on some form of occupational therapy, and on a number of wards odd patients were attempting to knit, sew or do jig-saws on their own. A few were reading comics or looking at picture books, but in every case they constituted a minority of patients on the ward, and when questioned

[1] It is difficult to be entirely accurate since it is possible that in some wards we missed seeing some activity at the time of our visits.
[2] Also used as a day room.

about their activity they usually evinced no real interest in what they were doing. On a children's ward, in the middle of the afternoon we found fifty older children wandering round aimlessly or sitting making noises, despite the fact that there were six staff actually on duty on the ward. There were no toys, books, games, pictures or ornaments in evidence and the staff stood around talking to each other.

On the men's wards the position was in some ways even more depressing since men do not normally have sedentary hobbies such as sewing or knitting. A few read comics, but if they were doing anything at all it was generally playing billiards or watching television.

We were not normally in a position to spend much time with patients on the wards, and therefore were not able to observe their interaction with each other for long periods. Sometimes the events we witnessed seemed significant, for example the following report by a research worker:

> The ward housed 61 severely subnormal males and all but 15 of them were out of the ward at industrial training. The visit took place at 2.30 p.m. and there were four staff actually on duty on the ward for the 15 patients. Rain was coming in through the window on to the patients who were sitting individually or in groups of two or three in armchairs arranged in rows. A doctor visited the ward and occupied the charge nurse thus leaving three nurses available for the patients. The door of the day room was open and led to a central corridor where all three nurses were sorting linen. For a period of 15 minutes no staff came into the room or checked on the patients. The patients communicated by gross gestures or by touching each other, rather than by speech. For several minutes two patients stood holding hands, looking away one from the other and making noises. Occasionally patients shouted to each other, repeating the same sounds over and over again. Some talked incoherently to themselves or rocked abstractedly backwards and forwards. A patient took a handkerchief out of his pocket, paused, threw it on the floor in front of another patient who looked at it, then picked it up, gave it back to the first patient who blew his nose on it and put it back in his pocket, all without expression. Patients repeated the same gestures over and over again, very slowly, so that to the untrained observer it seemed as if nothing was meaningful or that their minds were quite vacant.

Only on very few wards was the patient's physical appearance neglected, although the need for variation to reflect individuality was not always appreciated. For the most part the women sat on the wards in clean pinafores, their hair cut short (and regularly fine combed), and if the men appeared less well turned out, it may simply have been that they had no overalls to hide the ill-fitting clothes underneath, nor did the badly-laundered thick hospital shirts with open collars and braces, lend themselves to an air of neatness.

Quite apart from the practical problems involved in the sheer day to day handling of so many patients, we feel that one important reason for lack of staff/patient involvement lies in the attitude of medical and administrative nursing staff. As we suggested earlier, nurses generally suffer from low morale, due to such factors as isolation, lack of involvement in decision making, poor communication, and the doctors' lack of interest in the nurses' work.[1] Whilst administrative nursing staff recognize (sometimes only reluctantly), that traditional nursing skills are not required to any great extent in subnormality hospitals, they have not as yet encouraged more junior nurses to develop and substitute other skills. Thus the traditional emphasis on cleanliness, tidiness, orderly behaviour, etc. predominate and since little more is expected of nurses, little more is given.

One way of encouraging nurses to take an interest in patients' activities (as opposed to their physical care) might be to encourage them to know more about the patients on their ward, though it is unlikely that this could be made feasible with present organizational forms. At present by no means all nursing staff have access to patients' case notes as is indicated in Table 8.3 :

Table 8.3

ACCESSIBILITY OF PATIENTS' RECORDS (PERCENTAGES)

Availability	*Patients affected*
Case and personal records available to all staff	26·4
Case and personal records available to trained nurses only	6·0
Case notes only available to all staff	27·7
Case notes only available to trained nurses only	16·3
Only selected notes kept on ward (at doctor's discretion)	7·4
No case notes kept on ward (i.e., in medical records office)	7·4
No ward office, but notes easily accessible	2·9
No ward office, and notes not easily accessible	5·9
TOTAL	100·0
No information	40
No. of patients	3,038

The main reason given by senior nursing staff for withholding information from more junior staff was the question of confidentiality. In two subsidiary units of one hospital even the matron did not have access to all the notes, these being kept at the main hospital.

Whilst not all trained nurses had *full* information about patients,

[1] See Chapter 6, especially p. 127 ff.

most had access to case notes; on the other hand for approximately one-third of the population studied, unqualified nurses had no access to any part of the patient's record. However, as many matrons and chief male nurses pointed out, even when allowed to do so, not many nurses availed themselves of the opportunity to read them.

Patients' access to medical superintendent

We have already pointed out[1] that infrequent visits by medical superintendents to subsidiary units often resulted in their having little or no personal contact with the patients. Even in the main units of the various hospitals the extent to which patients had access to the medical superintendent varied considerably, but in general we think superintendents were under the impression that they were more accessible to patients than was actually the case. Most superintendents claimed that patients could write a letter asking to see him, and this he then arranged, or more usually, he arranged for them to be seen by the doctor actually responsible for treating them. One superintendent who always referred any special requests to the responsible medical officer, suggested that the fact that doctors were ignored by patients when they did ward rounds indicated that they were satisfied with the amount of personal contact they had: 'If patients do not see the doctor often enough, they crowd round him when he visits the ward, here we are just ignored'. Approximately 73 per cent of sampled patients were in hospitals where formal application had to be made, and in view of the difficulty experienced by many patients in communicating verbally, let alone in writing, this requirement appears somewhat unrealistic, particularly since in most cases it was necessary for the nursing staff to help with the letter. Once this becomes the practice, a form of censorship is implicitly built into the situation, and patients are often asked by senior ward staff why they want to see the superintendent and then gently talked out of it. Again this procedure exemplifies the nurses' need to control patients, and suggests that staff may conceive of them as acting like misguided children.[2]

Just over one-fifth of patients were said to have frequent and easy access to the superintendent, but we think that this was an unrealistically high figure, and so far as we could tell it was a 'privilege' reserved for those higher grade patients who had jobs in and around the administrative offices, or those on daily licence who were usually better able to communicate both verbally and in writing.

[1] See Chapter 6, p. 120 ff.
[2] The superintendent is very much the 'father' in this situation. Patients who misbehave are threatened in much the same way as in families where mothers control their children by threatening to 'tell Daddy'. Similarly, fathers must be protected from too many demands, 'don't bother Daddy now, he's busy' (tired), etc.

Social control

The efficiency of any large scale bureaucracy is dependent upon the smooth running and orderly activity of all its departments. Little tolerance can be extended to behaviour which is likely to be disruptive to the life of the ward and even the mildest of disturbed behaviour must be 'treated' before it spreads to other members of the community; usually this is achieved by the use of sedatives.

Although medical superintendents generally disliked the idea that punishment might be regarded as a form of 'treatment', there was no doubt that sanctions played an important part in maintaining a quiet and orderly regime. Sometimes the medical superintendents themselves believed in punishment, but more often they said they allowed punishments to be carried out because the nursing staff demanded it. One said he did not think it had any therapeutic value, all it did was 'protect patients and staff'. In this particular hospital three methods of control were used, one of them, stopping the patients' money, was used 'because the staff think I ought to do *something*. I don't think it makes much difference. When I'm driven to stop it I do, but under duress'. Another superintendent expressed much the same view in different terms; asked if he thought sanctions or punishments had a therapeutic value, he replied:

I'm trying to evade it – I want to say 'no', but when you work with matrons and chief male nurses they say 'yes'. Another factor that influences one is the patients themselves; *they* want those who do wrong to be punished. One feels a certain amount of discipline has to be imposed, it's like dealing with a lot of children. I'm anti the word 'punishment'; I don't like to hear doctors or nurses using it, but maybe I'm not facing up to things. It *does* work, but whether because it's the right thing to do, well . . .

In the antiquated, overcrowded, poorly staffed conditions that we have described on so many wards, nurses feel the need to give priority to the maintenance of order, or the situation might easily deteriorate to one of generalized disorder.[1] The question is simply whether punishments are the best way of achieving order. The 'misbehaviour' of a single patient means that probably all the nurses available on the ward must stop attending to their other duties in order to cope with the immediate crisis. Subnormal patients tend to be great imitators of each other's behaviour; a low grade patient was burned to death during the period of our visit to one hospital and at the inquest it was assumed that someone had thrown a lighted cigarette out of a window. On the same evening a female patient set light to some curtains in one of the day rooms and there was considerable anxiety amongst the nursing staff who felt the problem remained largely unresolved.

[1] This feeling may well reflect an emphasis in the training of nurses.

They believed that the patient who caused the first fire still had matches in her possession.

Signs of 'bad' behaviour are met with immediate action – there is not time to 'talk about it' (though one superintendent maintained that he dealt with all misdemeanours in this way), or to try and find out what lay behind the patient's disturbance. The custodial function of the nursing staff is reinforced and the medical superintendent is a more or less willing conspirator, depending upon his personal views.

In one hospital visited the medical superintendent said that if patients absconded he made them contribute from their pocket money or savings towards the cost of bringing them back. The Hospital Management Committee objected strongly to this method but he had the support of the administrative nursing staff and so continued to use it, even extending its use to making them contribute towards the cost of repairing broken windows. This same superintendent commented that one method of punishment that he used was to break off a good relationship with a patient: 'I become very unpleasant; this is what the patient dislikes most'.

The three types of punishment mentioned most frequently were stopping parole, stopping entertainments or similar privileges, and reducing pocket money. All these methods were used very extensively. Less frequent, but nevertheless used a great deal, were sending patients to bed early, and sending them to a locked or refractory ward. Some superintendents gave 'pep talks' but this applied mainly to higher grade patients and in particular to those in hostels.[1]

Many superintendents mentioned drug therapy: 'There's no seclusion, if they are violent we use drug therapy'. It is interesting to note this widespread use of drugs as an alternative to sanctions (often at the instigation of the nursing staff who 'recommend' to the doctor that a patient be sedated), since it suggests that the use of tranquillizers and similar drugs may be more custodial than therapeutic; the idea is to quieten the patient and stop 'bad' and disruptive behaviour, not to cure him, nor to find out why he behaves in this way.

The fact that patients were in some cases sent to refractory or locked wards as a form of punishment may be of particular importance. At the time of our visit, 2·2 per cent of the sampled patients were in refractory wards, of whom just over two-thirds were in locked wards.[2] In addition to those wards specifically labelled 'refractory' a minority of others were also kept locked at all times, and some were partially locked, that is they were locked at certain times of the day, or alternatively certain parts of the ward (usually the dormitory) remained locked. Fourteen per cent of our sample were in wards locked at all times and 2 per cent in partially locked wards; many children's wards were locked either at the main entrance

[1] This latter group were also threatened with being returned to the main hospital.

[2] Chapter 5, Table 5.3, p. 82.

or at the gate of the play space surrounding the ward. We were told of a number of instances where children had, in the past, run off and been drowned in a nearby lake or river, or had been killed on the road. Nurses on wards with active children felt safer where there were locks to prevent accidents of this kind.

The locking of wards may still be arguable, though it should be pointed out that few hospitals practise this more than minimally. There was one extreme exception however, where the proportion of patients in locked wards was as high as 41·3 per cent, almost all of them being in the main unit where the proportion rose to 56·1 per cent. In many cases in this hospital both adults and children were netted into their cots. In another hospital handcuffs were issued to nurses in order to take patients from a locked ward to another department, but these were said to be used only very occasionally and we saw no evidence of their use.

Parole

In the preceding section we pointed out that one of the most frequently mentioned methods of social control was that of stopping parole. This term refers to the degree of freedom extended to *all* patients to leave the hospital grounds unaccompanied by staff, and not simply to those who are compulsorily detained. There has recently been a considerable amount of criticism of the use of the word 'parole' in subnormality hospitals, and we were often told by nursing staff that they were discouraged from using it (it was never clearly specified from where the objection came). However it was generally felt that no equivalent term could be found to replace it, though some staff agreed that it carried an unpleasant echo from prison procedures. Parole differs from 'leave' or 'licence' in that it extends only to short outings to nearby towns or villages and does not normally include being away overnight.

From Table 8.4 it can be seen that there is almost no difference in the parole status of male and female patients.

It might, perhaps, be thought surprising that as many as 42 per cent of sampled patients were confined to the ward in which they lived, a figure which far exceeds the proportion limited in mobility by physical handicap. The information given to us does not appear to be unreliable[1] and it seems likely that it never occurred to anyone to get these patients out, other than in groups supervised by a nurse.

More of those with a relatively high IQ were allowed out, though this may not be a reliable observation in view of the paucity of the

[1] See Chapter 4, p. 69. We think it unlikely that the figure is unreliable since it approximates so closely the information on patients' occupation (see later in this chapter), which shows 48 per cent of patients with no occupation or working on their own ward. We feel it may be justifiable to assume that most of the patients in these two groups are confined to the ward.

o

Table 8.4
PAROLE STATUS BY SEX (PERCENTAGES)

Parole status	Male	Female	Total
Confined to ward	41·7	42·2	42·0
Allowed to walk in hospital but not grounds	6·6	9·0	7·6
Allowed to walk in hospital and grounds	33·1	30·4	31·9
Allowed to go outside hospital (accompanied)	0·6	0·8	0·7
Allowed to go outside hospital (unaccompanied)	18·0	17·6	17·8
TOTAL	100·0	100·0	100·0
No information	5	13	18
No. of patients	1,664	1,374	3,038

data on intelligence. Amongst *adults* known to have IQs of 50 or more, 20 per cent were confined to their own ward, and 42·5 were allowed outside the hospital on their own or with other patients. Comparable figures for those known to have IQs of less than 50 are 37 per cent confined to ward and 18 per cent allowed outside the hospital alone, or accompanied by other patients.

In view of the rigid regulations about segregation based primarily on fears of pregnancy,[1] and to which reference has been made at various points in the report, we thought it likely that similar attitudes might affect the degree to which patients were allowed parole. Certainly in what was probably the most rigidly segregated hospital we visited, only a very small proportion of patients were allowed parole (approximately 9 per cent of the total adult population). However this was an exceptional case, and it is in fact difficult to determine the extent to which attitudes regarding patients' sexual behaviour affected the granting of parole. One factor which complicated the issue was the fact that we were unable to determine where the *real* decision was made – whether by medical or nursing staff; although *officially* a medical decision, we feel it may well have been a question of rubber stamping a nursing decision, as was so often the case with regard to patients' occupation.

In hospitals where the superintendent considered that sexual relations constituted a problem for patients on parole, but not if they remained in the hospital, 11 per cent were allowed out unaccompanied, as compared with 18 per cent where the superintendent considered this not to be a problem at all. However 24 per cent of patients went out unaccompanied in hospitals where the superinten-

[1] Although staff usually referred to sexual behaviour generally in discussion, it appeared that their fears related specifically to pregnancy.

dent considered patients to be generally promiscuous whether on parole or not, so that it seems likely that attitudes to sexual behaviour are no more than a minor determinant in deciding upon parole status.

The whole question of granting parole may rest upon the general philosophy of individual superintendents; compare, for example, the view expressed by one superintendent: 'There are no sexual problems, they are delightfully promiscuous', with another who commented: 'Unofficially we can't stop them having girl friends, but we don't encourage it since it would lead to a new generation of subnormals'. In this latter case both the superintendent and the hostel warden said that they would condone homosexuality rather than have patients molesting girls.

The views of matrons and chief male nurses were often far more punitive in such matters than were those of superintendents. One chief male nurse told the research worker that 'slackness of staff shows up immediately in illegitimate births' (among patients) and the matron of a small children's unit commented that they were 'highly sexed and do have problems'.[1]

Patients at work

It might be thought that all adult patients able to be active would be at work away from the ward during the day, but our evidence would suggest that this is not the case. As is shown in Table 8.5 below approximately 48 per cent of adult patients had no occupation or worked only on the ward; since over 83 per cent of the total sample were fully ambulant it is likely that a considerably higher proportion of patients could have been occupied elsewhere than on their own wards. Occupational therapists often expressed the view that more patients would benefit by attending the department if it could be arranged, and certainly many of the patients to whom we spoke on the ward would seem to be suitable for occupation of some kind.

Cross[2] in his survey of hospitals in the Birmingham region found that 6·9 per cent of males and 8·2 per cent of females worked on daily

[1] Views on this matter vary; Saenger, G.: *The Adjustment of Severely Retarded Adults in the Community*. Albany: New York State Interdepartmental Health Resources Board (1957) shows that the great fears of sex activity on the part of the mentally retarded have little basis in fact. Walker, N., and McCabe, S. ('Hospital Orders' in *The Mentally Abnormal Offender*. A Ciba Foundation Symposium, ed. de Rueck and Porter, Churchill, 1968, pp. 219–34) reporting on a sample of 330 subnormal male offenders dealt with by Hospital Orders in England and Wales from 1963–4 found that whilst most were convicted of aquisitive offences, approx. 28 per cent were convicted of sexual offences (statistic derived from Table 1), and this group accounted for two-thirds of all the sex offences in the total sample (969) which included schizophrenics, and those suffering from personality disorders and depressive illnesses. The authors point out, however, that very few of the sex offences committed by subnormal persons were against small children.

[2] *op. cit.*

Table 8.5

OCCUPATION OF ADULT PATIENTS BY IQ (PERCENTAGES)

Occupation of adult patients during week of survey	IQ					Total
	Untestable	Under 50	50–69	70 and over	Not tested or no information	
None	58·6	24·0	9·2	11·2	35·7	31·4
Domestic work or OT on ward*	12·8	18·4	19·6	14·7	15·9	16·6
Utility or domestic work in hospital or grounds	7·6	27·6	34·5	35·3	22·4	23·6
Occupational therapy†	12·3	14·7	11·2	11·2	11·0	12·5
Industrial training	4·1	9·8	12·9	14·7	9·8	9·4
Working outside hospital (daily licence)	0·6	2·6	11·2	12·9	2·7	3·9
Attending school (over 16)	3·9	3·0	1·4	—	2·5	2·7
TOTAL	100·0	100·0	100·0	100·0	100·0	100·0
No information	1	2	—	1	4	8
No. of patients	487	882	357	117	833	2,676

* In some cases patients spent half the day doing domestic work on their own wards and the other half in the OT department. In these cases the morning occupation was recorded if there was no time differential.
† Although separate figures for OT and IT are given here, the distinction is not always so clear as was discussed in Chapter 7 regarding specialist departments.

licence compared with our figure of 3·9 for both sexes. Our findings do, however, approximate closely those of O'Connor and Tizard[1] in their London survey where they gave a figure of just over 4 per cent in daily domestic service.[2]

The proportion of patients on daily licence varied considerably from hospital to hospital, depending to some extent upon the degree of its physical isolation. Patients who went out to work were more often men than women and most frequently lived in the ancillary units; these were often situated nearer centres of population and generally speaking housed the less severely physically disabled. Most of the men worked on farms and most of the women were in domestic service; very few were employed in factories, a finding which is also confirmed by O'Connor and Tizard.

Whilst most of those who worked on their own ward had an IQ of less than 50, it would be a mistake to assume that all the others who worked there but for whom test results were not available *necessarily* had a similarly low IQ. This may be important since information obtained informally from nurses, as well as our own observations, suggest that in many cases it would be more accurate to describe these patients as unemployed, since they did little or no real work. Amongst these working around the hospital generally, or in the grounds, the higher grade female patients often worked (and sometimes lived) on children's wards where they cleaned and helped to look after the children. O'Connor and Tizard[3] hypothesize that in hospitals where there are a high proportion of low grade patients, few of the high grade patients are sent out on licence and they suggest that one reason for this may be that they are needed to help run the institution. We have no precise information on this point since we are dissatisfied with the data regarding classification based on IQ, but certainly our observations would appear to support the hypothesis. One Medical Superintendent in discussing allocation to jobs said: 'They have depended on older patients looking after younger ones. They are needed there to keep the hospital going, or so they say'. When questioned about the meaning of 'they', the reply was ambiguous, and although in this hospital the responsible Medical Officer was said to make the decision, the implication appeared to be that nursing staff put pressure upon medical staff to provide help with the care of children. A great many of the female patients who worked round the hospital were employed either in the kitchen or the laundry; relatively few were in the sewing room. So far

[1] *op. cit.*

[2] The percentage of the total hospital population on daily licence in 1950 was 9·7 per cent (Ministry of Health *Annual Report for 1950*, Command 8342, HMSO 1951). It is possible that the gradual reduction in the number might be associated with the 1959 Mental Health Act, as a result of which a large number of those who in the past would have been on daily licence have now been discharged into the community.

[3] *op. cit.*

as the men were concerned, most of this group worked on the gardens, but a sizeable proportion worked alongside tradesmen as painters, bricklayers, shoe repairers, etc. Virtually no women were given outdoor jobs.

Medical Superintendents were asked what criteria were used as a matter of general policy in selecting adult patients for specific jobs, and who normally made the decision. In almost 40 per cent of cases we were told that the preference of the patient was the main consideration. This we consider to be something of a distortion and our observation led us to believe that patients are very rarely consulted in any meaningful way, with the possible exception of the higher grades. It seems doubtful whether such a high proportion of patients would choose to do domestic work if the choice were entirely theirs, and we believe that their 'preference' can only be expressed within a very limited framework, i.e. the patient can 'choose' between the laundry, the kitchen or general cleaning, though even this choice may be restricted when any of these departments are full. For such patients freedom of choice would not normally extend to occupational therapy or industrial training; furthermore we think patients are induced to show certain preferences, as for example where the Medical Superintendent commented: 'They are offered more money if they don't like a particular job'. Another Superintendent said that patients were allowed to request certain jobs, but that he 'didn't necessarily take any notice of them'. A third said: 'Most people go automatically to occupational therapy or industrial training'.

Nor could female patients do what is regarded as 'male' work, for example, gardening, farmwork, woodwork, etc., though it was occasionally possible for male patients to work in the kitchens, normally regarded as the prerogative of females. This division of work tasks reflects the very strict staff attitudes to segregation that we found to exist in almost all hospitals. Only in five hospitals were patients encouraged to mix; in most of the others they were allowed to do so at socials, some hospitals encouraging this and others keeping strict supervision of the situation. A few occupational and industrial therapy departments were mixed, as was discussed earlier[1] possibly because training staff did not share the nurses' fears about integration. In one hospital where the chief male nurse allowed patients much more freedom than did the matron, the former admitted that he could do so with no fears, since he was confident that matron would never become more liberal minded!

Apart from the patients' own preference, the criterion most often mentioned was their mental capabilities (about one-third of the sampled patients), and certainly a slightly higher proportion amongst this group were involved in occupational therapy or industrial training, although the total numbers were relatively small.

Only in very few instances did hospitals have any kind of unit for

[1] Twenty-nine out of 130 (see Chapter 7, p. 142).

assessing work suitability; fewer than 4 per cent of adult patients in our sample were in hospitals providing such facilities. For patients living in hostels attached to hospitals, the type of work depended largely upon the facilities available in the area. The decision was normally the responsibility of the hostel warden, though he had little or no say in the patients sent there from the hospital.

With regard to work allocation in the main hospitals, the responsibility for decision-making was nominally that of the medical staff, although in subsidiary units the decision was most frequently made by the matron or chief male nurse. In one hospital the Superintendent specifically mentioned that the psychologist's advice was 'quite often given'. He did not indicate whether it was taken. From our observations, however, it would seem that even where the medical staff are *officially* responsible for the decision, it is mainly a question of rubber stamping the proposals of the nursing staff. If more workers are required on a specific task, names are put to the Medical Superintendent (usually at the morning meeting of senior staff) and these are automatically agreed. Similarly if patients misbehave or are felt to be in some way unsuitable in their job, the administrative nursing staff make proposals for their transfer and these are confirmed.

This situation may account for the fact that in terms of the distribution of various tasks and occupations it appeared to make relatively little difference who made the decision. In those hospitals where all staff were said to be concerned in the decision-making process there were rather fewer patients who were not working at all. In those where the decision was made solely by nursing staff, most either did no work (36 per cent), or worked in and around the hospital or grounds (36 per cent). On the other hand where the decision was made by nurses only, fewer patients worked on their own wards (8 per cent) as compared with approximately 16 per cent where others were also involved in the decision-making process. However where a patient worked may not be related so much to the rôle of the person(s) making the decision but rather to the opportunities available for alternative types of work. Thus in the 119 subsidiary units visited, only 62 had occupational therapy or industrial training departments (some of these had both), a situation which considerably reduced the opportunities available for patients to do work other than that of a domestic nature. In such cases size may be less important than the subsidiary status of the unit, in other words it is often the main unit that provides auxilliary services, rather than its subsidiary units, but if the unit is autonomous, even though small, it may provide them. The largest proportion of patients in occupational therapy and industrial training departments was to be found in hospitals of between 1,000 and 1,800 beds (approximately one-fifth); but if one considers only occupational therapy then size makes little difference and, except in the very small units about 12 per cent of patients attend. The major difference relates to industrial training where very few patients in the largest hospitals (over 1,800 beds) attend, and similarly very few of the small units make such provision.

Hours of Work and Pay Whilst it must be borne in mind that about one-third of the adult population were not working, of those who *did* work some 26 per cent did so for between 25 and 34 hours per week and a further 22 per cent for 35 hours or more. Although relatively few patients worked in the community, most of those who did so worked a normal working week of about 40 hours, and for this they received a wage which was negotiated with the hospital administrators. Deductions were made for board and lodging and the amount of money they retained for their own use varied from hospital to hospital, though one pound was usually the minimum. The balance was generally credited to the patient's account.

Apart from those on licence, patients who worked the longest hours (usually in excess of 35) were those who did utility or domestic work in the hospital or grounds: the cleaners, gardeners, artisans, laundry and kitchen workers, etc. Most were paid between five and ten shillings per week though a fair proportion received between ten shillings and a pound for this type of work.

Those doing occupational therapy or industrial training worked on average for about 30 hours a week and pay was likely to vary from two shillings and sixpence to five shillings per week and though a small number earned up to ten shillings, the rate was more likely to be under two shillings and sixpence.

Patients who worked on their own wards varied enormously in the amount of time they spent working; a few worked either extremely long or extremely short hours, but for the most part the distribution was about equal between those working 15 to 24 hours and those working 25 to 34 hours. Pay appeared to be completely arbitrary and in no way related to the number of hours worked, or to the type of ward work undertaken.

Illustrated in diagrammatic form, the pattern of reward money follows a normal distribution save that 5 per cent of patients are not paid at all.[1] (See opposite.)

Medical Superintendents were asked upon what criteria decisions regarding pay were based. Apart from those who were not paid, or who were paid in kind, or those at the other end of the scale who earned over one pound, the major factor in deciding pay was said to be the amount of effort expended.

For the most part, however, the whole question of reward money seemed to be quite haphazard; one Medical Superintendent himself used this expression commenting: 'It's very unsatisfactory . . . pay is

[1] This pattern is quite different from that obtained by O'Connor and Tizard in their London survey. Theirs was a steeply falling curve with 42 per cent earning one shilling or less and 2 per cent earning sixteen shillings or more.

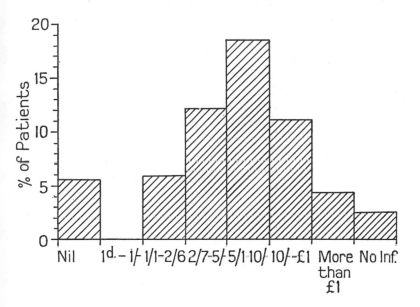

quite haphazard and bribes are given to patients to stay in unpleasant jobs'. Another Superintendent adjusted patients' pay so that they were unable to buy more than five cigarettes a day. Yet another said he 'dangles open rewards as a carrot to inspire patients to work'. In another hospital the Superintendent said that patients were paid according to the old classifications: three shillings for idiots, six shillings for imbeciles, twelve shillings for IQ up to 60, and the others get a maximum of sixteen shillings. However, from our data on this particular hospital, it was apparent that only part of the money is given to the patient, the rest was compulsorily saved. 'Good behaviour' was mentioned quite frequently, as was the value of the patient's work to the hospital. In some units the monies were 'pooled' and spent on patients as a whole to provide day trips, clothes, entertainments, etc.

It was our intention to exclude pocket money from this particular question and to obtain information about reward money only. In this we were not wholly successful for a number of reasons: firstly in some hospitals no distinction was made between these two sources of patients' income. One hospital had a combined system whereby all pocket money had to be spent in one week, otherwise less was given the following week; all reward money was credited to the patients' account. Secondly, nursing staff were often unaware of the amount given, although they were responsible for signing for it in the Finance Office and for seeing that it was distributed to patients. They rarely kept a note of the amount, nor did they usually know which was reward money as distinct from pocket money.

Even more than in the case of criteria for job selection we felt that decisions about reward money were completely fortuitous. In the two hospitals where elaborate scales or systems of pay existed in theory, in practice these were not put into effect, largely because no one had time to do so.

Just as training personnel were rarely involved in decisions about jobs, so was this true about pay. In no instances were they alone responsible for the decision; on the other hand medical staff were *always* involved. In only about one-quarter of cases were all the staff concerned with a particular patient said to discuss the matter jointly; for the majority of patients the decision was made either by medical staff alone (20 per cent) or jointly with nursing staff (27 per cent). When the decision was made by all staff, the criterion for pay was most usually 'amount achieved'; where medical or nursing staff decided either singly or jointly, the main criterion was 'amount of effort expended'; where medical and training staff were jointly involved the criterion was most likely to be 'appreciation of money'. Patients needs and the amount of responsibility involved proved to be minor factors in assessing rates of pay. Again as in the case of criteria for job selection, we do not place too much importance on these findings as we think the answers given by Superintendents reflect a formalized situation which rarely exists in practice. Whilst the initial decision at time of admission (or when the patient's case is reviewed) may be made in the way they suggest, any subsequent changes are likely to be brought about quite fortuitously, and to depend upon one individual, be it nurse, therapist, doctor or trainer, approaching the Superintendent and asking if a particular patient could have more or less reward money.

Leisure activities

One of the forms of social control mentioned frequently was that of stopping entertainments and similar privileges. But our observations indicate that as a form of social control, prohibiting attendance at these functions may well have a very limited deterrent value, since a high proportion of patients do not in any case attend. Furthermore, in view of the infrequency with which activities take place in some hospitals, patients must find it difficult to link the prohibition with 'being naughty' (as staff usually refer to it), possibly many days, even weeks earlier.

The leisure activities of patients consisted largely of entertainments in the form of films, socials, dances and outings, and we shall now briefly discuss each of these activities in turn.

(a) *Films and Dances* All but four of the main hospitals provided films, and rather more than half of the ancillary units also did so; in addition about one per cent of patients were allowed to visit local cinemas and dance halls. Films were usually shown weekly or fortnightly, and although the number of patients attending varied considerably from hospital to hospital, only in very few places did less than one-third attend, and in many cases as many as three-quarters of the patient population did so.[1]

Dances were held in all but one of the main units but in only approximately a third of the subsidiary units. They took place fortnightly or monthly, usually during the winter months only. So far as the subsidiary units were concerned, they were often single sex affairs, though occasionally arrangements were made for patients to be taken by bus to the dances at the main hospital. We were frequently told that films and dances, particularly the latter, have become less popular now that television is readily available on the wards. Certainly the number attending dances was considerably smaller than in the case of films – in only 16 units did the number attending exceed 50 per cent of the patients, and it was usually between 30 and 45 per cent. The fact that a higher proportion of males than females usually attended may again reflect the keener desire on the part of male nursing staff to involve patients in treatment or training, to which we have referred in other situations. Great play was made on female wards of the way in which patients attending dances liked to dress in their 'best' clothes. Possibly the fact that male patients were less concerned about their appearance meant that it was less trouble to the staff to get them ready.

(b) *Social clubs* Thirty-nine per cent of sampled patients were in hospitals which made no provisions (other than films and dances) for patients' recreation, and another 5·1 per cent were able to attend recreational activities outside the hospital.[2] Facilities in those hospitals having a social club are set out in Table 8.6:

---

[1] Except where stated otherwise the figures quoted in respect of films, dances, socials, outings and holidays refer to the total population of the hospitals visited and not to the sampled patients.

[2] This includes one hospital where the League of Friends for the whole Group ran a club in the town which was used by parole patients from five hospitals in the Group, including the one under discussion.

Table 8.6

PATIENTS' SOCIAL CLUB FACILITIES (PERCENTAGES)

Facilities for social clubs	*Patients*
Special buildings (sole use)	13·8
Hall or room (sole use)	3·2
Hall or room (part-time use)	38·1
Attend social club facilities outside hospital	5·1
No social club	39·8
TOTAL	100·0
No information	27
No. of patients	3,038

Clubs were mainly run either by nursing staff or by specialist staff (i.e. recreation organizer,[1] teachers, occupational therapists, etc.). A very few were run by the patients themselves; one was a joint staff/patient club and one was run by the local WRVS.

(c) *Outings* The highest proportion of patients to go on day outings organized by the hospital appear to do so from those hospitals with between 1,000 and 1,799 beds (86 per cent). In the hospitals over that size only approximately one-third of patients go on such outings and in the smaller ones about a half do so. Furthermore in hospitals where a high proportion go on outings, they also tend to go regularly (i.e. monthly or even more frequently), and at the other end of the scale, in hospitals where fewer than 25 per cent of patients go, it tends to be on rare occasions only, for example to a Christmas pantomime or a day at the seaside. One of the reasons for this may be that the larger hospitals are often provided with special buses, often the gift of some voluntary organization, which can be used for carrying crippled patients from wards to specialist departments, as well as for day outings. However this does not offer a satisfactory explanation as to why the proportion should be so small in the very large hospitals.

We also asked about outings organized by outside bodies, but although these did occasionally take place, the numbers were insignificant.

Patients also went out in small groups with nursing staff, particularly on shopping expeditions which sometimes included tea. Nurses expressed fears about patients becoming jealous of each other so they took care to ensure that different people went each time, and groups rather than individuals were taken.

---

[1] Most recreation organizers were in fact nurses seconded for special duty.

(d) *Church attendance* No systematic information was obtained about religious activity in the hospitals, nor about the work of the chaplains. We asked whether patients could attend church in the community if they so desired, most hospitals confirmed that they could, but in the larger hospitals it was rarely thought to be necessary since both Church of England and Catholic services were usually held weekly or more often on the premises. In the smaller units arrangements could be made for Catholics to attend churches outside in the community, but we were given the impression that very few patients showed any inclination to do so.

(e) *Open and sports days* In all but the smallest hospitals an Open Day was held annually, although in one subsidiary unit the matron said that she had stopped it because she felt the public were 'just coming to watch the antics of the patients'. For the most part however, this was the day around which the whole social life of the hospital centred – at any rate if the staff are to be believed. Unfortunately these Open Days do not appear to have stimulated increased contact between relatives and staff during the remainder of the year.[1]

Summary

The data presented in this chapter draws attention to two important aspects of hospital life: firstly, and most clearly, to the great disparity between institutional life and the life led by the majority of adults in the open community. The seal is set at the outset with the failure to look upon admission to hospital as being of concern to the family as a whole. There are undoubtedly a certain number of cases where the family deliberately rejects its subnormal member and is glad to be relieved of the burden of caring for him (her), but such total rejection is probably rare and parental feelings are normally ambivalent. The ritualized exclusion of the relatives symbolizes a denial on the part of the hospital that relatives have feelings and concerns about the patient, and at the same time it establishes the future pattern of relationships between the hospital and the relatives about which we shall say more in the next chapter.

The second factor which we believe emerges from our findings is the ambivalence of all levels of staff in relation to their custodial role. The patients are constantly referred to as 'children' by the majority of nursing staff, and this is further symbolized by their attitude to punishments and sanctions. Stopping entertainments or parole, sending patients to bed early, reducing pocket money, these are all methods which would normally be acceptable as a means of social control with children. Yet the great majority of patients in the hospitals studied were adults, and the behavioural norms expected

[1] See in particular Chapter 7.

of them were those of adults. In other words they are expected to behave as grown-ups, but treated as children.

This involves a redefinition of the patient's status: irrespective of his chronological age he is defined as a child and the hospital is defined as being *in loco parentis*. Not only is this redefinition socially regressive, but it has the expectation, subtly understood if not explicitly stated, that patients are children and, moreover, children for ever.

Chapter 9

RELATIONSHIPS BETWEEN THE
HOSPITAL AND THE COMMUNITY

HOWEVER much it may appear so from the inside, subnormality hospitals are not 'islands unto themselves', but part of a wider community. In this chapter we shall discuss their links with the outside world under three main headings: firstly, the formal contact that the hospital has with the Ministry, the Regional Hospital Board and the Hospital Management Committee; secondly we shall refer to the more informal contacts that they have with voluntary organizations and those members of the public who show an interest in their work; and thirdly we shall discuss the contact between patients and relatives and indicate the ways in which the hospital fosters or puts constraints upon such relationships.

Formal contacts

The limited time which we spent at each hospital gave us very little opportunity to assess in any depth their relationships with the Ministry of Health, and we shall therefore confine our remarks to the Regional Hospital Board and the Hospital Management Committee.[1]

(a) *Regional Hospital Boards* Apart from occasional Committee meetings attended by the matron or chief male nurse regarding matters of nursing policy, only the medical superintendent and the Group secretary normally had regular contact with the Board. Group secretaries were not interviewed by the research team, but medical superintendents were invited to discuss the extent to which they felt consulted by the Board in relation to matters of policy.

In the very largest hospitals the overwhelming majority of superintendents said either that they were only consulted on minor matters, or alternatively that they were consulted and their views ignored. One superintendent replied: 'Inadequate – they're very touchy, but I'm not going to be quoted as being derogatory. They consult me, but the results bear very little relationship to the discussion. At a personal level I'm very friendly with them'. Another superintendent of a large hospital, asked the same question, replied: 'No', and he asked the interviewer to underline it three times: 'Our Board is a very dreadful

[1] A more detailed discussion of Hospital Management Committees will appear in Chapter 10.

Board, superintendents' meetings are held twice a year', and he went on to describe how his patients were moved to other hospitals without his being consulted. A similar view was expressed by another superintendent under the same Regional Hospital Board '. . . We have access and can make our view known, but things still occur affecting this hospital which it is not possible to agree with, or to comprehend how the decision was reached, so that one tends to feel one wasn't consulted . . .'. In a smaller hospital the superintendent commented: 'Oh yes, they're very good. Not that they take the slightest notice of what I say, but they do consult me'.

None of the superintendents in the very large hospitals expressed unqualified satisfaction, but those who were also members of the Board's Medical Advisory Committee agreed that their views were taken note of, *because of their position on the Committee*, not because of their role as a superintendent of a hospital.

In the medium-sized hospitals (1,000–1,800) beds, about half the superintendents expressed themselves as wholly satisfied, and the remainder were equally divided between those who were satisfied because they were members of the Medical Advisory Committee, those with reservations, and those who felt they were not consulted at all.

In hospitals with fewer than 1,000 beds just over half the superintendents had reservations about the matter and the remainder could be roughly divided between those who were satisfied and those who felt they were not consulted at all.

Looked at in terms of patient population, only approximately one-third (32 per cent) were in hospitals where the superintendent was satisfied with the degree of consultation, and almost one-quarter of the patients were in hospitals where the superintendent claimed not to be consulted at all on questions of policy.

(b) *Hospital Management Committees* Immediate responsibility for the hospital's administration lies in the hands of the Hospital Management Committee, a body comprised of approximately 15–20 people chosen by the regional hospital board to represent the local community. Four or five of the members will be doctors, two or three of these being members of the staffs of the hospitals which comprise the group. They usually meet once a month and from the membership of this committee various sub-committees are appointed: finance, general purposes, house committees, etc.

The Ministry of Health issue a *Handbook for Members of Hospital Management Committees*, in which it is stated that one of their responsibilities is to see that 'hospitals are well administered in the best interests of the patients'. In practice their overriding concern was with finance, where necessary acting as a 'buffer' between the hospital and the Regional Hospital Board. This concern with finance was perhaps not surprising in view of the fact that most members of the committee had no medical expertise[1] and little knowledge or understanding of mental subnormality. A medical superintendent addressing the Annual Conference of the National Association for Mental Health in 1966 described what he called a 'typical' committee: 'Sixteen members of whom nine were over 60 and four were over 70 years of age. None were under 50 and four had been members since 1948'. Although we did not obtain details of the age structure of Management Committees, our observations and the views of superintendents and administrative nursing staff would tend to support the view that committee members are mainly elderly, and while age was not necessarily the main cause for the dissatisfaction of those interviewed, it was often mentioned.

Our observations suggest that the extent of the power exercised by Management Committees within a particular hospital is determined by the kind of relationship existing between the medical superintendent and the chairman of the Hospital Management Committee. Virtually all the power of the committee is vested in the chairman, and unless he is both knowledgeable *and* very active in hospital affairs, his powers could be (and frequently were) effectively eroded by the medical superintendent, in direct relationship to the extent that *he* wished to exercise power. There is a parallel here with the ability of senior nursing staff to limit the effective rôle of medical staff by informal methods such as blocking lines of communication.

Superintendents and administrative nursing staff were asked whether the Hospital Management Committee understood the needs of the hospital.

We believe that the large discrepancies between the views of superintendents and those of nursing staff reflect both the 'deference' of the latter, and their unwillingness to criticize the Management Committee to the research workers. Furthermore since the degree of contact between the superintendent and the Hospital Management Committee was much greater than that between the administrative nursing staff and the committee, the former were in a much better position to assess the attitudes of individual committee members. Whilst it is possible that some superintendents may be prejudiced in their views about Management Committees, our observations in the intensive study tend to bear out many of their complaints.

Almost all superintendents were critical, some extremely so: 'How do you expect half-wits looking for OBEs to run a hospital. They are rigid in their attitudes and do not take kindly to progress . . . if a patient dies they will not ask what he died of, but they will turn the place upside-down to find a missing chicken'. Another superintendent said he thought their understanding was limited 'by experience and intelligence'. A superintendent who said he got on well with the

[1] Medical members of the board do not normally play a very active part, but they serve a useful function for the medical superintendent since they will tend always to support his view, at least publicly.

P

Table 9.1

EXTENT TO WHICH HOSPITAL MANAGEMENT COMMITTEE
UNDERSTANDS HOSPITAL'S NEEDS (PERCENTAGES)

Whether HMC broadly understands the needs of the hospital	Patients affected	
	Superintendent's views	Matron's/CMN's views
Yes	38·7	61·8
Yes, with reservations	30·8	12·9
Some members do	3·3	9·7
No	24·3	12·1
Other	3·3	3·5
TOTAL	100·0	100·0
No information	—	400
No. of patients	3,038	3,038

chairman felt that too many members wanted power 'they tend to put their own position before the needs of the hospital, they're too much concerned with their own prestige'. And as a final example, one superintendent complained: 'They are too steeped in local government management; they are lay people with the minimum of medical people. They assume all the duties of a management committee but do not bear any of the responsibilities'.

So far as the nursing administration were concerned, one chief male nurse complained that *general* hospitals are 'the apples of the management committees eyes. They don't bother to understand the mental subnormality hospital'. The matron of the same hospital said that the Management Committee only visit once a year. However this appeared to be exceptional and most main units were visited monthly, though in subsidiary units there was usually an annual visit, with the House Committee meeting more frequently. One matron of a very large hospital said she didn't expect the committee to understand 'but they are a conscientious body of people who don't get paid'. Hospital size was a relevant factor here and nursing administrators in the smaller units were most likely to be satisfied with the degree of understanding shown by the Hospital Management Committee. At the same time it must be recognized that they were likely to see the members less frequently.

Apart from their understanding of the hospital's needs, superintendents were asked about the extent of the Management Committee's activities. Their replies are set out in Table 9.2.

Table 9.2

EXTENT OF ACTIVITY OF HOSPITAL MANAGEMENT COMMITTEE
(PERCENTAGES)

Superintendents' views of extent of activity by HMC	Patients
Active	50·2
Pay statutory visits only	21·5
Activity discouraged by medical superintendent*	22·6
Other	5·7
TOTAL	100·0
No information	69
No. of patients	3,038

* In such cases the superintendent discourages committee members from performing any functions other than statutory visiting.

It was almost solely in the largest hospitals that superintendents said they did not encourage the Management Committee to play an active part. However this may simply be because in the smaller hospitals (fewer than 1,000 beds) the Committees rarely did more than pay a formal monthly visit and attend committee meetings. Their activity may also have been restricted by lack of encouragement from the medical superintendent, but whereas in the larger hospitals the superintendents felt free to say so, in the smaller ones they preferred to imply that it was the committee who voluntarily restricted the amount of contact.

Administrative nurses were asked about the nature of the relationship they had with members of the Management Committee. About half the patients were in hospitals where such staff said they had a very good relationship, rather more than a quarter were in hospitals where the staff saw them at committee meetings, or on rota visits only. In most of the remaining instances the relationship was said to be good with some members, or they had reservations.

It was almost always in the largest hospitals that relations were described by nursing administrators as 'very good'; since these were also the hospitals where the medical superintendent did not encourage the Management Committee to play an active role, one wonders whether relationships were good just *because* visits remained very formal and the amount of contact was minimal.

Informal contacts

(a) *Interest of voluntary organizations in the work of the hospital* In spite of increased state provision there has been a growing recognition of the need for voluntary action in all fields of social welfare.[1] '... Vigour and abundance of voluntary action outside one's home, individually and in association with other citizens, for bettering one's own life and that of one's fellows, are the distinguishing mark of a free society. They have been outstanding features of British life ...'.[2] One might expect this to be particularly relevant in the subnormality hospitals where nurses complain of staff shortages and many patients are known to lack contact with relatives.[3]

Matrons and chief male nurses were asked to identify local organizations, groups, or individuals who showed an active interest in the work of the hospital. We do not claim that a complete list was obtained in this way, but Table 9.3 gives some indication of the type of organization involved in such voluntary activity.

The intensity of their involvement varied considerably; for the most part organizations were concerned to raise money for amenities and equipment; some, such as the local schools, undertook to visit patients regularly, and many others provided entertainment. The WRVS and church organizations were primarily concerned with providing tea for visitors, or in the case of the latter, with decorating the chapel and conveying patients to and from churches in the community. Local Mental Health organizations sometimes arranged holidays for patients, although more usually this was organized through the national body. Near one hospital a local chain store remained open late one evening each week so that the more severely subnormal patients could go shopping.

Without wishing in any way to undervalue the contribution made by these organizations – often one which made a great difference to the 'homeliness' of the institution – we nevertheless observed that there appeared to be little real contact between the patients and the community in terms of personal relationships. It was much more usual to find such contact in small subsidiary units where the matron or chief male nurse often made real efforts to link the unit with the local community. Rarely did we hear of patients being invited to join outside clubs, or to visit private homes, nor were many visited personally in the hospital.

(b) *Leave* The contacts with the community which we have so far discussed could be described as 'hospital-centred' rather more than 'patient-centred'. We shall now examine the extent to which patients have contact with their friends and relatives and the conditions under which they do so.

---

[1] In the penal field, see, for example: *The Place of Voluntary Service in After-Care*, HMSO (1967).

[2] Lord Beveridge: *Voluntary Action – a Report on Methods of Social Advance*, George Allen and Unwin (1948).

[3] Details will be given later in this chapter.

Table 9.3

INTERESTED LOCAL ORGANIZATIONS

Type of organization	No. of times mentioned*
Friends of the Hospital	59
Rotary/Inner Wheel/Round Table	28
Women's Institute/Young Wives/Townswomen's Guild/Mothers' Union	28
WRVS	25
Religious Organizations	19
Mental Health Organizations	17
Local Schools	16
Local Firms	16
TOC H	13
Local Dramatic Society/Dance Band/Sports or Social Club	10
Other	9
Brownies/Guides/Youth Organizations	6
Other Charitable Organizations	5
Red Cross/St John Ambulance	5
Private Individuals	4
British Legion/RAF Association	3
Total number of persons interviewed	141

* Both matrons and chief male nurses were asked the question and this table covers both sets of answers.

Despite the fact that nowadays very few patients arc in subnormality hospitals under compulsory orders, a number of formalities must still be gone through before leave is granted. Although many of these procedures are undoubtedly intended to safeguard the patient's interests, the fact that some hospitals are much more rigid than others in their observance, suggests that there is still an element of 'hangover' from the old days when the majority of patients were compulsorily detained.

Only approximately 3 per cent of sampled patients were in units which had no special requirements, 90 per cent were in units which required a letter from the relative or friend to whom the patient was going, just over half in units which required that the patient be medically examined before leaving and a third in units where a form had to be filled in by the staff. Only 9 per cent of patients were in units where the local GP was informed of the patient's intended visit, and this occurred when it was thought that additional drugs might be required. Twelve per cent of patients were in units where a social worker was asked to visit the home before the patient's first period of leave, in order to make sure that it was a 'suitable' place.

In most hospitals we were told that approximately three days' notice was asked for, in order to prepare the patient; in at least one hospital a period of fourteen days was insisted upon and in another, seven days, the reason given in this latter case being 'to arrange National Assistance'. Where compulsory patients were concerned there is a statutory requirement that the police in the area to which the patient was going be informed.

(c) *Holidays*[1] For the purposes of this research only holidays of one week's duration or more were included, two distinct categories being considered: those organized by the hospital, and those organized by relatives or friends of patients. The most striking fact which emerged is that relatively few patients went on holiday at all; in most hospitals the figure varied between 10 and 25 per cent in a year and the number was roughly the same whether organized by the hospital or by relatives. The main difference appeared to be that in the larger hospitals a greater proportion went on 'hospital' holidays, and in the smaller hospitals the emphasis was on holidays organized by relatives. Furthermore rather more patients tended to go from hospitals where visiting opportunities and arrangements for leave were least restrictive. This may have arisen because some of the larger hospitals were able to support holiday homes exclusively for their own use; they were open all the year round, and suitable groups of patients were sent for a week or two at a time. This arrangement served an additional function in that it freed their beds in the hospital for short term care cases.

However, an analysis of the kind of arrangements made by different hospitals in relation to the proportion going, showed that, whilst it may have been easier to organize when they had their own holiday home, this type of arrangement was not widely used and the great majority of patients went on holiday as a result of private arrangements made between the hospital and individual landladies. Also widely used were special camps, often organized by voluntary societies.

(d) *Patients' contacts with relatives and friends* In an earlier chapter[2] we set out the extent to which patients were known to have relatives, and it was pointed out that just over 13 per cent of sampled patients were believed by nursing staff to have no relatives, mainly patients aged 50 or over. We are concerned here with the extent to which patients *having* relatives had contact with them, or with friends.

These data were obtained from the nurse in charge of each ward, and some nurses found it difficult to provide accurate information, though where they had been working on one particular ward for

---

[1] The formalities for granting leave referred to in the preceding section would also apply to patients going on holiday with relatives or friends.
[3] See Chapter 4, p. 64–5.

many years they did not experience many problems of this kind, and they not only knew their patients well, but knew about their families in considerable detail. In some hospitals a list was kept on the ward giving details of when the patient was last visited and by whom, as well as when they last went home to stay. This practice was by no means general however, and in many cases the latter information was available only from the records office; thus sometimes answers given by nurses depended upon the reliability of their memory.

Relatives' visits to the hospital[1]

Over 37 per cent of our sample had been visited within the preceding four weeks; a further 19·7 per cent had been visited within the past year (though not within the past month) making a total of 57 per cent visited at least once during the year. As might be expected, there was a progressive decline in visiting associated with age of patient and length of time they had been in hospital. Whereas 52 per cent of those in hospital for between one and three years had been visited in the four weeks preceding the research visit, the proportion of patients who had been in for twenty years or more and who had been visited within the four week period dropped to 21 per cent.

Amongst patients under the age of 30 a slightly higher proportion of males than females were visited, but in the other age groups the position was reversed and more females received visits[2] (see Table 9.4).

We did not, in the national sample, analyse the distance relatives had to travel in order to reach the hospital, since this would have required considerably more work than the resources of the research budget would allow.[3] We did, however, endeavour to obtain this information for the two hospitals studied intensively and found some slight indication that relatives living at a considerable distance from the hospital appeared to visit patients more frequently than those living nearer. Although the two hospitals were polar extremes in terms of geographical isolation, the amount and frequency of visiting indicated that this was not a major factor affecting visiting, although the transport facilities were incomparably better in the hospital situated near a large urban centre.

In order satisfactorily to explain these findings it would be necessary to control several variables and investigate the social circumstances of each family, but the fact that the majority of visitors came

---

[1] Although we refer to 'relatives' throughout this chapter, friends are also included, since we did not specify the relationship of the person visiting.

[2] Amongst those aged 60 or over the difference is too small to be meaningful.

[3] To do this would have meant checking each patient's personal notes in the general records office, and having ascertained the next of kin's address, assessed the distance from the hospital. Furthermore we know, from the intensive sample, that it was not always the next of kin who visited, so that the information would have been of doubtful value.

Table 9.4

AGE AND SEX OF PATIENTS NOT HAVING BEEN VISITED IN
PREVIOUS TWELVE MONTHS (PERCENTAGES)

Age	Not visited		
	Male	*Female*	*Male and Female*
0–15	20·7	22·1	21·3
16–19	25·7	32·6	28·4
20–29	29·6	32·5	30·8
30–39	44·2	38·6	41·9
40–49	53·0	35·4	44·8
50–59	62·6	40·7	51·9
60 and over	57·1	58·2	57·7
All ages	43·4	38·5	42·7
No information	6	5	11
No. of patients	1,664	1,374	3,038

by car suggests that there may be a socio-economic bias which affects visiting, although we have no firm data on this point.

Approximately one-third of patients in all sizes of hospital had received no visits in the year preceding the research visit. A further one-third had been visited within the past year but not within four weeks, and once again hospital size was not a major factor, although rather more in the very small hospitals had been visited. However size did appear to make a considerable difference to the *pattern* of visiting as distinct from the *amount* of visiting. Amongst patients visited within the preceding four weeks there was a marked and progressive decline according to size of hospital: only approximately 18 per cent of those in hospitals of 1,800 beds or more had been visited within this period, as compared with approximately 36 per cent of those in hospitals with between 1,000–1,799 beds and almost 45 per cent in hospitals with under 1,000 beds.

It seems likely that factors affecting visiting are unrelated to sheer distance, or to the convenience of public transport, but related rather to the age of the patient, the amount of time he has spent in hospital, the size of the hospital, the attitudes of the staff towards visitors and perhaps predominantly to the feelings of the relatives for the patients. This latter is, perhaps, an aspect that is not widely considered. If the lack of community or domiciliary services is one of the major precipitating factors in hospitalization, and we have some reason to believe that this is the case, then the relative is likely to have ambivalent feelings about visiting. The visit itself may involve a long and probably tedious journey, and coming face to face with the patient in hospital may be a reminder of the failure of the community at large to be able or willing to care for him/her.[1] On the other hand there may be the rationalization that the patient is well cared for in hospital and the relatives need not therefore worry unduly about what is happening. It could be this that makes long periods between visits emotionally tolerable for the relative.

Patients with parents *and* siblings alive were visited most frequently, the visiting often being shared by different members of the family. On the other hand almost 10 per cent of those who received visits had no known relatives, suggesting either that they were visited by friends, or alternatively that the staff did not know they were relatives. Sixty per cent of patients who had siblings alive, but no parents, received visits.

We attempted to see whether there was any connection between level of intelligence and frequency of visiting. Whilst the findings must be interpreted with great caution in view of the unreliability of data relating to IQ, the information set out in Table 9.5 indicates that there appears to be no marked connection. Because of the relatively small number of patients in the sample with IQs of 70 or over, we have grouped these together.

Going home

Perhaps the clearest evidence we have of the degree to which patients entering hospitals for the subnormal are cut off from the community lies in the fact that three-quarters of the sampled patients never went home. Information about home visits broken down by age groups is set out in Table 9.6.[2]

From this table it will be seen that of those patients who did go home, irrespective of age, considerably more had done so in the preceding month than any other period (it will be remembered that this was also true of relatives visiting the hospital). A disproportionately high number of children under 16, compared with adults, suffered from multiple handicaps as well as from severe physical handicaps,[3] and this may explain why so many in this particular age group never went home. The fact that there was a slight but progressive decline in the number going home from the age of 16 onwards may reflect the ageing of relatives and their consequent inability to cope with their subnormal child, either through infirmity or through death; on the other hand there may also have been a gradual atrophy of familial ties and obligations through lack of reinforcement, since

---

[1] Much has been written about the guilt of the parents *vis-à-vis* their own inability to look after their mentally subnormal child as well as about the guilt they feel at having given birth to such a child, but we think little has been said about this present aspect.

[2] It should be noted, however, that 5·5 per cent of the patients had been in hospital for less than one year.

[3] See Chapter 4, p. 72.

Table 9.5

DATE OF LAST VISIT BY IQ (PERCENTAGES)

Date of last visit	IQ						
	Untested or no information	Untestable	Under 50	50–59	60–69	70 and over	Total
Visited within preceding four weeks	39·6	44·7	33·5	33·2	32·6	40·5	38·4
Visited between four weeks and one year	21·4	16·4	22·5	24·0	12·4	21·5	20·1
Not visited in past year	39·0	38·9	44·0	42·8	55·0	38·0	41·5
TOTAL	100·0	100·0	100·0	100·0	100·0	100·0	100·0
No information	25	7	16	3	5	2	58
No. of patients	1,005	593	951	232	134	123	3,038

Table 9.6

AGE BY FREQUENCY OF HOME VISITS (PERCENTAGES)

Last visit home*	Age groups							
	Under	16–19	20–29	30–39	40–49	50–59	60 and over	Total
Under one month	10·6	16·2	13·5	9·7	8·4	6·3	3·7	9·2
One to three months	5·3	8·3	8·3	6·4	5·4	5·7	2·9	5·9
Three to six months	5·3	4·8	5·3	3·7	3·4	3·1	1·5	3·7
Six months to one year	4·7	4·8	4·4	3·3	3·0	1·0	2·2	3·1
One year or more	3·1	1·3	1·9	2·4	1·4	2·0	1·0	1·8
Never goes home	71·1	64·6	66·4	74·5	78·3	81·9	88·8	74·9
TOTAL	100·0	100·0	100·0	100·0	100·0	100·0	100·0	100·0
No information	2	3	9	10	7	6	4	41
No. of patients	362	232	533	465	505	497	414	3,038

* At the time of the research visit.

little appeared to be done by the hospital staff to encourage contact between relatives and patients. It is interesting to note that amongst older patients, going home was by no means confined to those who had recently entered hospital. Fifty-seven per cent of patients over 50 years of age had been in hospital for 20 years or more and 16 per cent of them went home from time to time. Eight per cent of patients in this age group had been in hospital for four years or less, and 20 per cent of these went home.

A true picture of the extent to which patients have contact with their relatives must necessarily bear in mind both visits *from* relatives and visits *to* them. Approximately half of the 75 per cent of those who never went home had not received a visit during the preceding twelve months. Approximately one-fifth had been visited between four weeks and a year ago and some 30 per cent had been visited within the preceding four weeks. Thus approximately 37 per cent of the patients in our sample had neither been visited in the past year nor gone home, a much higher proportion than those found to have no relatives (13 per cent).[1]

We had thought that there might be some relationship between the parole status of the patient and the amount he or she was visited or

[1] See Chapter 4, p. 65.

went home. This proved to be the case only in relation to the latter group as is indicated in Table 9.7:

Table 9.7

CONTACT WITH RELATIVES BY PAROLE STATUS (PERCENTAGES)

	Parole status		
Contact with relatives	*Confined to ward*	*Confined to hospital grounds*	*Allowed outside hospital grounds*
Patients receiving visits	53·4	57·8	50·2
Patients going home	16·8	23·1	38·6
No. of patients*	1,269	1,194	559

* There were a further 16 patients about whom we have no information.

The fact that almost 17 per cent of patients who were confined to the ward whilst in hospital, were nevertheless able to go home reinforces our earlier suggestion that patients may be confined to the ward because it has never occurred to anyone to let them out, or because of the shortage of nursing staff which tends to result in patients being dealt with in groups, rather more than because of the severity of their physical and mental handicap.

In an earlier chapter we indicated that the presence of a social worker in the hospital made little or no difference to the degree of contact between patients and relatives.[1] Other factors which might be thought to affect the extent of such contact are the flexibility of visiting hours, the availability of the doctor to see relatives, and possibly the degree of involvement in hospital affairs by the Parents' Association or League of Friends.[2] We shall examine each of these factors in turn:

(a) *Visiting hours* Table 9.8 sets out the regulations regarding visiting as they affected the patients in our sample.

Almost all visiting appeared to take place at weekends,[3] so that provided the stipulated visiting days included a Saturday or Sunday (as was invariably the case), restrictions relating to specific days made little difference.

[1] See Chapter 7, p. 161.

[2] Although these are separate organizations we found a considerable amount of overlap in their activities *vis-à-vis* the hospitals. Furthermore some hospitals had one but not the other so that we have tended to treat them as interchangeable in our discussion.

[3] It was only in exceptional cases that members of the research team saw relatives around the hospital from Monday to Friday.

Table 9.8
VISITING HOURS (PERCENTAGES)

Permitted visiting times	*Patients affected*	*Patients visited in past four weeks*
Any time	60·7	35·5
Every afternoon *or* evening	5·8	12·0
Weekends only	11·2	36·2
Some afternoons or evenings	19·4	26·1
By appointment only	2·8	31·3
No. of patients	3,038	3,038

In most hospitals where visiting was said to be 'at any time' there were usually a host of qualifications. In the first place the hope was always expressed that relatives would inform the hospital authorities of their intention to visit,[1] the reason given for this being to ensure that patients were available and not out at work or at school. The way in which the arrangement actually worked had unfortunate results since it often meant that patients were kept on the ward, possibly for a whole day, in order to await a visit which might not take place until late in the afternoon. Similarly dental appointments, and those with chiropodists, speech therapists, etc. were often cancelled for the same reason. Had patients been allowed to continue with their usual routine it might have given the relatives an opportunity to see them engaged in some purposeful activity instead of sitting dressed in their best clothes waiting for their visitor. It would also have given the staff of the departments concerned the opportunity to meet the parents, a matter about which they so often complained.[2]

Children under 16 could generally be visited at any time, but as in the case of adults, in practice they tended to be visited only at weekends. Staff attitudes to parents varied widely; the superintendent of a very large hospital commented: 'Officially the visiting hours are Wednesday and Saturday afternoons but anyone who wants to come another day is welcome. But they must ask. Sometimes if people come too often and they are rather obnoxious I'll tell them off. There are certain people who are a perfect nuisance'. Another superintendent of an equally large hospital with similar visiting arrangements commented: 'All my staff have been instructed to make visitors welcome and have been taught the psychology of parenthood. They have also been taught that the parent is never wrong. We have one visiting

[1] There is no evidence to suggest that unheralded visitors were ever turned away.
[2] See Chapter 7 for a discussion of this problem.

room on the female side which is very attractive, and where there are very young children visiting, they see the patient in there, privately, rather than on the ward or in the general visiting hall'.

These represent 'official' views, we know little of what went on when parents *actually* visited, though from our limited observation visitors were generally tolerated with polite indifference. There appeared to be little or no attempt by nursing staff to take advantage of such visits to learn more about their patients, nor to try and encourage the relatives to be more involved in the process of training and social integration. The fact that relatives had handed over the care of the patient to the hospital staff seemed to be interpreted as a final act, henceforth their care was regarded as the sole concern of the staff, and relatives were seen as 'visitors'. There was little evidence of antagonism or unfriendliness, and some of the sisters and nurses tried to counsel and help relatives. Many nurses expressed the view that visits upset the patients, but we think perhaps they were more concerned lest visits upset the orderly routine of the ward.

In most hospitals, particularly the larger ones, a special building was provided for visits, and teas were often served by some voluntary organization such as the League of Friends or the WRVS. Such an arrangement minimized the amount of contact possible between relatives and nursing staff and reinforced the 'visitor' role to which we referred above. In these hospitals only non-ambulant patients could be visited on the ward, though as an alternative to the visiting hall some hospitals had 'visiting rooms' near the main entrance to each ward or villa.

Many of the larger hospitals provided a fortnightly or monthly bus service from the nearest railway station, but this was not widely used, most visitors travelling by car.

(b) *Doctor's accessibility to relatives* Only 3·5 per cent of patients were in hospitals where a doctor was always on duty during visiting hours, though it was by no means certain that relatives knew he was available should they wish to see him. The great majority of patients (89 per cent) were in hospitals where it was necessary for the relatives to make an appointment to see the doctor (including the medical superintendent). In approximately 3 per cent of cases other arrangements were made, for example a doctor was on duty during visiting hours once a month, or, as in another hospital, the superintendent claimed that relatives could telephone him at any time.

Where the patient lived in an ancillary unit at some distance from the main hospital the situation was particularly difficult since it inevitably meant a special journey to the main unit if a relative wished to see the doctor responsible for the patient, or the medical superintendent. If the ancillary unit was not one which was regularly or frequently visited by the doctor, he might know relatively little about the patient's day-to-day activities or his response to the regime. As a result, relatives of patients in subsidiary units saw almost exclusively nursing rather than medical staff.

The fact that in so few cases were doctors on duty to see relatives made it impossible to relate this factor to the extent of visiting. Nor did the presence of a doctor in any way indicate that relatives used the opportunity to discuss patients with him. One medical superintendent commented that in six years he had only seen one relative: 'No one wants to come and see the medical superintendent'. Another said he thought most relatives were not at all interested: 'Once a patient is in hospital, he is out of the way'.

The superintendent of a large hospital where a doctor was always on duty during visiting hours said that they aimed to do a great deal of counselling: 'Mental retardation is a family problem. It [counselling] is a very important service and helps when they come to visit'. He was one of a very small group who offered such a service; most superintendents considered it desirable, but said that they had no facilities. Sometimes relatives were referred to the Local Authority Mental Welfare Officer, and very occasionally to the hospital social worker if one were employed.

(c) *Parents' Associations or League of Friends*   A third factor which we suggested might influence the extent of visiting was the presence of an active Parents' Association. In practice it often proved difficult to obtain reliable information about these associations – in many hospitals the superintendent was not interested and had only the vaguest notion of how many parents belonged. Where this was not the case, and superintendents were relatively well-informed, the size of membership was no guide to the number of parents who participated in hospital affairs; as in so many associations there appeared to be a small group of activists, but the majority were nominal members who did little more than contribute financially and attend such functions as Open Day.

There was an almost direct *inverse* relationship between unit size and membership of the Parents' Association. If units with under 100 beds (which usually had no association) are excluded, the smaller the unit the more likely was it that there would be a high proportion of parents belonging to the Parents' Association – whether actively or not. Thus the only units in our sample where *all* parents were members had fewer than 1,000 beds. Similarly units of more than 1,800 beds were more likely to have no association.

Furthermore it was in units with between 300 and 999 beds that the activities of both the Parents' Association and the League of Friends were most widespread. Whereas in the larger hospitals both these organizations were primarily concerned with providing material comforts (television, outings, holidays, pocket money, toys, film projectors, etc.) and with fund raising for hospital amenities for both patients and staff, in the medium size units other, more personal activities, such as arranging lectures or discussion groups for parents, and visiting patients who had no relatives at all were likely to be included.

We referred earlier to the fact that some of the biggest hospitals have no Parents' Association, and it interesting to compare the reasons given by two medical superintendents whose hospitals were in the same area:

First superintendent:

> Because of socio-cultural, and economic patterns in a working-class area. They haven't the time or the money or the culture. They complain that it's disgusting that we haven't a Parents' Association or League of Friends, but when I sent out six hundred letters asking them to form one, one Jewish gentleman and one wealthy lady replied saying they couldn't come themselves but they would send money. The others said they couldn't come because they had to work.

Second superintendent:

> Reason? Our catchment area – the distance they would have to come and the general factor – the shortage of all types of worker in this hospital. [League of Friends?] In the past many local people visited the hospital and it appears some had keys to the hospital. It was necessary to control these privileged people who came, and so we find a certain resentment in the past to the existence of a mental hospital in the area. It was politically difficult to form a Friends of the Hospital because of the apparent number of factions that existed. To get over this I introduced the WVS who are doing many of the things that the Friends would do . . .

Letter writing and the use of telephone

Two other matters which might conceivably bear some relationship to the amount of contact patients had with their relatives were letter writing and the use of the telephone. In almost all cases we were told that stationery was provided for any patients who wanted it, and that both staff and other, higher grade, patients helped those unable to write. We have no data about the number who actually did so, nor did we see any evidence of letter writing on the wards, though patients often showed us with great pride the cards and letters they had received from relatives and friends.

With regard to the telephone, 43·3 per cent of patients had no access to the telephone at all.[1] Thirty-eight per cent could use the public telephone box in the hospital if they wished, but no one gave

---

[1] Telephones having an outside line were not normally available on wards and staff wishing to use the telephone had to make their calls from the general office or use the public call box.

them any instruction. A further 13·7 per cent received instruction 'when possible', often in school or evening classes. Patients who worked outside the hospital, or those who were allowed town parole could, of course, use public telephone boxes and in one hospital the chief male nurse specifically sent patients to town in order to practice making 'phone calls to him. In one hospital where patients were not encouraged to use the telephone, the matron told the interviewer that the question had made her think, and that they would, in future, start training patients.

There was no connection at all between patients' freedom to use the telephone (with or without instruction) and the amount of face to face contact with relatives.

Summary

In many of the preceding chapters we have suggested the sheer impossibility of providing more than basic physical care for most of the many thousands of patients in subnormality hospitals today. Patients who are not physically ill or totally disabled appear to be confined to their wards largely because there is nowhere else for them to be and scarcely anyone to train them. On the ward they cannot be helped individually partly because nursing staff are busy performing the work of ward maids or nursery maids and partly because their role as nurses has not been redefined by medical or senior nursing staff.

Yet in this chapter we have indicated just how little seems to be done by the hospitals to ease the load by encouraging contact with the community outside. In any institutional setting there are natural barriers to communication between 'inside' and 'outside'; the hospital erects others – by being physically remote, by providing no satisfactory environment for functionally meaningful visits, by restricting parole and so forth. The fact that 37 per cent of patients in the sample had neither been visited in the past year nor gone home indicates a high degree of isolation, yet little appears to be done to encourage more contact between the patients and their relatives.

Hostility is fortunately rare, but neutrality commonplace; yet with counselling and encouragement there might be greater willingness on the part of those outside to take patients home for periods and so relieve pressure on nursing staff. If parents were allowed on the wards to help feed and look after their children, or permitted to go into the schools and training departments, they would see the positive side of hospital life, and staff might benefit from a feeling that their work is appreciated by parents and relatives.

Similarly, if more encouragement were given to organizations like Parents' Associations and Leagues of Friends, people would surely be found who were willing to involve themselves in the day to day activities of the hospital. Undoubtedly many people are glad to have

Q

the excuse not to involve themselves, to avert their heads as they pass the hospital gates, and there are certainly parents who do not want to visit their children. But we believe that the reluctance of the community to become involved with the life of the hospital is part of a two-way process. There is an unconscious resistance by staff at all levels to allowing the outside world to impinge upon the world of the institution and to allowing patients to leave the hospital and see the world outside for themselves. Either happening may disrupt the social equilibrium of the regime in which a vital component is 'order'. 'Order' is a very fragile thing, achieved only as a result of long and patient efforts on the part of the staff, and although easily disturbed, it can only with difficulty be re-established. Furthermore staff develop a proprietorial interest in their patients and for many of them responsibility, care and control are indivisible.

Chapter 10

BLACKBRICK AND CLOVERFIELD[1]: A STUDY OF TWO SUBNORMALITY HOSPITALS

THE aim of this chapter is to supplement the preceding account of a national sample of hospitals with a more detailed discussion of two particular hospitals which were studied intensively.[2] We have concentrated particularly upon the formal objectives of the institutions and the extent to which these are being met; this will inevitably involve discussion of the physical and relational difficulties existing within the hospitals and will, we believe, both emphasize and highlight many of the problems to which attention has already been drawn in the preceding chapters.

In selecting primarily the formal structure of the hospital for study we recognize that insufficient attention has been paid to the informal aspects of hospital organization, and in particular to the question of patients' relations with each other and with staff. To include this area of hospital life would have necessitated selecting a small number of wards and treatment units within each hospital and spending a great deal of time in them, since, unlike general hospitals, prisons, or institutions for old people, verbal communication is extremely difficult with the majority of subnormal patients in hospital, and until one has learned to understand both their words and their behaviour, any interpretation of relationships and feelings can be dangerously misleading.[3]

We shall begin by a discussion of the organizational structure of the two hospitals, then go on to consider the extent to which they possessed clearly defined formal objectives, and how far these objectives accorded with the policy statements made by the Ministry of

[1] In order to maintain confidentiality the names of hospitals and subsidiary units are, of course, fictitious.

[2] The findings of this section of the survey are based largely upon informal methods of observation and discussion (see Chapter 2, p. 37 ff.).

[3] A study of the informal structure would of course make a very valuable contribution to the understanding of subnormality hospitals and might well raise important queries regarding some of the findings of this study. In institutions for offenders the inmate subculture is able to modify the formal structure in important ways and this may well be true of the patient subculture in subnormality hospitals. See for example, Miles, A. E.: 'Some Aspects of Culture Amongst Subnormal Hospital Patients', *Brit. J. Med. Psychol.* (1965), 38, 171.

Health. We shall then examine the ways in which the objectives are carried out in the treatment and training of patients, and discuss those aspects of hospital life which seem to impede the achievement of stated aims.

The physical setting

In many respects the two hospitals selected were polar opposites in that the areas they served differed widely in terms of their economic and social characteristics. One, Blackbrick, is situated on the fringe of a major conurbation, drawing both its patients and its staff from a vast metropolitan complex that has inherited all the worst features of the Industrial Revolution: physical congestion, bad housing and atmospheric pollution. Despite a post-war programme of urban renewal, it has been affected by population changes and a range of social problems associated with the influx of immigrants.

The other hospital, Cloverfield, is situated in the verdant surroundings of a rolling countryside, far removed from smoke, grime, and congestion and away from any major centre of population. Unlike Blackbrick, Cloverfield draws its staff and patients from a vast area more than a hundred miles long and sixty miles wide, spread over six counties. It serves both a large rural population and a number of important industrial and market towns that happen to be located within the borders of its catchment area.

Both hospitals are comparatively large institutions, holding approximately 1,000 patients. Like many of the hospitals studied, neither of them is located on a single site, but the differences between them in this respect are important. Blackbrick consists of one main unit housing some 700 patients, and a second, smaller hospital eight miles away for approximately 200 male patients; the remaining patients are distributed between four much smaller units, Beeches, Firs, Pines and Bellevue all within fairly close proximity of each other and of the main hospital from which they are administered.[1] There are no children in any part of the Blackbrick complex.

The situation is quite different at Cloverfield: here roughly 400 patients live in the ten wards comprising the main unit. At Springbush, some forty miles away, about 300 patients are accommodated in five male wards and one children's ward; a further 175 patients live sixty miles from Cloverfield at Bedwell where there are three female wards and a male annexe. There is a hostel for 14 male patients at Chalk Hill, situated on the outskirts of a small village twelve miles from Cloverfield; and at Southwell, twenty-two miles from the main hospital, there is one ward for 65 patients. Finally

---

[1] These are habitually referred to as 'hostels' although in fact they are run by nurses as though they were wards of the main unit.

Northridge, two miles away, provides a special children's unit accommodating 30 children and 6 females.[1]

Problems arising from the dispersal of units

Since this pattern of dispersal was common to most of the hospitals visited, some special attention was paid to its relevance in this more detailed study. The consequences are important in understanding the effectiveness of the hospitals in terms of their social cohesion and administrative efficiency.

In terms of management, such groupings are often far from ideal; for any institution to maintain a sense of social solidarity and administrative purpose there must be manifest opportunities for communication, and while distance may to some extent be overcome by the telephone, this can provide no substitute for the infinite variety of face to face contact which stems from physical proximity.

The hierarchical structure which characterizes institutions such as hospitals reinforces the social distance between various levels of staff, and by virtue of the uneven distribution of authority, has an in-built tendency towards the isolation, and even alienation, of the lowest ranks of staff. This tendency is accelerated by the physical dispersion of the units of the hospital, since communications between staff are likely to diminish in direct proportion to rank. That is to say, the extent of inter-unit communication at the upper level of the hierarchy is less likely to be affected by dispersal than that at the lower levels, simply because the latter have no formal need to maintain contact with their peers in other units.[2] It does not necessarily follow, however, that communication will be maintained at a higher level on the administrative plane, and one of the characteristics noted at Cloverfield in particular was a lack of co-ordination between the units comprising the hospital. The economies of scale achieved by having in common such services as laundries and engineering staff are lost unless these activities are geared to the needs of all the units of the group. The tendency is for specialist staff to see the problems of the units in which they are themselves located as being the most important. The immediacy of perception is an important determinant of action.

Formal organization

As in all National Health Service Hospitals, ultimate authority for the provision of services is vested in the Ministry of Health, but the Ministry is in London and remote from the everyday life of the

[1] Since the research was carried out, a further rural property has been acquired, situated 16 miles from Cloverfield. The Medical Director, Group Secretary and newly established Principal Nursing Officer moved there in the autumn of 1966 but at the time of writing (December 1967) three are still no patients.

[2] See also discussion in Chapter 6, p. 125ff.

hospital. Real external authority is vested in the Regional Hospital Board who are charged with administering the services within their area. But to most of the staff at Cloverfield the Board seemed equally remote, mainly a body to be held responsible for the lack of financial support necessary to run the hospital in the way that they thought proper. At Blackbrick the Regional Hospital Board appeared to give the hospital a good deal of freedom in deciding how its financial resources were to be allocated, although all capital work had to be approved by the Board. The medical superintendent thought that perhaps there was too much freedom since it was possible for money to be wasted by bad administration. Nevertheless a certain inflexibility is imposed by the accounting system of the hospital service which does not allow funds to be carried over from one financial year to the next. A striking example of how what is bureaucratically convenient can be therapeutically disruptive arose over the renewal of central heating on some of the villas. Clearly it would have been most convenient for this work to have been done during the summer, but the Board was unable to allow funds to be carried over until the following year and the hospital secretary thought that money would not be made available for the same project again, so the work was done in mid-winter with maximum inconvenience to both patients and staff.

An example of apparent bureaucratic ineptitude concerned the kitchen boiler which had been fitted some nine months earlier. The boiler was designed to operate at 150 psi but the safe limit for the system to which it was coupled was only 80 psi. Prior to the fitment of a reducing valve, the only thing which prevented the boiler from blowing up was a thermostat, which was potentially fallible and which was, therefore, constantly watched by one of the engineering staff. A reducing valve had been ordered and was actually on the site, but it could not be fitted as the Regional Hospital Board had not authorized the expenditure. The hospital secretary had attempted to get authorization for nine months and had repeatedly written to the Board, quoting a warning from the insurance company to the effect that the boiler was dangerous. Finally, the *Hospital Management Committee* took the decision to proceed with the repair and wrote to the Board informing them of the step taken. This produced the desired money and authorization. One result of this delay was, however, that serious faults had developed in the system which by then required immediate attention; but the work was not being carried out because it could not be decided whether the contractors were responsible or not and therefore no decision could be taken as to the financial liability.

The Hospital Management Committee at Blackbrick

The Hospital Management Committee acts as an agent for the

Regional Hospital Board and is responsible for the management and control of the hospital. In cases such as the one just described they acted as an intermediary between the hospital administration and the Board, and when maintenance work is in progress this relationship can be a crucial one. In general terms the managers are responsible for the engagement of all staff below the rank of registrar (the Regional Hospital Board is responsible for those above). At Black-brick three members of the Management Committee were doctors, nine were local persons eminent in social and political life, and eight members of the hospital staff attended in an advisory capacity. The chairman was the squire of a small village near one of the units (Crossways) and his family had had close connections with it when in the past it had been a private institution. Although he did not play an active part in policy making, long years of experience with Cross-ways gave him a competent knowledge of hospital business and a kindly, if paternalistic, concern for the welfare of the staff. The Committee itself was described by the hospital staff who attended as a 'rubber stamp'. This is scarcely surprising given that members of the Hospital Management Committee are essentially seen as visitors to the hospital community rather than participants in its daily life; hospital staff – like those in penal establishments – think of the institution as a closed world that can *only* be understood by those whose lives are largely encompassed by it. During the period the research worker was in the hospital the Committee set up three new sub-committees and these appeared to make an important improve-ment in that members of the full Committee became much better informed. At Crossways there is a separate hospital secretary res-ponsible to the Group secretary at Blackbrick, and also a separate house committee.

The main Committee was largely passive,[1] service on it for the most part being literally a 'public service' such that any member of a local socio-political elite would regard as normal. The relative passivity of the Committee encouraged the dominance of the permanent staff, of whom the medical superintendent was far and away the most powerful. At Blackbrick the traditions of a strong medical superintendent died hard and although the previous incum-bent had been retired for almost fifteen years, his views were still quoted with reverential approval. He had particularly disliked the Committee structure and had described administration by committee as 'democracy with the accent on the mock'.

Some years previously the then Chairman of the Hospital Manage-ment Committee had made an unheralded visit to the hospital. The erstwhile medical superintendent summoned him to his office and pointed out that although, as Chairman, he was free to visit the hospital, he, as medical superintendent, had the right to be informed

---

[1] Most members remained completely silent throughout the meetings attended by the research worker.

of the visit and to accompany him round the hospital. This tradition had been maintained by the present superintendent so that members of the Committee paid only formal visits to the hospital. Having no independent sources of information, Committee members learned only those things which were fed to them by senior staff, a crucial state of affairs when the access of patients to the Committee is in any case limited, and relatives appear to take little active interest in what goes on in the hospital.[1]

The senior staff used the Committee's structural authority to take up matters with outside bodies, such as the Regional Hospital Board, and on one occasion with the Ministry itself. Being effectively in charge of the Committee, the medical superintendent was not likely to bring examples of discord or conflict amongst his staff to the notice of the Committee for discussion. The rest of the staff did not question this state of affairs, partly out of loyalty and partly because of their consciousness of their own inferior status in the hierarchy. In Committee, they did not see themselves as policy makers, but as executives. They may have had doubts about the wisdom of some decisions affecting therapeutic services, but they did not publicly question the superintendent's actions. On one occasion at a meeting of the Management Committee at Crossways, the hospital secretary attempted to disagree openly with the medical superintendent about arrangements for an Open Day. This was dealt with by the medical superintendent suggesting that they talk about the matter after the meeting as it was not committee business. After the meeting, when only the Chairman, medical superintendent, chief male nurse and research worker remained in the room, the dispute became heated, to the embarrassment of the Chairman who, when appealed to by the secretary, declined to intervene on the grounds that the wishes of the medical superintendent, as chief officer of the hospital, should be deferred to.

Thus a tradition of personal autocracy established before 1948 persisted until the present time. That the medical superintendent *should* dominate and control is part of the tradition of Blackbrick and one which the senior nursing staff and the lay administrative officers in particular accept as legitimate, even if they do not always agree with the nature of the decisions which stem from the exercise of such power. Representatives of the Medical Advisory Committee did not attend any meetings of the Hospital Management Committee during the research period. This may have been partly due to the fact that the superintendent did not easily delegate authority to medical staff, and partly to the fact that there was a good deal of conflict between the doctors. The individual tradition of command which has thus

[1] This was possibly made worse by the fact that there were no children; the Parents' Association was said to have about 100 members, of whom 40 were said to be active, but of the 1,000 patients in the hospital fewer than 10 per cent were known to be without relatives.

become an integral part of the Blackbrick staff culture is reinforced by the fact that the present medical superintendent is a man of eminence in the field of subnormality outside the hospital. The Management Committee, because it has a low level of motivation for involvement in the details of decision making, and because it is at a distinct disadvantage in having minimal contact with the hospital except through the superintendent, is in no position to challenge his supremacy. Thus in no sense does the Committee really 'manage', and the scope of its activities are narrowly defined by the hospital staff. It may be concerned with making decisions about grants to the staff social club, or special awards to the lower ranks of the hospital staff, but beyond this kind of topic its policy-making role is largely to approve the decisions that have already been taken by the medical superintendent.[1]

The Hospital Management Committee at Cloverfield

The situation at Cloverfield is complicated by the existence of so many subsidiary units. The Hospital Management Committee is centred on Cloverfield itself, where there is a Group Secretary and a deputy who have responsibility for Cloverfield, Northridge, Chalk Hill and Southwell. This Hospital Management Committee has three sub-committees (nursing services, finance and general purposes, and medical advisory committee), and in addition two house committees whose meetings are held in rotation in the various subsidiary units. Springbush and Bedwell share a separate house committee: there is a hospital secretary based upon Springbush who is administratively responsible to the Group Secretary at Cloverfield.

As at Blackbrick, all the committees at Cloverfield as well as those at Springbush and Bedwell were dominated by decisions made by the hospital staff, but this was achieved by manipulative skills rather more than at Blackbrick where it resulted from a combination of a medical superintendent with a dominant personality and the disinterest of the Committee members. At Cloverfield in any area of disagreement, medical and nursing representatives supported each other against the Committee members and in most cases were supported in turn by the administration, although sometimes the administration preferred the role of neutral and unbiased mediator. Many of the senior staff felt that the committee machinery was a façade, since all major decisions had already been taken in someone's office beforehand, the main skill involved being that of giving the Management Committee the impression that it was making its own decisions.

[1] In an earlier chapter we referred to attempts by the Ministry of Health to limit the power of medical superintendents, and we have suggested that the extent to which this was achieved varied greatly from hospital to hospital. The fact that at both Blackbrick and Cloverfield the superintendents retained considerable power will be discussed later in this chapter in the section dealing with administration.

As at Blackbrick much time was spent discussing the smallest details; relatively few members of the Committee contributed anything to the discussion.[1] The first half hour of one meeting was spent talking about the inadequacies of a boiler recently installed in one of the units. Senior nursing staff and administrators felt that the people on the Committee were far too old and had been members for far too long. It was thought that they tended to use appointments to the Management Committee as a means of self-advancement for social, business or political ends. Most of the members were said to visit the hospital only rarely and almost never went on the wards. Some attended meetings only infrequently, some came but never spoke, and some appeared quite uninterested. On the other hand a few did try to take an interest in all the activities of the hospital. Unfortunately the chairman was not seen by the research worker and his deputy chaired all the meetings we attended, and we were therefore unable to assess the chairman's role in the situation.

Having very briefly indicated the organizational structure of the hospitals, we will now consider their formal objectives.

Formal objectives of the subnormal hospital as defined by the Ministry of Health

Only very shortly before our visit to Cloverfield and Blackbrick, the Ministry of Health had sent out a circular – HM (65) 104 – entitled 'Improving the Effectiveness of the Hospital Service for the Mentally Subnormal'.[2] This was the first time that the objectives of such hospitals had been officially set out and made readily available to the staff. The circular was accompanied by an enclosure which pointed out that the considerations which applied to an earlier circular relating to the effectiveness of hospitals for the mentally ill, applied equally to hospitals for the subnormal. The general aim of hospital care, in the words of the enclosure, is: 'wherever possible to enable the patient to return to life in the community, either independently, or with help from the local authority, or from other sources'. It goes on to state, categorically, that 'patients admitted to hospital because they are mentally handicapped generally have emotional, social or physical problems as well'. Seven categories of patient who might be admitted to a hospital for the subnormal are then listed:

(i) those requiring constant nursing care;

---

[1] At the meetings attended by the research worker fewer than six people usually contributed to the discussions.

[2] The implications of this circular will be further discussed in a later chapter, but we found the statement of objectives contained therein to be a useful framework against which the findings of our intensive study could be evaluated. See also Stewart, R., and Sleeman, J.: *Continuously Under Review*, Occ. Papers on Social Administration, No. 20 (1967). This report studies the response of RHBs and HMCs to a Ministry Circular relating to out-patient departments.

(ii) those in need of special methods of diagnosis;

(iii) those requiring hospital treatment for a condition other than subnormality but who cannot be admitted to other hospitals;

(iv) those with marked physical disabilities who cannot be cared for at home;

(v) those with severe behaviour disturbances making them unsuitable for care in the community;

(vi) those requiring special security conditions;

(vii) those requiring short-term care.

The emphasis throughout the pamphlet is in the direction of admitting to hospital only those patients who cannot be cared for elsewhere, and ensuring that only those for whom no other provision is possible remain in the hospital.

The hospitals' reaction to the circular

(a) *Cloverfield* At Cloverfield, at the time the study began,[1] the distribution of the circular had barely reached committee level. By April it had been discussed by both the Medical Advisory Committee and at a session of the Hospital Management Committee itself, at which the medical director maintained that it reflected credit upon the Cloverfield Group since there was nothing in the circular that was not already part of their hospital policy. In other words, it was suggested that there was nothing in the circular that was *inconsistent* with the formal ideology of the hospital as perceived by the upper echelons of the hierarchy. To senior medical staff the circular appeared as a reinforcement rather than a spur. The question revolved around the degree to which there was a perceived margin between the goals of the hospital and actual performance.

The circular was later criticized by some of the senior nurses who said that its faults lay in that it pre-supposed a full establishment of staff. Furthermore much of it was considered to be unrealistic and unrelated to the facts of life in subnormality hospitals; for example to speak of bringing patients *back* into the life of the community was considered largely irrelevant and meaningless, because most of them had never *been* part of the community outside.

Certain hospitals within the Regional Board had duplicated the circular and were using it in training programmes for staff; this did not appear to be the case at Cloverfield and until the final stages of the research, the document had not been seen by either the social worker or by the union officials, the latter maintaining that they did not know of its existence. This may reflect the ineffectiveness of communication within the organization – the hospital authorities being responsible for its dissemination among the staff – and/or the relative isolation of the union officials. The Regional Hospital Board

[1] The research workers were in the hospitals between January and April 1966.

recommended that the circular be fully discussed and, since it represented government policy, that it be used in every way to improve conditions in the hospitals within the Group.

The major problem that arises with all formal communications of this type, is that, being despatched from the Ministry in London, they inevitably appear remote to the hospital staff as a consequence of their very generality.[1] In institutions such as the subnormality hospitals, the need to maintain the operational efficiency of the institution may make abstract thinking appear as something of a luxury, and concrete recommendations a pipe dream. HM (65) 104 states, for example, that each child needs to have toys and possessions of its own, and that a large stock of play things should be available for use by all children on the ward. Simple, solid play equipment should also be provided, such as swings, climbing frames, chutes and roundabouts. Children at Cloverfield simply did not have enough space in which to play, and given the nature of the accommodation it is difficult to see how conditions which might obtain in some new and gleaming purpose-built unit could be achieved here. Even at Northridge, a highly specialized unit for 30 children, there were only two playrooms.

The staff generally were well aware that the new philosophy of subnormality hospitals required them to accept the view that all patients other than those who are chronic cases with poor prognoses, ought eventually to be discharged. Some nursing staff were of the opinion that if this were so, they ought to be more involved in the after-care of patients, since they considered they knew as much as anyone about them, and thought the relationship between nurses and their charges ought not lightly to be discounted. One senior official explicitly made the point that there were parallels between the hospital and the prison, in that patients were often brought miles from their home area, and put into unwieldy units within the institution. Apart from the shock of being transferred from one type of environment to another, there was often the specific deprivation of the mother. In his view, 90 per cent of admissions need not take place, were there adequate provisions within the community. The person closest to the patient, whether it be relative, nurse, trainer or teacher was the most important factor in rehabilitation and it was necessary for this person to create a warm and affectionate relationship which most patients desperately needed. Such views, of course, while being wholly within the spirit of the circular, are open to criticism on the grounds that they appear rather more like slogans, coined in the atmosphere of the psychology of deprivation, than specific formulae on which an actual programme of treatment might be based. They reflect, too, the gulf between

---

[1] For a similar view see Stewart and Sleeman, *op. cit.*: 'There is too the feeling that circulars are produced by people who are well away from the scene of conflict, who are not aware of the local difficulties and are out of touch with the realities of the situation' (p. 16).

reality and desire which is likely to characterize the thinking and the expression of most staff in institutions which are in the process of having their social 'charter' re-defined and their objectives re-allocated from the sphere of care and custody to treatment and eventual discharge.

(b) *Blackbrick* The medical superintendent of Blackbrick had been personally concerned with the preparation of Circular HM (65) 104 and was therefore wholly committed to it, and saw it as a powerful lever for introducing change into the hospital, authoritative by virtue of its coming from the Ministry.

Possibly because of the superintendent's known involvement, the circular was to some extent a current topic of conversation amongst senior staff. In general its appearance was welcomed, but there is little way of knowing how far this was merely an expression of polite compliance.

Both matron and chief male nurse claimed to welcome the circular, but they appeared more concerned with its practical consequences in terms of the decisions and changes being made by the medical superintendent, rather than with the principles of the circular itself. In the superintendent's view the hospital did not fulfil its training function adequately, and one of his first steps was to remove responsibility for the training schools[1] from the nursing administration and to combine the male and female schools under a new department which was to have parity of status with the nursing hierarchy.

Matron and chief male nurse were both worried about this change since it deprived them of a sphere of authority, and they accepted the change more out of deference to the views of the medical superintendent than through any belief in the rightness of the decision.

Nursing staff generally were not at first encouraged by the matron or chief male nurse to read the document, but this changed when rumours about pending changes, particularly those in the training department, began to circulate lower down the nursing hierarchy – the implication being that the changes would then be seen as relating to the circular. However the nursing staff continued to see the changes as acts stemming from the person of the medical superintendent and not as any implementation of ministerial policy.

Medical staff tended to define their roles rather narrowly, so that they were more concerned with their daily activities than with the objectives of hospital policy. They played no part in the training school which was the most rapidly developing department in the hospital. The medical superintendent believed that the two broad aims of care and training were compatible in the same hospital, on the other hand the senior psychologist disagreed and suggested that

---

[1] Although referred to as 'schools' by the hospital staff, these are in fact training departments; the type of work carried out by patients in these 'schools' will be referred to later in this chapter.

the minority of high grade patients suffered through living in an institution geared to the needs of a greater number of lower grade patients, and he would have preferred to have had the two groups catered for separately.

As at Cloverfield, the lower echelons of the nursing hierarchy seemed infinitely more concerned with the day to day problems of the hospital than with any sophisticated discussion of principles. Thus the view of the hospital and its effectiveness is bound to look different on an over-crowded ward first thing in the morning and in the relative isolation of the superintendent's or the matron's office. The lower one's status the more the reality of the situation (i.e. what is being achieved) impinges upon one's perception of the objectives of the institution. By contrast the higher one's status the more divorced one's perception of objectives becomes from the reality of the situation. This has important implications in terms of achieving change within the institution; it suggests that a prerequisite to changes in the behaviour of subordinate staff towards patients is improved communication regarding the objectives of the institution. (There then arises the question of who is to ensure that the behaviour of staff remains consistent with the newly understood aims.)

It also seems relevant to induce staff to see administrative acts as rational rather than apocalyptic. At the lower levels only the students and those who had recently completed training appeared to consider the wider aims of the hospital as a whole as opposed to the limited aims of their particular role. In training the therapeutic role of the nurse is emphasized, but once they become settled on the wards conflict is likely to arise when they question the more conservative and custodially oriented views of the senior staff with whom they have to work.[1]

Having briefly summarized the Ministry's policy and staff reaction to it, let us now examine how far the objectives set out in the circular are shared by those working in the two hospitals studied.

Formal objectives as seen by staff

(a) *Cloverfield* The medical staff at Cloverfield saw the most important function of the hospital as providing psychiatric treatment for the patients in addition to ordinary physical care. The medical director, in particular, felt strongly that the hospital had a clear duty to concern itself with mentally disturbed patients who were also deemed to be subnormal; he believed that such patients could and should be cared for within the hospital's framework of activities; each patient represented a challenge and the hospital had a legitimate duty to provide psychiatric as well as physical care for these patients.

[1] For a similar situation in relation to new recruits to the prison service see Morris, T., and Morris, P.: *op. cit.*, p. 95.

Whilst the need to provide long-term custodial care was recognized, a further objective was the provision of short-term care for the young chronic-sick in order to meet specific social, medical or economic needs. If possible the hospital should also provide day centres for children who would return to their own homes at night. Both these latter objectives were considered to be a service to the community, but in effect the geographical isolation of all the component units of Cloverfield, and the huge catchment area, made it difficult to talk in meaningful terms of a relationship between the hospital and 'the community'.[1] 'Intellectual subnormality' by itself was not considered by medical staff as an intrinsic reason for admission to hospital, and only those who could not be treated elsewhere ought to be admitted.

Besides physical care, doctors maintained that the hospital ought to provide occupation for patients in order to further their social training with a view to rehabilitation. It should ensure that patients had a balanced existence, in which therapy, work, training, recreation and pleasure all played a part. In other words the requirements of the patient had to be modelled on the life of a normal person. It was recognized that there are factors which limit the possibility of a subnormal person from having complete satisfaction in respect of the basic essentials of man's existence – work, play, and the experience of affection – but this was no reason for not aiming towards them.

Not all patients could be helped equally: for severely handicapped patients the task of the hospital was to prolong life and nothing else, but there were many others whom the hospital could help and stimulate, provided that the right kinds of staff were available.

Where Northridge was concerned, being a unit for disturbed children, the objectives were necessarily more specific, the intention being to provide a therapeutically organized environment in an atmosphere less like a hospital unit than a children's home. The consultant in charge expressed the view that mental subnormality hospitals have a long tradition in the training of children which the psychiatric hospitals do not possess. This view has a great deal of substance in so far as the earliest treatment of subnormals was essentially pedagogic: because the mortality rate of the grossly subnormal was high, those who survived tended to be trainable. At the same time the long period of custodial negativism which characterized mental hospitals from the 1880s to the 1940s effectively precluded treatment for patients of any age, most of all for the young, in respect of whom diagnostic techniques were probably most imperfect.

From the foregoing it will be seen that at least the attitudes of the medical staff at Cloverfield appeared to be closely aligned to the

---

[1] For example see Chapter 9 where reference is made to the large number of voluntary organizations in the community who perform services *for* the hospitals, but nevertheless the amount of actual personal contact between patients and the community is very limited.

treatment ideology of the Ministry Circular which assigns a special role to the subnormality hospital. We shall explore later whether attitude corresponded with practice and whether any failure to achieve these goals was due to shortages of staff, money, and geographical remoteness as suggested by the medical staff, or to more complicated characteristics of hospital organization and training.

The views of non-medical staff were, however, not so uniformly in accord with what may now be regarded as the 'official' view of the role of the subnormality hospital. The social worker, for example, expressed the view that all that could be done for the subnormal was to treat them decently because they did not 'appreciate anything'.

The views of the nursing staff varied greatly: in their attitudes to the psychiatric care of mentally disturbed patients, many of the nursing staff showed antagonism and were in direct conflict with the views of the medical staff, and in particular with those of the medical superintendent. At least one nurse thought that higher grade disturbed patients ought to be sent to a government detention centre. In the case of the severely subnormal and the physically handicapped there was a general feeling that all that could be done was to aim at custodial care in its simplest form. In most other cases it was the role of the hospital to recognize the needs of patients in terms of food, clothing, entertainment, employment and limited contact with the outside world, since except for a very few it was felt there could be no question of their having an independent existence. There were also the institutionalized high grades whom the nurses considered it would be unfair to turn out of hospital after so many years.

However not all nurses shared this pessimistic and limited view. Some saw rehabilitation and work towards eventual discharge as a realistic goal to be aimed at wherever possible. Others placed stress on character training and habit formation which would make for better standards of behaviour in later life. Those who aimed at eventually returning their charges to the community recognized that there were environmental problems for which the hospital could not make proper provision, in particular the question of sexual behaviour.

In general the attitude of nurses was that there was no single function for the hospital: it had to protect and care for the subnormal both with regard to their physical disability and their subnormality, since they were 'less privileged' persons in society. At the same time they should be provided with an environment in which they could express themselves and there should be a stress on association with normal people.

Ancillary staff – engineers, workshop instructors, maintenance men, etc. – saw the function of the hospital rather differently: they considered that persons who were not sick ought to be cared for in the community, not in a hospital. However, once admitted to hospital patients ought to be kept occupied with work of some description otherwise 90 per cent of their time was wasted. They distinguished between *patients* who needed positive treatment, and *persons* who needed work. The prime object of the hospital should be to teach patients to look after themselves to the best of their abilities, although it was recognized that some patients could never function adequately in society. There was a large and important role to be played by day centres and sheltered factories or workshops. Some ancillary staff were critical of the fact that the objectives of some of the training units were still unrealized; this, they maintained, resulted from poor classification of patients which was thought to create difficulties for the staff.

(b) *Blackbrick* Blackbrick is unlike Cloverfield largely because of its different historical development. From 1948 onwards it had been under the direction of two superintendents who had clear-cut views as to the aims of the hospital and who both accepted that it should be directed towards care, treatment and training, instead of merely custodial care. Since then, too, the hospital has had the services of a psychological specialist who has played an important part in building up the training school, so that there is within the hospital plenty of experience of a dynamic policy as opposed to the heritage of institutional inertia which is to be found in most of the hospitals visited.

In the view of the medical superintendent there was a paramount need for the hospital to provide training; in addition he saw the function of the hospital as providing nursing care for the severely disabled, and a curatorial role for those patients who do not need medical care, yet who could not as yet be cared for by their local authorities. This latter role he considered far from essential for the hospital, indeed one which was a relic of the old attitudes towards subnormality which he felt unfortunately lingered on amongst some of the older nursing staff, particularly on the female side. He said he was constantly trying to find ways in which nursing staff could be encouraged to play a more therapeutic and less passive, authoritarian role.

The superintendent's views were supported by the hospital secretary who was strongly of the opinion that the presence of so many patients who were being provided with social care in the absence of local authority provision was deflecting the hospital from its proper therapeutic purpose.

On the nursing side the staff at Blackbrick appeared to divide into two main groups. The first were the older, more senior personnel, many of whom, especially on the female side, had worked at Blackbrick for years, often since before World War II. Their views were formed in the days when Blackbrick was a Colony, and many of the subsequent changes were seen as a falling away from an ideal, rather

R

than a new and more desirable view of treatment in mental sub-normality.

On the other hand there were the younger, more recently trained staff, whose outlook was essentially professional. They had a thera-peutic rather than a custodial bias, but were frustrated by a lack of opportunities to practice the therapeutic role they had been taught.

Charge nurses, sisters, and their deputies found some difficulty in handling abstract concepts about treatment and training, and tended to define objectives in terms of keeping patients clean and tidy, habit training and creating a happy family atmosphere. But there were few indices of success by which performance could be evaluated, although those who were given over to the idea of training could draw satis-faction from seeing the improved skills of the higher grade patients in their care. Those looking after long-term patients felt that they too ought to get results, but on finding that in many cases this was not possible, they tended to become discouraged and to discuss the activities as 'pointless'. Only on some of the high grade villas was there any very articulate expression about aims on the part of senior nurses. But here there was constant resort to the aim of 'getting patients out' even where there were great misgivings about the quality of after-care.

To sum up, one might say that at Blackbrick in spite of the extent to which some of the most senior staff (including administrative nursing staff) were publicly committed to the aims of therapeutic rehabilitation, commitment to an *active* therapeutic ideology was accompanied by anxieties, especially on the part of the nursing staff. Attitudes ranged from near cynicism to frustration and doubt. The medical superintendent commented: 'There is a lot of insecurity in the hospital. Really we are just drifting and barely scratching the surface'. Frustration must be related to such objective features as overcrowding and staff shortages, but there is also the problem of resistance to change and the inertia to which we referred earlier and which is particularly difficult to overcome when the custodial function is so much easier to achieve.

This is well illustrated by the situation at Crossways, which caters exclusively for low grade male patients and where the objectives were straightforward – to keep the patients 'comfortable' and 'happy'. One of the main difficulties mentioned by senior nursing staff was that of preventing both staff and patients from getting 'bored'. However the lack of conflict over the objectives of the unit resulted in considerably less frustration and doubt, and a greater sense of security and cohesion was observable.

From the foregoing it will be seen that even in terms of ideology there were many on the staff of both hospitals who did not share the objectives of the Ministry. Nevertheless without a systematic enquiry involving all members of staff, it is virtually impossible to assess the degree of concensus or conflict between the views of staff at different levels and those of the Ministry. To do so it would be necessary to establish the degree of emphasis given by individuals to particular hospital functions. For example it would seem that the superintendents of these two hospitals, as was the case with almost all the others visited, agreed with the Ministry about the *overall* functions of the subnormality hospital. Where they differed from the Ministry, and amongst themselves, was about the proportion of patients suitable for any specific form of treatment such as short-term care, living or working in the community, suitable for training or education, etc.[1]

Some indication of the discrepancy between the ideal and the reality may emerge from the following discussion of the services available for patients.

The treatment and training of patients

(a) *Cloverfield* Distinct efforts were made to make life as tenable as possible for the patients at Cloverfield; there were, for example, frequent parties for which the nurses spent a lot of time and effort preparing food; the industrial unit arranged outings for patients, there were many little social clubs in the various units, and staff/ patient football games took place as well as matches against local village teams. In one unit the staff ran a patients' art club – it was limited to community singing, dancing and a few individual performances – but it helped to establish a uniquely effective relationship between the staff and patients. A summer pantomime was also planned with the willing co-operation of staff, patients and relatives. Such work undoubtedly encourages self-expression among the patients, many of whom were formerly completely withdrawn and severely disturbed. Unfortunately the organizational restrictions and the often conflicting aims of the hospital leave a vacuum in the lives of the patients which the efforts of the staff are able to fill only partially.[2]

For severely handicapped patients with a poor prognosis, the staff showed, within their general limitations of time and ability, a high degree of devotion and care. From the point of view of *nursing* care little more could be done for such patients and the staff often involved themselves in dealing with the anxieties of relatives.[3]

The demand for beds for the young chronic sick is high and there

---

[1] See, for example, our earlier discussion of hospital function in relation to patients living in the community (Chapter 6, p. 113 ff.).

[2] Nevertheless our observations suggest that more joint activity of this kind took place at Cloverfield than in the majority of hospitals visited, and it was certainly distributed more evenly throughout all the wards.

[3] This is not to say that more could not be done about the medical, educational, psychological and social problems of the patients.

are hopes at Cloverfield for the acquisition of a new unit to accommodate them. In addition to their subnormality, such patients constitute an essentially paediatric rather than a psychiatric problem, whilst in sociological terms they present the hospital with its most serious ideological problem: by emphasizing the function of care, and underlining the futility of hopes for improvement, the presence of chronic patients runs counter to the general direction of the hospital's affirmed intentions.[1] All wards had television except for the two children's cot and chair wards, and radio was arranged through the rediffusion system controlled from the nurses' office. Newspapers and comics were available on all wards, though in many instances the provision of the former appeared to be more of an advantage to the staff, and there was nothing to suggest that television and radio programmes or reading matter were chosen with cognizance of the abilities, needs and interests of the patients.

Many nurses thought that the policy of 'free expression' advocated by the medical director was too lenient, as were his sanctions which were in effect no more than reprimands, whereas they would have preferred the withdrawal of privileges. Where there was bullying by high grade patients of other patients, one explanatory hypothesis put forward by the staff was that this was a legacy that patients had learned from the example of bullying staff of the 'old school'. Although it would be quite untrue to say that there was no evidence of any kind of bullying by staff, it would equally be naive to assume that it never took place.

The treatment of disturbed patients, as we indicated earlier, was a constant source of conflict between medical and nursing staff. The ward staff, with an investment in order, were not always able to interpret and understand the behaviour of patients, and frequently what was reported came into the simple category of misdemeanours such as window breaking. The medical director was not altogether happy about the way in which awkward adolescents, 'erring high grades' and some detained patients were transferred to low grade wards where they had to assist with feeding, cleaning, and toileting the most helpless patients. The method was nevertheless used by the staff as a sanction to buttress their authority.[2]

Psychopathic and psychotic patients were said to demand a great deal more time than other patients, or at least those staff trained only in subnormality nursing perceived it this way. Drug therapy was one form of control, but some nurses took the view that such patients required more outdoor activity – which of course they claimed that staff shortages precluded! The staff were unclear as to the

---

[1] We have since learned that a further unit for the young chronic sick has in fact been opened but this is situated in yet another very isolated unit at a considerable distance from Cloverfield.

[2] In most subnormality hospitals this practice is quite usual, though not necessarily used as a form of sanction.

desirability of separating disturbed patients by putting them in separate wards, which might then become pockets of trouble; on the other hand it was also felt that they exercised a bad influence on other patients, encouraging them to get up to mischief.

At times it was considered necessary to seclude patients or restrain them physically, but this practice was not universally used through-out the hospital. There were 21 wards (excluding Chalk Hill hostel and Northridge) and on twelve of these there was no seclusion book, nor were any patients put into side rooms; strong or restrictive clothing was not used, nor were there railed airing courts attached to these wards.[1] Certain patients are difficult; at night they may throw things out of windows and in one ward restraints had to be used to stop patients eating the paintwork in the sanitary annexes and the day room. Not all nurses held the same view on restraints; one, for example, an RNMS in charge of a ward of adolescent boys, stated his disapproval of sending boys to bed during the day or to seclusion for bad behaviour, and also of the excessive use of tranquillizing drugs. Another nurse, an RNM in charge of a sick and infirm ward said that he had not seen a strait-jacket in use for over 17 years, and he thought that drugs were the answer to the problem of disciplining difficult patients. It could, of course, be argued that the ethical problems can be as great in using drugs as in using strait-jackets. A charge nurse suggested that patients under regular sedation developed 'completely different characters' and this hampered the nurses from discovering the true personality of the patient. Yet accurate assessment of personality was, he felt, important in the training and re-habilitation of both the mentally ill and the mentally subnormal.

The pattern of relationships between staff and patients is in some respects one which contains a high degree of ambivalence and even apparent inconsistency: on the one hand the staff spend an enormous amount of time simply caring for patients and going to great lengths to make them happy, while on the other hand they may resort to a whole series of what are fairly crude methods of controlling refractory behaviour. Certain nurses perceived this contradiction, and felt that seclusion and the use of physical restraint undermined the confidence of patients in the nursing staff.

Cloverfield has two schools, one a junior training centre in the grounds of Cloverfield itself and the other forms part of the children's unit at Northridge. The school at Cloverfield caters for children from outside as well as hospital patients and is run by the local authority. A lack of communication between the teachers and the hospital staff was a major source of criticism on both sides, but neither side seemed to have the initiative to do much about the situation, and most contacts were quite formal and limited.

[1] On five wards nylon strong clothing was used, on three children's wards restrictive clothing was used, and one ward used side rooms for extra bed space and changed patients round if the seclusion of any patient was necessary.

The gulf between the teachers and the nursing staff at the Cloverfield school was made wider by resentment on the part of the nurses that not only did the teachers work a five-day week, but that at times of school holidays they left the scene, leaving behind bored and restless children to be amused and occupied by the nursing staff.

The situation did not, of course arise at Northridge since this was a therapeutic community in which all members of staff shared; staff conflict was minimal within this unit since there were frequent staff meetings and case conferences, and a recognition of the need to break down the hierarchical system. Everyone was considered to have a therapeutic role, including the handiman and gardener. Children returned to their homes during the school holidays in order to help parents gain confidence in handling them. During term time there were two play therapy groups and two classes.

On an adult female ward at Cloverfield a Social and Maturity Training Programme was in operation, the aim being to lead patients towards a more competent standard of living by encouraging them to attend social functions in the hospital, to go out on shopping expeditions, to understand the importance of personal hygiene and appearance, and to take an interest in the various common skills.

At Chalk Hill Hostel the warden encouraged patients to take as full a part in the activities of the community as they could, attending local events in the village, visiting the local pub, and so forth. In the hostel itself whist drives and darts competitions were held which outsiders from the local community were encouraged to attend.

In general both doctors and nursing staff felt that there was a need for greater integration of the sexes, though with some reservations; some thought integration should be limited to social occasions such as entertainments, others felt that eating and working together were an essential feature in the training of any patient. Within the hospital there was said to be a certain amount of homosexuality amongst patients; one nurse explained that this was largely condoned since it was recognized that it in some measure compensated for the deprivation of ordinary heterosexual relationships which was stifled in hospital life. On the other hand since the world outside condemns homosexuality, staff recognized that this variation might well confuse patients when they are discharged or on leave (of absence). Doctors felt there should be a day centre which would provide a half-way house and through the integration of patients at work and play, patients might be better prepared for life in the community.

A substantial amount of time at Cloverfield was taken up with an attempt to train patients to deal with incontinence, although it was recognized that there will always be a small proportion of patients who will never respond to any form of training.

At Springbush there was a Habit Training Unit, but the unit there is not regarded as successful by the staff themselves. The original intention had been that the patients would be divided into small groups in the charge of a trainer, the object being to upgrade patients as they progressed towards bladder control. The work of the unit began with the best of intentions and its failure had a demoralizing effect on the staff. Elaborate progress charts had been prepared, but these were not kept up; the interest of the staff had been lost and the status of the ward, which was initially high within the informal ranking system of Springbush, had gone down. The reasons for failure are complex, but one of them is the fact that medical staff did not seem to have heeded staff warnings regarding the imminent breakdown of the scheme as the number of patients increased and the number of staff decreased. Nor do there seem to have been any attempts to extend staff involvement by using female staff, or by linking the training to other activities, such as occupational therapy.

Occupational therapy exists on quite a modest scale in the Cloverfield group. We have referred above to the Social and Maturity Training Programme at Cloverfield itself which undoubtedly served a definite purpose, but at the other units the possibilities of occupational therapy had not been fully exploited. Some occupational therapists worked on the wards, but this seemed to help the nurses rather than train or interest the patients, and there was a tendency for the therapists to be overloaded with patients in order to relieve pressure on the nursing staff.

There were units for play therapy and handicrafts at Cloverfield, Springbush and Northridge. On the children's cot and chair ward play therapy was the concern of cadet nurses, and there was a happy atmosphere in which higher grade children responded well to the attention and affection that all levels of staff gave them.

At Springbush there was also a therapist attached to the cot and chair ward, but in common with many aspects of life at Springbush, this compared unfavourably with the services at Cloverfield. The children were very low grade and there was little actual space in which they could play. The therapist often became no more than an extra pair of hands on a ward preoccupied with feeding the children and changing their clothes.

Two other groups at Springbush also received a form of play therapy; in one case twelve patients came (in two groups of six) for an hour each morning to a hall where some could play with toys, others did jig-saws and one or two attempted some writing, but these patients could well have benefited from more individual attention over a longer period, and it seems likely that there was a potential here which was not being developed.

Another larger group was run by three untrained nurses who followed a similar programme with rather more patients and for a rather longer period. There was no co-ordination between the two groups and at the time of the research both presented a somewhat aimless picture; it was almost a question of the wives taking patients off the wards in order to give their husbands a rest.[1] The only possible benefit appeared to be the presence of women as 'mother figures' in what was otherwise an exclusively male dominated environment.

The medical officer at Springbush expressed strong views about the acute need for a speech therapist and a physiotherapist in the Cloverfield Group. In his view most of the children in the hospital had normal vocal chords, and their failure to speak resulted from no one having taught them to do so. Similarly with physiotherapy, he felt there were many children who were bedfast or in wheelchairs who would benefit materially from physiotherapy. The only physiotherapist in the Group worked part-time at Cloverfield, and it was generally felt that a full-time therapist would have plenty of work in the Group as a whole.

The pharmacist was also only part-time although great stress was laid upon the use of drug therapy. He came only twice weekly to Cloverfield and maintaining any check on drugs was difficult because of the long lines of physical communication between himself and all the various units. Communications between the pharmacist and individual units varied, and at Springbush the staff did not even accompany him into the dispensary when he made checks. He felt his role was reduced to that of storeman, since drugs were issued to wards on the basis of estimated weekly requirements, and not on an individual basis for each patient, as had been his experience at other types of hospital. Methods of controlling drug expenditure were crude and he believed that savings which could be made by employing cheaper but equally effective drugs were not being effected. He, like many of the part-time staff, was excluded from active participation in the general social system of the hospital, and perceived of himself as an outsider.

(b) *Blackbrick* At Blackbrick only about 30 out of a total of approximately 1,000 patients are confined to bed or chair,[2] most of them are old or chronic sick and are housed in the hospital block. Others who might be expected to gain little benefit from the training provisions of the hospital are mainly a legacy from the past; some, if they were younger, would no doubt be discharged, and they remain in the hospital largely because this is their only home;[3] their presence tends to perpetuate the old Colony tradition. The medical superintendent estimated that up to half the patients could be discharged to the care of the local authorities if suitable hostels had existed. Unlike Cloverfield, which prides itself on the provision of short-term care, there are only very few such patients at Blackbrick, usually no more than half a

---

[1] At Springbush most of the trained nurses were male and their wives worked as assistant nurses or SEN's.

[2] It will be remembered that Blackbrick does not have any children.

[3] Approximately 22 per cent of the patients have been in hospital for 30 years or more, this compares with a figure of only 5 per cent at Cloverfield.

dozen, and there are no special facilities for them. A small proportion of patients (approximately 6 per cent), mostly young males, are in the hospital under the terms of a legal Order.[1] They are not physically restricted, although they cannot discharge themselves and can only go home under special provisions. Some villas have single rooms where patients may be secluded, but no villas are locked and the hospital has numerous exits from which any patient may leave the hospital unobserved.

There is some evidence to suggest that over the years the intellectual level of Blackbrick patients has declined, if only because of more modern and liberal views regarding the release of those patients embodied in the Mental Health Act of 1959. On the other hand this is impossible to demonstrate with any convincing statistics owing to the gross inadequacy of the hospital records, which even now are kept in a very disorganized manner.

The staff universally believe a decline to have occurred even though the hospital still contains a relatively high proportion (compared with most subnormality hospitals) of the higher grades of patient. If there has been a decline, or even if it is felt to exist, it may go some way to explaining why many of the older and more experienced staff are pessimistic about training and therapy, and identify their task in terms of care. Even where there has been a commitment to the idea of training, it is believed by many nursing staff that, in part resulting from a declining interest by the senior psychologist (he has moved his interest to developments outside the hospital) the 'great days of training are over'.

At Blackbrick, treatment by means of drugs is freely administered in the form of tranquillizers, anti-convulsants and sedatives to over one-third of the patients, drugs being used as a means of controlling behaviour as well as for treatment in a strictly medical sense. In practice sanctions were quite often used as a punishment, in particular putting patients to bed early. The medical superintendent disapproved of this, believing that difficult behaviour was a 'symptom of stress and required treatment not punishment'. But the administrative nursing staff who might have acted as agents of the superintendent by cautioning a charge nurse who disciplined patients in this way did not do so because they were nearer to the realities of ward life.

There are separate training schools for males and females, the male school accommodating some 150 patients at the time of the research, of whom 117 were severely subnormal. Patients are engaged on a variety of repetitive assembly tasks under the general supervision of female nursing assistants. There is some mixing of male and female patients as a result of overcrowding in the female training school.

The purpose of the work is of marginally therapeutic value, and is

[1] The figure for Cloverfield is 2 per cent.

largely designed to provide low grade patients with some useful occupation. A few have managed to acquire some dexterity and so have been transferred to undertake the more difficult work on the first floor of the building. Here there were 36 patients, mostly young men considered as being potentially able to earn their own living outside. Several of the nursing staff had industrial experience and under their tutelage patients learned to operate lathes, a drilling machine, and to do some spot welding. Two of the staff have served apprenticeships as fitters and they were capable of breaking down work tasks with the aid of jigs in order to simplify the processes for patients. In addition to light engineering there is some joinery, and two relics of the old days of the Colony crafts remain – tailoring and upholstering.

The female training school offered a more limited range of work. About 100 women and girls attached saucepan menders to cards or sewed together pieces of chamois leather to make mop heads. A few operated sewing machines. The abler patients are given social training in small groups by a teacher and nursing assistant under the supervision of the senior psychologist, with a view to remedying or ameliorating the various inadequacies that psychological testing has revealed.

There is a need for the total environment of the hospital to support the work of specialized training by giving patients the opportunity to develop the wider social skills that they will need outside. One place where this can be done is the canteen, where they can be customers yet not be penalized for their inadequacies by being cheated or ridiculed. They also have dances throughout the winter, frequent outdoor games in summer, a social club for patients under 25, a Darby and Joan group at which the older patients have tea and play bingo. There are also film shows and television, the latter being sometimes a mixed blessing since it is on almost non-stop in the day rooms; one patient at Crossways preferred to escape the cathode tube image by sitting alone in an ill-lit lavatory, quite absorbed in reading seed catalogues!

More research work is carried out at Blackbrick than is the case in most subnormality hospitals, mainly because of the presence of a psychologist who has a substantial reputation in the field as an authority on the training of subnormal patients. Research is principally in relation to high grade patients for whom the prognosis for return to the community as self-supporting or partially so, is good.

Two of the villas which have been extensively and expensively converted and modernized are also to some extent experimental and one is devoted to severely subnormal cases. The number of patients has been drastically reduced (from 60 to 38) so that staff have much more time to spend with them and the general atmosphere is good compared with the physical congestion of other villas. It is hoped that under these improved conditions the behaviour of patients will also improve, reducing, among other things, the level of incontinence.

The other renovated villa is for high grade girls and conditions have been made much more congenial and less institutional.

Neither of these villas is experimental in any scientific sense, but they constitute rather crudely empirical attempts to improve the standard of care for selected groups of patients.

At Crossways, where most of the patients are low grade, they are mostly off the wards during the day either in the various training shops or doing music and movement. Some do weekend work for the local residents, such as sweeping up leaves, and many go down to the local cafe where they sit for long periods and appear to be accepted by the local community.

Most staff eat together in the dining hall. This has great advantages in terms of informal communication, and enables trainers to get to know the nurses and gives the nurses an opportunity for learning what goes on in the shops.

Staff appear to have much greater knowledge of all the patients at Crossways than at Blackbrick where there is a tendency to know well only the high grades, and it was noticeable that staff at Crossways seemed able to understand patients where the research worker was unable to do so, or even when they said nothing.[1] The habits of patients are very regular and charge nurses sought the reason for any deviation, since it was considered to be a possible symptom requiring attention. There was a good deal of bullying of patients by others, as well as of stealing. Many patients were said by staff to sleep on their clothes and took their money with them to the lavatory.

Administration and staffing

(a) *Cloverfield* Cloverfield, as we have already pointed out is not a homogeneous entity, but essentially a group of local units separated in distance such that organization and administration on a *hospital* basis depends upon a sociological fiction and formal channels of communication and command. Chart I illustrates the structural paradigm of each separate unit of the hospital. In broad terms there is a distinction to be drawn between the lay administration, the medical staff and the nursing staff: overall the medical director presides.

Whereas the total picture of command is confused by the distinctions between the three hierarchies, particularly in relation to the overlapping that exists in areas of shared interests, the hierarchy of the nursing staff (Chart II) is simpler and conforms more closely to

---

[1] This type of situation confirmed our belief that any study of inter-personal relations involving subnormal patients would require a quite different methodological approach.

Chart I

FORMAL CHAIN OF COMMAND[1]

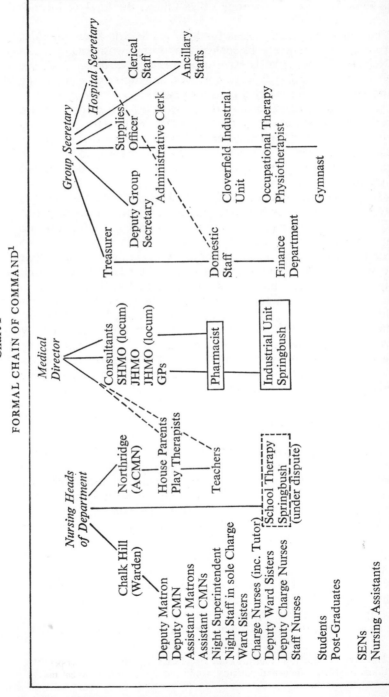

FOR ALL UNITS

MATRON (Cloverfield)
- Deputy Matron
- Assistant Matrons (2)
- Unqualified Tutor
- Charge Nurses / Ward Sisters / Night Sister
- Deputy Charge Nurses
- Deputy Ward Sisters
- Staff Nurses
  - SENs
  - Nursing Assistants
  - Cadets
- *Assistant CMN (Northridge)*
  - Ward Sister
  - SENs
  - Nursing Assistants

ACTING CMN (Cloverfield)
- Assistant CMNs (2)
- Charge Nurses
- Night Charge Nurse
- Deputy Charge Nurses
- Staff Nurses / SENs
- Nursing Assistants
- *Warden* / Relief Warden
  - Students
  - Post-Graduates

CMN (Springbush)
- Deputy CMN
- Assistant CMN
- Night Superintendent
- Charge Nurses
- Deputy Charge Nurses
- Staff Nurses
  - SENs
  - Nursing Assistants

ACTING MATRON (Bedwell)
- Acting Deputy Matron (Unqualified Night Sister in Sole Charge)
- Ward Sisters
- Acting Ranks
  - SENs
  - Nursing Assistants

MATRON (Southwell)
- Deputy Matron
- Unqualified Ward Sister / Sister / SENs
- Nursing Assistants
  - Domestics

KEY: – – – – – Delegated Responsibility

the less complicated model that is found in other institutional settings' such as penal institutions, military units, or ships at sea. It is, moreover, both more explicitly bureaucratic and authoritarian, with fewer ambiguities in the definition of responsibilities at each level.

The administration of Cloverfield as a whole may be divided into two main areas of concern, the first centring around the continuous series of routine and contingent decisions which have to be made in order to keep the hospital functioning on a day to day basis, and the second around the implementation of therapeutic programmes, or treatment policy.

The units are dispersed over a wide area, so that it would not be unreasonable to make an analogy with a larger scale political structure. Cloverfield itself may be regarded as the 'metropolitan centre' of an empire, the constituent parts of which have a measure of self-government, but overall responsibility is vested in the medical director at the centre. He himself sees the units functioning autonomously, and independently of the centre, enjoying parity of esteem, irrespective of size. In some ways this view was quite unrealistic: Cloverfield itself, by virtue of its size and the concentration of the central administrative staff and the training school was, if nothing else, *primus inter pares*. But in formal terms, he, the medical director, was in charge of all the units and in fact attempted to make his position felt. He was conscious of his overall position which was made formal and explicit in the legal status of the constituent parts of the hospital as a whole, 'the Cloverfield Group'. His policies were in evidence in all the units, and their implementation was normally left to the doctor in charge of each individual ward. The standard of medical staffing both in actual number and in quality varied by unit and it might fairly be said that the influence of the medical director was in inverse proportion to the effectiveness of the ward medical authority on the spot. This was particularly true at Northridge where the consultant in charge ran a unit which was virtually autonomous.

Contingent problems were referred to the medical director, but because of the inadequacy of communications, including those by telephone, doctors in units away from Cloverfield were delegated more authority. Thus it might be said that the hospital was modelled, at least from an administrative and political view, like the French empire; units, however remote, are assumed to belong to a whole and to participate in a common process of decision making, irrespective of the extent to which physical distance and inadequacy of communication make for acute practical problems.

Medical matters apart, administrative procedures and decision making constituted a severe problem in the three larger units. Demarcation difficulties and the identification of areas of jurisdiction, together with lack of co-ordination between the administrative and the nursing staff in the Group as a whole, meant that there were constant clashes of personality and professionalism. It must be recognized that these remarks do not apply to the highly autonomous units of the hostel at Chalk Hill, the children's unit at Northridge, and the adult female unit at Southwell. However, the remaining units all suffered severely from unco-ordinated administration.

In an earlier section of this report[1] we dealt at some length with the Ministry of Health's attitudes towards the administration of mental subnormality hospitals, and in particular to the respective roles of the medical and lay administration, and we pointed out that the Ministry gave to the Regional Hospital Boards and Hospital Management Committees the task of deciding upon the administrative organization of any particular hospital, a situation which has led to uncertainty and dissatisfaction affecting not only the organization of the hospitals, but through this the treatment that patients receive.

This is quite apparent at Cloverfield where the major issue is the failure of the system of tripartite administration to enjoy any more than formal legitimacy. The nursing profession as a whole respect the medical profession; the latter constitutes a 'priesthood' with sacred knowledge, while the former stand in a position of reverent acolytes. Hence what the doctors say has, for the nursing staff, an air of authority which depends perhaps less upon the concept of bureaucratic authority than upon the charisma of the doctor's role. In the last analysis the lay administration, lacking as they are in medical knowledge, and therefore not sharing in the charisma of the medical staff, are often seen by the medical and nursing staff merely as clerks who have been translated into positions of power. This is logical in the sense that the administrator and the clerk are both concerned with administration and its execution rather than with treatment. It does not follow of course that the nursing staff will put into operation all the demands of the medical staff, even where these are expressed, and to the extent that the medical director is unable to make a significant impact on the working of a particular unit, the nursing staff will see themselves as having a right to autonomy, even if they do not actually enjoy it, and to challenge the directives of the lay administration.

Matters that concerned either the nursing staff or the administrators alone were dealt with at Cloverfield by the respective heads of the departments, but where there was an overlap of interests (e.g. laundries, maintenance, etc.) altercations took place both at an open and a disguised level. To some extent the outcome of such disagreements was affected by the fact that the three elements in the tripartite system have differential opportunities of expressing solidarity. Nursing and medical staff, because of their ancient establishment in professional terms, and the mystique of their craft, have a source of solidarity which is not yet paralleled among administrative staff. Administrators are, as yet, still under-professionalized, and depend upon their structural powers alone to survive in dispute. At Clover-

[1] See Chapter 3, p. 52 ff.

field itself the lay administration appeared to function reasonably well, partly because the arrival of a new Group secretary was viewed as an improvement upon the previous state of affairs. At Springbush and Bedwell however, the lay administration was found to be engaged in open conflict with the nursing staff, a fact which seriously eroded the morale of the staff as a whole.

Even among the nursing staff themselves, all was not always well. Nursing administration within the Group as a whole tended to be unco-ordinated. With the exception of periodic meetings of the Nursing Services Committee and various other *ad hoc* meetings and social events, there was little inter-unit communication of any kind. The medical director quite openly expressed his preference for a principal nursing officer and a fully integrated nursing service for the Group as a whole, but this appeared to threaten the staff in certain units who had fears for their autonomy.

Individually, units can clearly function well in terms of nursing administration, but much depends upon the extent to which resources are sapped in conflict with the lay administration. At Cloverfield itself the male side functioned adequately, if not dynamically, under three nursing administrators who had between them many years of service. On the female side there were four such administrators who were inclined to delegate less responsibility, with the result that the work was more rigidly performed. At Springbush there were three nursing administrators and superficially there appeared to be a good deal of devolution of authority. On closer inspection however, it is doubtful whether the two junior members of the administrative trio exercised any substantial degree of autonomy since all decisions had to be approved or countersigned by the chief male nurse. At this unit senior ward staff suffered from a frustrated sense of loyalty in the conflict between nursing and lay administration; in addition they were severely hampered by a series of restrictive standing orders. At Bedwell, where severe conflict between nursing and lay administration also existed, the situation was not so acute in that there was only one member of the nursing administration and he had been able to consolidate the nursing staff and reduce disputes among them.

Staff recruitment clearly played an important part in the maintenance of stability in the hospital community at Cloverfield. Patterns of recruitment in turn emphasized the status distinctions between various levels of staff. Professional and specialist staff were recruited by means of advertisements in the press and professional journals, whereas the unqualified and unskilled staff were recruited essentially on a local basis and by means of personal contact through existing members of staff. The extent to which this applied varied as between one unit and another, depending upon its geographical location and the consequent condition of the labour market. The main unit at Cloverfield itself drew its unskilled staff from the neighbouring village which had a population of some 2,500 people. As far as the village itself was concerned, virtually all those who could be recruited had been, and the paucity of public transport precluded people from other, more distant villages, from seeking employment at Cloverfield. In addition to this, the area is one in which there is a generally pronounced rural/urban drift of population. At Cloverfield there were a substantial number of husband/wife appointments among the staff, particularly among the trained nursing staff. In some cases there were wives willing to work as nursing assistants although after two years of full-time and five years of part-time service they had been assessed as SENs.

At Springbush the situation was most extreme in that practically all the trained nursing staff were male while their wives worked as untrained nursing assistants or State Enrolled Nurses. This is probably the most geographically isolated of all the units, having to all intents and purposes no public transport and with the nearest settlement being hamlets some three to four miles away. The recruitment pattern at Springbush was also unusual, in that almost all its staff had been recruited from other subnormality and psychiatric hospitals and as a result they tended to be more knowledgeable and less parochial in their outlook, with experience in psychiatric as well as subnormality nursing. As opponents of the lay administration they were to that extent the more formidable. The possibilities of work and participation for both husbands and wives on the nursing staff at Springbush makes for a degree of cohesion and solidarity which showed itself in the conflict with other types of staff.

(b) *Blackbrick* In terms of the formal structure, the administration of Blackbrick is similar to that of Cloverfield (see Chart III) though simplified because the hospital really consists only of Blackbrick itself and Crossways (the remaining units are literally on adjoining grounds) and even these two are within a few miles of each other. Nevertheless Crossways is viewed by the medical superintendent as a completely separate hospital, one which he regards as having better staff, better staff/patient relations, and a better atmosphere. Being a single sex unit (and therefore having only one nursing hierarchy), it is housed in one building, with only one dining hall, and the workshops are contained within the building; as a result there is a much greater degree of integration than at Blackbrick.

As in Cloverfield, the medical superintendent has overall responsibility for the running of the hospital, but the introduction of the tripartite system has again made some inroads into the traditional structural supremacy of the superintendent, in that there are now three hierarchies, with the nursing administration subdivided into two parallel and autonomous hierarchies – male and female.

The tendency of tripartitism in most hospitals has been to limit the power of the medical superintendent by giving greater autonomy to other sectors of the staff. At Blackbrick, the process of change has

s

Chart III

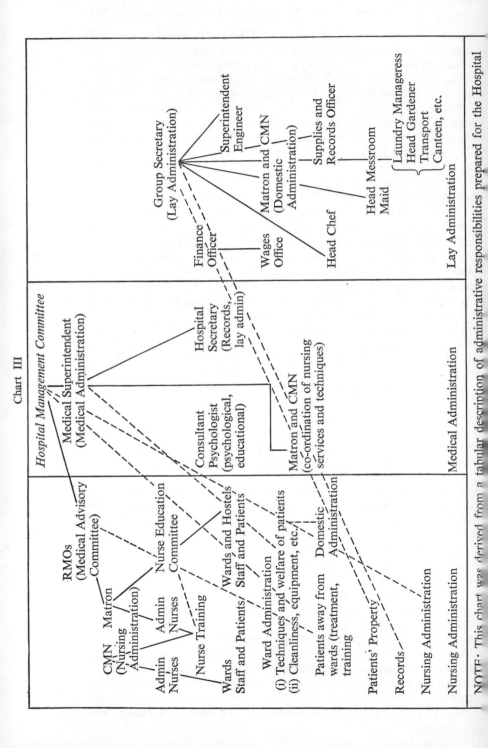

NOTE: This chart was derived from a tabular description of administrative responsibilities prepared for the Hospital

not been made easier by the fact that the medical superintendent holds certain views that are in direct conflict with those of many of the medical staff. He sees mental subnormality as being primarily an educational rather than a medical problem, and ideally would like to see the hospital divided between pedagogic and nursing care. Because he did not want Blackbrick to become what he called a 'doctors' hospital' he tended to define the doctors' role as narrowly as possible, frequently mentioning that several doctors had actually left the hospital because 'no one took any notice of them' (sic).

In his relationship with the nursing heads it was apparent that despite the tripartite system his traditional primacy was essentially unchallenged. So confident did he feel of the loyalty of the nursing staff that he did not think it necessary to make out a case for taking away from them the responsibility for the training schools, he merely went to the Management Committee, received the official *imprimatur* and presented his nursing colleagues with instructions which he expected them to carry out.

The nursing administrators themselves eschewed the role of policy makers, partly because being inured to the old traditions of the Colony, they did not see this as their role at all. As mentioned earlier, when asked about the objectives of the hospital and ways in which change might bring them nearer to realization, both matron and chief male nurse were reluctant to express their own views and echoed those of the medical superintendent. The Group secretary was also content with the role subordinate to that of the medical superintendent.

There were, of course, ways in which although the authority of the medical superintendent could not be disputed, its effectiveness could be minimized.[1] The existence of separate hierarchies of administration meant that there was a multiplicity of levels between the medical superintendent and 'front line' staff. Communication with junior levels of the nursing staff was limited by the need to channel everything through the chief male nurse or matron, whose areas of autonomy have been relatively extended. In this way information could be distorted or blocked altogether on the way down. In consequence the lowest levels of nursing staff tended to have a stereotypical image of the medical superintendent which emphasized the social distance between them. Because he was rarely seen on the wards at Blackbrick – all his personal patients being at Crossways – ward staff saw him as a vindictive tyrant of unpredictable moods who demanded impossible standards of perfection; they had little opportunity to check this image against reality simply because they had hardly any direct contact. Had he made such contact, he would have offended the nursing administration who saw mediation as an inalienable right. He himself was not fully aware of this situation as was demonstrated by his belief that his attendance at ward meetings

[1] See, e.g., p. 231 *supra* in relation to the use of sanctions.

as an aid to training junior staff, contributed to a better understanding between himself and the nurses. In fact the junior nurses knew exactly what was expected of them in these discussions, and were subsequently told by senior nurses to forget all he said after he left the ward – *they* were in charge of the patients, and *they* knew what was best.

The superintendent recognized that when he was away the hospital 'went into neutral'. It seems likely that he did not fully appreciate the gulf that existed between the various autonomous sectors of the tripartite administration; in order to carry through any policy decision it had to be sustained by continuous pressure from the top since conflict and confusion of aims precluded any consensus about the direction of change. In many matters such pressure was not sustained over a long enough period partly due to the many demands on the superintendent's time.

The position of the medical superintendent at Blackbrick illustrates the degree to which traditional, as opposed to bureaucratic, authority is effective only in so far as it is systematically executed. Autocracy is nothing if it is not accompanied by single-mindedness and sustained application. On the other hand the tripartite system was ineffective partly because of the extent to which the traditional system lingers as legitimate in the eyes of many of the staff, and partly because it did not incorporate a division of labour which was clearly defined. In an efficient bureaucracy, roles are strictly defined and behaviour in contingent situations is anticipated by a system of formal rules and restrictions. At Blackbrick there was no clear division of powers, but rather a series of overlapping jurisdictions, demanding co-ordination which could not always be relied upon to originate from the medical superintendent. Areas of overlap and ambiguity included, for example, the laundry, hospital transport, and the training school: although the nursing administration were directly responsible to the Management Committee, the matron and chief male nurse could find themselves dealing with medical or lay administration over all such matters.

At Blackbrick the behaviour of the nursing and lay administration can be seen as an amalgam of compliance on the one hand and resentment on the other. Too inhibited by respect for traditional authority to challenge outright, even on issues over which there was disagreement, they reacted by failing to mediate fully between the medical superintendent and their own subordinates.

The other medical staff were in a slightly different position. Their links with the nursing staff were at lower levels, in that without the sisters and charge nurses there was no way of knowing which patients needed to be treated. Because many patients are relatively or even totally inarticulate, often a physical disorder will only be revealed by a variation in the patient's daily behaviour which demands close and continuous observation by nurses. There is a bias towards physical methods of treatment, especially drugs, and the doctors tend to regard training and education as being somewhat outside their sphere of responsibility or concern. They knew nothing intimately of what happened in the training school and there were no formal means, such as case conferences, whereby they could become better informed. Nevertheless they were often jealous of their authority and were loth to share it with anyone else, such as the chief psychologist. The conflict between the responsible medical officers and the training staff tended to be perennial, for example the former might see that patients were taken off training before the latter were satisfied that the training had been sufficient.

The position at Crossways differed somewhat; here many more decisions are made by administrative nursing staff (who work in co-operation with the hospital secretary) since no medical staff are resident in the unit. All patients are in the care of the medical superintendent who visits daily and who knows the patients well, but in his absence his deputy has little knowledge of the hospital or of its patients.

Conflict between male and female nursing staff

One important difference between Cloverfield and Blackbrick was the extent of hostility at Blackbrick between the male and female 'sides' of the nursing administration which could be accounted for only partially by the shortage of staff on the male side, although the attractiveness of better paid employment in the city near Blackbrick made it particularly difficult to get men.[1] In terms of qualifications,[2] experience, and length of service, the female staff were of a higher overall quality than the male. The capacity to attract and hold staff more readily is a possible factor in the element of conservatism which was considerably more predominant on the female side. In order to keep male staff it was necessary for the administration to introduce certain innovations such as 'pairing', a system whereby two charge nurses worked on a ward on a shift basis. The older system, which continued on the female side, was for one sister to work a 12 hour day, seven days each fortnight, assisted by a deputy sister. The pairing system enabled the male nursing administration to improve both conditions and status, by raising deputy charge nurses to charge nurse level without contravening the pay scales. Furthermore, on the male side certain routine tasks such as the monthly ward stock check had been abandoned, thus reducing the volume of paper work to be completed by charge nurses. A great deal of autonomy was permitted at ward level, in contrast to the female side where the administration kept a much closer rein on subordinate staff.

[1] There was also a shortage on the male side at Cloverfield.
[2] Approximately 50 per cent of male nurses and 60 per cent of female nurses were trained in subnormality, psychiatric or general nursing, or had a combination of more than one type of training.

Greater female conservatism can also be explained in terms of the fact that there was a concentration of sisters with long service in the hospital. The average age of sisters was 51 and their average length of service 20 years. Corresponding figures for charge nurses was average age 41 and average length of service 12 years. A further important distinction between the two sides relates to the differential occupational status of male and female nurses. Male nurses have always been on the margin between the working and lower middle class, tending towards the working class, whereas nursing has traditionally been an occupational outlet for middle-class girls, both those who seek to marry (often doctors) and those who wish to make nursing a career.[1] Until well after the advent of the Health Service, the status of the matron was higher in overall terms than that of the chief male nurse.[2] This was also reflected in remuneration, and at Blackbrick the matron still had wider responsibilities in relation to domestic administration, the running of the nurses' home and the staff dining room.[3]

Traditionally, while female staff played a nursing role, the male nurse – known in the old lunatic asylum as an 'attendant' – was relied upon to provide physical coercion when dealing with difficult patients. The use of physical force effectively downgraded the male nurse from any professional status, and this role is still implicit, although drugs have long since taken the place of force in dealing with behavioural problems. Physical stature still seemed to be important in the minds of some male staff: once, when a new administrative staff member (who was some five feet eight inches tall) had to stretch on tiptoe to reach a file from a high cabinet, it was suggested to him that the office had not been furnished for dwarfs. The three oldest administrative nurses, including the chief male nurse, were well over six feet tall! This was not regarded in an entirely humorous manner since it was generally known amongst nursing staff that the chief male nurse took stature into account in deciding which candidates to recommend to the Appointments Committee when the post of deputy chief male nurse fell vacant.

The male staff resented what they saw as the old-fashioned pretentiousness of the senior female nursing staff; the latter retained as much social distance as possible between themselves and their subordinates, as part of their general authoritarian attitude. Female

---

[1] When, in 1895 it was proposed to open the register of trained nurses to men as well as women, the President of the Royal British Nursing Association commented, '. . . one can hardly believe that their admission will tend to raise the status of the association, while we foresee considerable trouble for the Executive Council from such members'. *Nursing Record* (1896), 2, p. 429.

[2] See also the discussion of the findings of the Bradbeer Committee, Chapter III, p. 55 *supra*.

[3] This is not true of all mental subnormality hospitals – in some cases a housekeeper or domestic supervisor is employed and is directly responsible to the Group or Hospital secretary.

nursing staff wore distinctively coloured uniforms which made rank immediately apparent; in contrast the male staff wore plain, all-white coats that were only marked with a name flash over the pocket at a late point during the research, when coats began to be stolen in large numbers. Male staff, although more informal in the super-ordinate/ subordinate relationship, prided themselves on being more efficient and business-like than the female staff. This self-judgment was confirmed by a number of independent sources, and it might be mentioned that the male staff rota, based on a purely mechanical system, was capable of being extended indefinitely into the future, whereas the female staff rota was worked out on a week to week basis; not only was this much more time-consuming, but it was organizationally vulnerable, and impossible for individual nurses to know well in advance when they would be off-duty.

Organizational efficiency was not, however, related to the standards of care on the male side; on the female side of the hospital patients were better clothed and groomed and generally cleaner. We have referred earlier[1] to the different role perception of male and female nurses, and this difference was abundantly clear at Blackbrick.

One reason for the comparatively poorly turned out state of male patients was that they did not have their own personal clothing,[2] clean clothing being pooled and re-issued by size. Charge nurses explained the impossibility of operating a personal clothing system in the following terms:

(i) sorting takes too long, and there is a staff shortage;
(ii) villas do not have enough storage space;
(iii) the laundry is slow and unreliable;
(iv) the inefficiency of the laundry would require enormous stocks to be held.

None of the charge nurses reflected, before giving these reasons, that a personal clothing system already existed on the female side, a possible indication of their ignorance of what went on elsewhere. It is true that the male staff are short-handed, but the storage space applied equally to male and female villas. What is significant here, we believe, is the clear evidence of discrimination occurring in the laundry in favour of the female patients' clothing because the laundry is closely linked with the female side, being near them physically and employing female-patient labour.

The laundry had in the past been controlled by a former matron and the present manageress shared a flat with the senior assistant matron who was also in charge of the sewing room where garments were repaired and, in the case of female clothing, marked with patients' names. The assistant matron had been at Blackbrick for 35

---

[1] See Chapter 6, p. 117 ff.
[2] Circular HM (65) states that this should be available for *all* patients.

years and was a staunch supporter of the ideology of the *ancien régime*. Even the chaplain bore witness to her fierce hostility to the male side and said that if ever a male director of nursing were appointed, she would no doubt resign.

But there were other reasons, apart from these personal ones, that suggest why female patients should be better clothed and groomed. Staff who see their role as being curatorial rather than therapeutic are more likely to spend a whole morning sorting socks than those who think that there are more important things to do, and a curatorial role is consistent with proficiency in the domestic arts which our society allocates so decisively to women.[1] More than this, the female staff go to considerable lengths to make the atmosphere of the villas cheerful and homely – a marked contrast to those on the male side – and this, among others, is a powerful reason for integrating male and female staff on the wards. The roles played by staff of both sexes are, in sociological terms, complementary, and neither is by itself sufficient to meet all the needs of patients.

An integrated nursing service

At Cloverfield a high proportion of staff agreed in principle that an integrated service would be beneficial to staff and patients alike, although there were some reservations from male nurses about the presence of women on certain low grade wards. Apart from one elderly male nurse who thought the female nurses should be of the 'dull, stodgy type' the views of most male nurses could be succinctly paraphrased: 'It would all depend on what she looked like'.

Staff who had previously worked in an integrated service thought the system worked well. Most specialist departments considered integration to be essential for the well-being of the patients. Children's wards were considered to get most benefit from mixed staff, and in wards where there was a senior male nurse over female staff, as at Springbush, this was said to work well, personal feelings were excluded and staff responded to discipline and respected the authority of the senior nurse.

The fact that the medical director had openly expressed his preference for the appointment of a principal nursing officer in order to streamline existing administrative nursing structure nevertheless caused some concern to senior staff about their own status and there were differing views as to the image that a principal nursing officer should project. Established female staff were inclined to reject the younger male principal nursing officer image, whereas the male staff saw these posts as being the trend of future developments and they were aiming their own ambitions in this direction.

---

[1] Two charge nurses on a male ward for severely subnormal patients and who played a largely curatorial role were spoken of by other male staff as 'fussing old women'.

Administrative staff saw the image of the principal nursing officer as an extension of themselves, that is to say, a strong, active personality, engaged on a fierce recruitment campaign able to improve the public image of subnormality; in effect a public relations officer with administrative and managerial training as well as the appropriate nursing qualifications.[1]

At Blackbrick, older and senior staff on both sides were fearful of the possibility of mixed staffing. Male administrative nursing staff did not want to have to take orders from women, and neither side wanted to be 'incorporated' into the other. Both sides thought this would happen if a member of the other sex were appointed as principal nursing officer.[2] Female staff thought there would be bad language from the men, and some even had fears of sexual advances. Young male staff did not, on the other hand, want to work under 'dragon-like' sisters whom they saw in a stereotypical image as reactionary and authoritarian.

Nevertheless both the chief male nurse, and with less enthusiasm, the matron, accepted the medical superintendent's view that duplication was wasteful and unjustifiable. The obstacles to unification lay in hospital politics rather than logic, for the stumbling block was the appointment of a principal nursing officer (or director of nursing as he/she was referred to at Blackbrick). If either the matron or the chief male nurse were appointed, it would have meant that one was subordinate to the other, and in view of their personal hostility this would have created a very difficult working relationship. A second possibility was the appointment of a third person from outside, but that person would be either male or female, so that the basic sex issue would remain unresolved. The third possibility would be to await the retirement of either the chief male nurse or the matron and appoint the remaining person, but since the chief male nurse was due to retire first, this would have meant a woman in charge, and on the whole there was less hostility among female nurses (apart from the most senior) to a man being in charge, than there was on the male side to being under the command of a woman. The medical superintendent wanted a man partly for this reason and partly because male staff at Blackbrick appeared both as more competent administrators and as more committed to the therapeutic aims of the hospital.

Staff problems affecting the treatment of patients

Undoubtedly the quality as well as the nature of the services offered

---

[1] The Salmon Report was being awaited at the time of the research, but was not published until after the study was completed. We have since learned that a male principal nursing officer has been appointed to this Group.

[2] We have since learned that the matron has in fact been appointed to this post.

to patients will depend greatly upon the relationships existing between staff at all levels. One doctor who regarded himself as instrumental in trying to reconcile the various factions in the hospital commented that until the question of poor staff relations at all levels was brought out into the open for discussion, 'the patients have to put up with second best attention'. We shall now refer specifically to some of these staff conflicts and indicate in what kind of ways patients could be affected.

(a) *Cloverfield* We referred earlier in this chapter to areas of conflict and overlap between the three hierarchies. At Cloverfield probably one of the clearest instances of disputed territory is the training units. Ideologically they do not fit easily into the pattern of the traditional hospital; their activities are not expressly concerned with 'care' such as is the undisputed province of the nursing staff. The training unit at Springbush was found to be in a particularly difficult state in this respect, in that its work had suffered in consequence of a long and protracted struggle for control. The consequences of the lack of stability and cohesion in the training units bore most heavily upon the patients, who were less able to benefit from the kind of regime on which the medical director and other specialist staff placed so much importance. A qualified engineer had very recently been appointed as industrial manager much to the chagrin of the nursing staff who wanted the appointment to be offered to a nurse. At the time of the research it was not possible to assess what the outcome would be: medical and administrative staff were very happy with the appointment, nurses were less sure, and some undoubtedly hoped that it would be a failure so that its jurisdiction might return to the nursing side. The administration of the unit was haphazard and somewhat chaotic: the chief male nurse kept a foot in the door by 'lending' staff rather than assigning them or seconding them. This meant that technically speaking the unit *could* be left without any staff at all.

At Bedwell the small industrial unit came under the Springbush industrial manager, but they had adjusted to this quickly and matron had seconded staff permanently to the department without dispute over jurisdiction. At Springbush there is an almost total absence of communication between the ward staff and the industrial unit. Nurses said that Standing Orders prevented them from having any communication except through the chief male nurse's office. The industrial unit felt that nurses were jealous of the department and were stubbornly determined to be uninterested in anything that the unit did or said. Industrial staff complained that patients arrived for work looking scruffy or untidy, sometimes they did not arrive at all and there was no explanation for their absence. Some nursing staff certainly disapproved of industrial therapy on principle and considered that the state should pay for the clothes and outings now paid for by patients' earnings. Others alleged that patients did not like going to the training units, and worried about their jobs. It was felt by the training staff that ward staff were glad to see the back of the patient in the mornings and therefore sent them more frequently than in the afternoons. The industrial unit also wanted to see more visitors and relatives, and for the latter to see patients in their everyday environment, rather than have them recalled to the wards if any visitors came, so that they could be 'scrubbed up'.

The chief male nurse still considered himself to be the head of the department even after the appointment of the industrial manager. The two small therapy groups to which we have already referred are destined to be incorporated into the industrial unit, but since the wife of the chief male nurse works in one of these groups, the matter of responsibility is further complicated by personal factors.

The whole picture of the industrial unit was rendered uncertain by the conflict of loyalties between training and nursing departments; the constant wrangling meant that ultimately it was the patients who suffered most.

It is interesting to note that at Cloverfield itself the industrial unit was run by a former charge nurse, a man well respected by all the staff and who had seen the department grow since its inception.

Another major area of difficulty which resulted in the patients discomfiture centred round the laundry services. Facilities at Cloverfield itself were said to have considerably improved with the appointment of a new manageress. Bedwell laundry, which also dealt with the 'best wash' from Springbush, was generally thought to offer the most satisfactory service, but worked at limited capacity as a result of the malfunctioning of the boiler and low water pressure. As in so many other areas it was the laundry (or 'cleansing station' as staff preferred it to be called) at Springbush that presented the major problem. There were voluble and bitter complaints about this from ward staff and judging by the appalling condition of articles returned from the cleansing station, these criticisms were justified. The cleansing station responded by pointing out that it was extremely hard to get staff (there were no women) and it was also said that since wards did not sluice soiled items it was surprising that anyone worked there at all, because the nature of the work was so distasteful. The procedure of the cleansing station was to sluice, rinse and dry, then put through the calender: the question of 'washing' hardly entered into it. Subsequent enquiries revealed that the ward staff had been instructed in Standing Orders *not* to sluice linen and that laundry workers were paid a bonus to do this themselves. The annual intake of soiled items is very high, 32,000 items compared with 5,443 sent to Cloverfield and Bedwell.

Ward staff were blamed for not being able to take care of their own clothes, for losses of stock, and for sending unmarked clothes, as well as for sending unnecessary alterations or repairs to the sewing room. It was felt by laundry staff that ward staff should not complain about clothing if their patients remained so incontinent that frequent laundering resulted in deterioration.

Domestic staff came under the jurisdiction of the lay administration and nursing staff frequently resented the fact that they could not get jobs done satisfactorily without first going through the matron and chief male nurse who in turn had to pass the request to the hospital secretary.

(b) *Blackbrick* In determining the level of care and the extent of training received by patients, the role of the charge nurses and sisters is of crucial importance, for despite inspections and subtle pressures from above, it was they and they alone who actually ran the wards and determined what should go on at 'ground level'. Here the nature of training was crucial; younger nurses trained in the newer approaches to mental subnormality with its emphasis on training and rehabilitation found themselves working on wards controlled by sisters and charge nurses whose thinking belonged to a former day. In addition they were hampered by conditions of overcrowding and by staff shortages, so that it would have been difficult for them to play a therapeutic role even if this had been encouraged by their superiors.

It seems likely that at Blackbrick morale was further lowered by the poverty of the ancillary services, such as the kitchen and laundry with whom the nursing staff had bad relations. Ancillary staff were of poor calibre and poorly paid, both of which facts are inter-related, bearing in mind that the hospital is located in an area with considerable alternative employment opportunities. The laundry, while it had excellent equipment, had to rely on comparatively inefficient female patient labour. In the kitchen not enough staff could be found to come to work early enough to cook breakfast. There was no properly qualified catering officer and some charge nurses complained that because of the incompetency of the catering staff they had to prepare special diets themselves. On several mornings each week ward staff had to prepare breakfasts and each villa had a store of groceries which were used to provide patients with 'cold teas'.

Any meetings of charge nurses (and complaints were more numerous on the male side because of the laundry) would be dominated by criticisms of the ancillary services, over which they had no control. They were frustrated by being constantly dependent upon inadequate services over which they had no authority, since ancillary staff were controlled by the hospital secretary. On the other hand charge nurses had little appreciation of the difficulties under which these staff worked, of which the most important was financial stringency. It is doubtful whether there is enough money allocated to Blackbrick to keep the buildings in good repair, and minor faults in, say, plumbing and lighting can be an irritant to nursing staff out of all proportion to the triviality of the technical fault. Blocked drains were another constant source of friction since it took much longer to get someone to come over than it did to do the job itself. Relations between nursing and ancillary staff seemed to limp from one petty crisis to the next.

Conflicts between the charge nurses and the maintenance workers, if they could not be resolved on the spot, had to be referred up to the chief male nurse, across to the hospital secretary, and down his hierarchy to the staff member concerned. This was not only a cumbersome procedure but one about which the chief male nurse complained in that it tended to jeopardize his good relations with those of comparable status in the lay administration. On the female side, more use of informal communication with ancillary staff was made by the sisters (they had a staff common room, which the male nursing staff did not have) but there was no evidence that this was any more efficient unless, as is the case of the laundry, close personal relationships also existed. Repairs and maintenance jobs for both male and female wards meant a tedious process of chits and requisitions: delays were normal, speedy results unusual; co-ordination in the matter of doing minor work could be non-existent. On one occasion when the floor of a ward had to be re-laid, the charge nurse, with the backing of the chief male nurse, insisted that the work be done during the week when as many patients as possible were at work off the ward. In the event the maintenance staff arrived early one Saturday morning when no charge nurse was on duty and all the patients were on the ward. Charge nurses complained that articles on requisitions sent to the stores were sometimes simply struck off the list. The shortage of face cloths was such that wards either received too few or none at all, but nursing staff were not told of the difficulties that led to the shortages. The decisions of ancillary staff were dominated by considerations of cost; this economic standard sometimes conflicted with the curatorial and therapeutic standards of nursing and medical staff. The supplies officer commented that subnormality hospitals were still 'in the Poor Law tradition' and received less money than other hospitals. In the past the matron and chief male nurse had not been involved in the purchase of clothes; today they were always consulted although sometimes their wishes were over-ruled on grounds of cost. Thus trousers with zip fastening fronts had been ordered, but as they required constant repair, considerations of cost had resulted in a return to trousers with buttons.[1]

Only when maintenance staff were actually on the wards performing tasks did they have any communication with nursing staff, so that they had little opportunity to build up a general mental picture of what principles ought to govern their activities in order to avoid conflict with the nursing staff. Trivial incidents, such as the issue of brown shoes to patients instead of black as in the past in order to prevent scuff marks on new floors was a case in point: there were still

[1] See also Chapter 3, p. 57, for information regarding in-patient costs per week in comparison with other types of hospital.

some black shoes on the wards, and patients found it impossible to work out whether black or brown shoe polish should be applied. They had got used to the idea that only one colour shoe and one colour shoe polish existed, and training them to discriminate was a lengthy procedure and time-consuming for the staff.

Other pressures on charge nurses and sisters arose from the kinds of patient in their care. With higher grade patients it was considered important – and not unconnected with the nurses' concept of personal success – to be therapeutic and get patients discharged. At Blackbrick a great deal of attention was focused on a small elite of patients, in whom the psychologist and training school staff were also primarily interested.

Charge nurses on wards with predominantly higher grade patients had therefore to be in constant co-operation with other specialist departments in order to get their patients 'moving', but communications were often poor so that frustration was felt by the charge nurses who saw all the therapeutic work being done off the ward. When patients returned, all that was left for nurses to do was care for them. There being less commitment to the therapeutic aims on the female side, this frustration was less acutely felt.

With the lower grade patients too, this frustration was less keenly felt by both male and female nursing staff, because care was obviously the more meaningful objective. Moreover there was a lower turnover amongst such patients and less paperwork, which resulted in the lower grade patients being less well-known to the higher levels of the nursing hierarchy. When the research worker was selecting the sample of patients for special study, the assistant chief male nurse was confidently able to say where the majority of high grade patients were located without having to refer to the wall chart. When it came to the low and lowest grades, he hardly knew any of them by name and actually referred to them as the 'low grades that nobody ever sees or hears of '.

Summary

Although throughout this chapter we have juxtaposed these two hospitals, Cloverfield and Blackbrick, any direct comparison between them is to be avoided because of the wide divergence of attitudes and the variety of treatments to be found in each hospital.[1] The existence of conflict was very obvious in both hospitals largely due to failure of communication, but equally each hospital had units where this was not apparently the case, for example, Northridge and Crossways.

---

[1] Nor did the research method employed lend itself satisfactorily to such comparison. The collection of non-factual and non-statistical data by two different people, even when carefully planned and with frequent meetings between workers as was the case here, did not result in strictly comparable material being recorded.

Furthermore, one might ask why it was that Crossways, an exclusively male unit, was less ridden with conflict than Springbush, also a predominantly male unit of roughly comparable size. The answer would appear to stem from the geographical isolation of Springbush both from any centre of population and from the main hospital. Staff were unable to get away from the unit, and since a relatively high proportion of married couples worked together, their home lives became almost an extension of their work lives. Such a tight, inward-looking community becomes easily prone to suffer from low morale, and as we have pointed out, there were many specific issues upon which it could feed; low morale had in fact become the norm at Springbush.

Crossways was situated near both a major conurbation and the main hospital, and although there appeared to be little contact with the latter, staff were by no means isolated from the wider community.

We do not suggest that isolation alone could explain the difference between these two units, but we do maintain that it was an important precipitating factor; the personal interaction of the staff undoubtedly contributed to the situation, and whilst Crossways enjoyed a general sense of security, supported by the attitude of the medical superintendent, the staff at Springbush lacked this sense of security and were much more riven by internal dissension.

In view of the fact that there are important differences amongst senior staff in their perception of the formal aims of the hospital, and particularly amongst different professional groups, the failure of communication is quite crucial, since it makes it impossible to ensure that treatment objectives, let alone the actual handling of patients, are in any way consistent within a particular hospital or subsidiary unit.

In both hospitals the advent of tripartitism has broken up the strictly hierarchical, bureaucratic system still to be found in some types of institution (in particular prisons), but the result has to some extent been to confuse the outlines of the power structure; the reality of patient handling is effectively decided by frontline staff and the role of the specialist staff, including the doctors, is minimized. At Cloverfield and Blackbrick the medical superintendent and medical director both remain in a unique position administratively, largely because of their control of their respective Management Committees, but both are less well able to control the activities of front-line staff now that the nursing hierarchy is autonomous, and policies which they determine are by no means certain of implementation.

At Blackbrick the situation is exacerbated by the frequent absence of the superintendent and by the unwillingness of his deputy to exercise authority, so that little effective follow-up of policy is undertaken. At Cloverfield the position is made particularly difficult by the dispersal of the units. In other words in both hospitals the superintendents are in control in so far as they can dictate policy, but they lack the power to ensure its implementation.

Although administrative nursing staff carry out regular ward rounds in both hospitals they are able to exert only minimal supervision, partly due to pressure of other work and partly because they are themselves aware of the inadequacy of these rounds as a method of effective control on ward activity. Just as the doctors tend to withdraw from their role as a result of their dependence upon nursing staff for information about patients requiring treatment, so the senior nurses tend to withdraw and leave the running of the wards to the nurse in charge. This situation is probably more acute in subnormality hospitals than in mental hospitals because so little medical treatment or skilled nursing care is needed. To be effective, supervision by doctors and nursing administrators would require their being on the wards far more frequently than at present, being involved in the daily treatment and handling of patients, observing their behaviour, supervising, advising and training the front-line staff. In practice, because of their diminished role, these senior staff tend to opt out of the situation.

However, as has been well documented in the extensive sample, this situation does not seem to occur in the subsidiary units, where the matron or chief male nurse is able to exert very considerable influence not only upon ward activity, but on the whole atmosphere of the unit and the morale of the staff. This may arise because of the smaller numbers involved, resulting in a more integrated community, but it is probably also connected with the fact that where there is no resident doctor, the administrative nursing staff assume far greater responsibility for all matters concerning the unit and, since they have more time for the purpose, they are much more actively concerned with the day to day handling of patients by their subordinate staff.

Dorothy Smith[1] has shown how, in an American state mental hospital, ward units emerge as 'pockets of information'; the front-line unit occupies a strategic position in the structure and is capable of discretionary action with respect to organizational goals. Dr. Smith continues: 'In a front-line organization, the locus of responsibility for organizational performance and policy making at the centre is peculiar in being divorced from the locus of organizational initiative in units at the periphery'. She suggests that policies devised at the centre tend to be in the form of statements of general principles, or rules to be followed at the front-line, rather than in the form of definite concrete objectives to be attained at some more or less specific time in the future.

We would largely agree with these findings in relation to subnormality hospitals, though not, as we have stated above, in connection with the smaller subsidiary units. However the type of policy

[1] Dorothy E. Smith: 'Front-Line Organization of the State Mental Hospital' *Administrative Science Quarterly* Vol. X, No. 3, December 1965, pp. 381–99.

formulation to which she refers resembles more closely those made by the Ministry of Health, and we believe that there are two kinds of power to be found in institutions for the subnormal. On the one hand there is the power exercised by the ward staff who effectively determine the nature of the patients' regime and who enjoy virtual autonomy in so doing; on the other hand there is the power of the hospital administrators whose exercised decision making enables the hospital to function as a viable organizational entity. Without the power and the authority of the latter, the activities and autonomy of the ward staff would simply not be possible.

We shall return to a general discussion of these organizational matters at the end of the report, meanwhile the next section will deal with those private homes, schools and voluntary hospitals included in the research.

T

Chapter 11

VOLUNTARY HOSPITALS AND HOMES

IN our discussion of National Health Service hospitals for subnormal patients, two themes in particular emerge: the first of these is the uncertainty experienced by all types of staff about their respective roles (and this primarily affects nursing staff because they are numerically the largest group, as well as the group most in contact with patients). Secondly, there is the disparity between the way of life in the institution and life in the community outside, a situation which is partly physical, but partly due to the fact that little attempt is made to articulate the two.[1]

But the mentally subnormal are also accommodated in voluntary hospitals, in residential homes, in mental nursing homes, and in private boarding schools; it might be thought that such establishments, being much smaller in size than National Health Service hospitals, and falling outside the scope of a nationalized service with its inevitable bureaucratic organization and procedures, would be less prone to the two problems referred to above.

In this chapter an attempt will be made to illustrate some of the main differences between state and voluntary provision, and in this way it should be possible to gain some idea of the extent to which the problems of role uncertainty and isolation from the wider community are also relevant in the voluntary homes, hospitals and schools.

By comparison with the National Health Service hospitals only a relatively short time was spent in each home,[2] and opportunities for observation of the daily routine, and in particular of interpersonal relationships, were therefore limited. Nor is the sample of homes entirely satisfactory from a methodological point of view,[3] and for this reason we will only draw attention to what appear to be quite major differences between them. Although use is made of statistical data, the validity of these differences is difficult to assess because of sampling problems.

Existing provisions

Official statistics do not always differentiate between the mentally ill

[1] See, for example, Chapter 9, p. 207 ff.
[2] For details, see Chapter 2, p. 33 ff.
[3] See Chapter 2, p. 30, and Appendix B.

and the mentally subnormal. Furthermore, homes open and close with considerable frequency, or alternatively they tend to vary the type of patient for whom they cater. As at 31 December, 1965 there were 90 registered mental nursing homes and 145 registered residential homes offering a total of 7,963 beds for the mentally disordered.[1] At that date 3,526 subnormal and severely subnormal persons were in receipt of residential care at the expense of the local authority, a considerable increase over the figure for 1964 which is given as 2,707 patients. According to the Ministry of Health Report, the number of elderly people in all types of residential care has risen steadily since 1961, and although there is no table giving a breakdown of patients by age, it seems plausible that the increase in subnormal patients may be partially accounted for in this way.

The Mental Health Act of 1959 distinguishes between 'mental nursing homes' and 'residential homes',[2] the primary difference being that nursing homes must provide 'nursing or other medical treatment'. It is important to bear this point in mind, since our findings suggest that this distinction is not so clearly observable in practice.

Another important difference lies in their administration, in so far as nursing homes come within the provisions of the Public Health Act (1936) and residential homes fall within the provisions of Section 37 of the National Assistance Act (1948).

The administration of these homes is very varied, they include special schools for the subnormal, village communities run by private Trusts and usually based on religious or educational precepts, homes belonging to religious Orders, and homes run by voluntary organizations or private individuals. All are registered with the Local Health Authority who are responsible for their supervision (in the case of schools this is the responsibility of the Department of Education and Science), but not for their administration.[3] The number of patients varies widely, some taking as few as two or three and others as many as 180. Individual homes or schools rarely accommodate more than 100 patients, and most house fewer than 50.

So far as *adults* are concerned, most of the homes differ from hospitals in that they accept either male *or* female patients, but not both, an important exception to this being the case of village communities; however it should be pointed out that the ancillary units of hospitals are also very often single sex establishments.

A number of voluntary hospitals and nursing homes have contractual arrangements with Regional Hospital Boards and financial

[1] Statistical information given here is derived from Ministry of Health Annual Report for 1965, HMSO, Command 3039 (1966). Where possible the figure for mentally subnormal patients has been recorded separately, but in many instances the Ministry do not distinguish between the mentally subnormal and the mentally ill.

[2] For detailed definitions, see Sections 14 (2) and 19 (2) of the Act.

[3] Hostels are provided by the Local Health Authority but these were not included in the sample. See Introduction, pp. 3–4, footnote 3.

responsibility for these beds devolves upon the National Health Service. We asked the secretaries of the Boards how the decision was reached as to whether a patient on the waiting list for hospitalization should enter a National Health Service hospital or a voluntary hospital/nursing home. Two Regional Hospital Boards have no such arrangement, and one uses it only in cases of emergency, the patient being transferred as soon as a National Health Service bed is available. In another area nursing homes are linked to individual subnormality hospitals and the physician superintendent decides where the patients should go. In the remaining areas the decision is usually made by the Board's consultant psychiatrist, and is based upon a combination of urgency and suitability. Since many of the voluntary hospitals and nursing homes are run by Roman Catholics, religious affiliations may play some part in their considerations.

There are also a considerable number of private hotels, boarding houses, etc., where subnormal persons are accommodated in conditions which vary widely. Such establishments are not registered with the Local Health Authority, and as no list of names is available, they have not been included in this research. Only establishments where 'the sole or main object is . . . the provision of accommodation . . . for persons suffering from mental disorder . . .' are obliged to register. Persons living in private hotels or boarding houses are normally paid for by the Ministry of Social Security, who *may* pay the money direct to the landlady.[1] However, if these subnormal persons are maintained by the Local Authority, it is technically an offence for them to be in a home which is not registered.

The homes in the sample

We have described in some detail the sampling procedure used to select homes.[2] Table 11.1 sets out the size of the 24 homes visited.

Half of the homes catered only for adult patients, in only one case, a small home for 23 patients, were both men and women accepted. There were four homes which took adults and children of both sexes, but in two of them the emphasis was clearly on children and the adults (approximately 10 per cent in each case) were there for special reasons. Of the remaining eight homes five took children only and three took adults and children of the same sex. All these homes were registered with the Local Health Authority but were run by voluntary organizations or individuals. Within the homes 511 patients were sampled.

---

[1] According to a private communication from the National Assistance Board (now the Ministry of Social Security), because of the difficulty in finding suitable homes they are ready to meet a rather higher charge than in ordinary cases of this kind.

[2] See Chapter 2, p. 30 ff., also Appendix B. The term 'home' is used throughout this chapter when referring generically to all types of residential establishment

Table 11.1
SIZE OF HOMES VISITED

No. of patients	No. of nursing homes*	No. of residential homes*
150 or more	2	—
100 – 149	5	1
50 – 99	3	5
20 – 49	2	1
10 – 19	3	—
Under 10	2	—
No. of homes	17	7
No. of patients	1,224	473

* One nursing home and two residential homes were run as boarding schools.

Finance

Two hundred and ten patients lived in six homes where they paid a fixed amount, the charges ranging from £13 2s. 6d. to £4 4s. 0d. per week. In four homes some of the patients paid, but with one exception the proportion doing so was very small. Another 162 patients living in four homes paid fees assessed on a scale to meet the income of the patient or relative and the remaining 841 patients lived in ten homes where no fees were payable.[1]

Where patients did not pay, the money was normally made available through the Local Health Authority or the Regional Hospital Board. One superintendent made a point of referring parents of potential patients to the Local Health Authority in order that they might obtain financial assistance, since a high proportion of the patients came initially through personal recommendation rather than through social agencies. In two instances the Ministry of Social Security contributed towards the care of some patients, and in one case the Ministry of Labour[2] did so. Where the establishments were schools, the Education Authority helped with fees where necessary, and in two instances the Greater London Council gave financial support.

In addition many of the homes were supported by private donations and Trust Funds, or in the case of religious foundations, by means of the Capital Fund belonging to the Order. Some of the village communities made a profit from the sale of goods made in their workshops.

[1] These figures are not weighted.

[2] These were registered as disabled employees, and as such the home – a village community – receives a deficiency grant from the Ministry of Labour in respect of those villagers who are registered as disabled but employable.

Waiting lists All but seven of the homes visited kept a waiting list, normally with fewer than 50 names, although in the case of certain homes specializing in particular forms of treatment the list was much longer. About half of the homes visited accepted temporary patients, the question of size or type of home not appearing to be a relevant variable here.

The physical setting

A major difference between the homes and the National Health Service hospitals was the fact that all but two of the former were housed on one site. One of these was run by a religious Order which had subnormal patients working in four separate convents, although the administrative care of these particular patients came under the auspices of only one Mother Superior. The other case was that of a village settlement, mainly for young people, which comprised two sites separated by only a short distance.

One of the serious disadvantages to which we referred in countless different contexts when writing about the National Health Service hospitals was the administrative difficulty of uniting separate units into a single entity which could be defined as a hospital. The isolation and alienation of the lowest ranks of staff which we found in the National Health Service hospitals and which was aggravated by the physical dispersion of the units had no counterpart in the homes. Whoever was in charge, be it Mother Superior, principal, matron or superintendent, they were resident on the premises and had sole responsibility for the day-to-day running of the establishment, a function that was clearly recognized by other staff members. To this extent the homes are administratively comparable with the *ancillary* units of hospitals, rather than the main units, and as we shall see later in this chapter, the similarity is confirmed by the kind of life the patients lead. In the homes, as in the ancillary units, patients often had a more homely environment, but tended to be less well provided with opportunities for treatment and training.[1] We do not suggest that no staff conflicts existed in the homes; to do so would be unrealistic. But in general it could be claimed that the physical setting did not provide the same structural opportunities for conflict that were found in the National Health Service hospitals.

Most of the larger establishments had a central Victorian mansion or stately home, often used with more recent buildings to house the patients. The smaller homes were mainly private houses dating from about 1900 and converted to their present use. As we shall discuss later in this chapter, with the exception of one home visited, few of the patients were crippled or severely physically handicapped, so that

[1] The fact that such opportunities existed in the main units of hospitals did not, of course, mean that all patients benefited from them (see especially Chapter 7).

the problem of nursing such patients in the kind of unsuitable buildings referred to when describing the National Health Service hospitals did not arise to anything like the same extent.

Nor, generally speaking, were the homes so isolated as the hospitals; whilst some were a long way from the nearest town, the sense of complete segregation from the wider community was by no means so apparent, although the village communities tended to prefer a way of life which insulated them from the world outside. It is possible that the degree of isolation in hospitals may have been partly due to the presence of patients who were more severely disturbed, both emotionally and physically, than those in homes, and because of this were less able to participate in activities in the surrounding community.

With two exceptions the general comments made by interviewers described the homes as: 'free and easy', 'happy', 'good-humoured', 'homely and pleasant.'[1] Similarly, interviewers were generally impressed by the standard of food and clothing. References to home grown produce and to well-cooked meals well served, were frequent. Most patients wore their own clothes with pinafores for protection when working; schools often preferred uniforms. Interviewers referred to smartness and cleanliness and only in one case was there adverse criticism, the appearance of patients being described as 'rather scruffy'.

Almost any residential establishment, be it boarding school, private hotel, or university campus, tends to reflect a certain institutional air. The mere fact that furniture and furnishings have to be provided on a larger scale than would normally be the case in a private home, creates a somewhat utilitarian impression. With one exception, however, we found that most of the homes had made considerable efforts to retain an element of homeliness and to try and reduce as far as possible the institutional image. Personal belongings were very much in evidence in all rooms used by the patients, and adequate provision of wardrobes, dressing tables, etc., replaced the communal storerooms attached to hospital wards.

Functions of homes

Although the functions of hospitals were thought by the staff to vary widely (depending often on the role that the respondent played in the institution), the presence of medical and nursing staff reinforced the definition of these patients as 'ill', and as requiring care and attention. This was less true in the homes because, although within the institu-

---

[1] It might legitimately be objected that these are merely subjective views; we would point out that the interviewers had previously been employed on interviewing in the hospitals and had therefore had a considerable amount of contact with institutions for the subnormal. Their positive statements may simply reflect the better conditions possible when catering for smaller numbers.

tions there was considerable overlapping of function, there was also more differentiation of function according to type of establishment; this may have been related to the fact that there was more differentiation between type of patient than was the case in the hospitals. For example, heads of schools invariably considered that they had a social training function, but only occasionally was this mentioned in residential homes and extremely rarely in nursing homes or children's homes. On the other hand all those in charge of nursing homes, and all but one of the heads of residential homes saw their function as providing a sheltered environment in which the patient could live and/or work, though such a function was mentioned at only one of the schools. Whilst heads of six homes mentioned the desirability of providing medical care, only three specifically mentioned the psychiatric treatment of mental and behaviour disorders.

There was a general feeling amongst the senior staff that there were many advantages in being independent of the state system. It was thought that this freedom presented an opportunity to provide more specialist care and treatment, as well as more individual attention. The latter was felt to be particularly important by staff in residential homes and in children's homes. Many of those interviewed thought that being independent allowed them to run their establishment more as a home than an institution; again this was particularly true of children's homes. Less red tape and formality were thought to be an advantage. Those nursing homes and children's homes which had a high proportion of patients coming from the Regional Hospital Board or Local Health Authority did not consider themselves to be really independent, but rather an extension of the National Health Service.

Internal arrangements

Only 2·5 per cent of patients in our sample slept in single or double rooms, and 32·8 per cent were in dormitories containing 30 or more beds. The latter were almost exclusively found in the larger homes run by religious Orders. About one-third of the patients were in dormitories containing between ten and 19 beds, these were most frequently found in schools and in the special 'village communities', the latter being normally divided into households.

Two-thirds of the patients had the use of only one day room, but unlike many of those in the hospitals these day rooms did not usually have a dual function as dining rooms. Both in terms of structural conditions and amenities the day rooms in homes, and to a lesser extent the dormitories, were better provided for than in hospitals. The main difference in the dormitories centred round the display of personal possessions and more originality in choice of decor and furnishings. However the difference was most striking in relation to amenities in day rooms, such as the provision of comfortable chairs, carpets, pictures, flowers, etc. In one large home miniature water fountains had been made by the staff and installed in the day rooms. Each of these rooms also had a small and well-equipped kitchenette leading off it where the patients (male) were encouraged to do simple cooking.

Sanitary annexes in homes were more generously provided than in many hospitals and almost invariably patients had their own individual toilet requisites.

The patients

In the homes sampled 38 per cent of the patients were male and 62 per cent female, and almost one-third were under the age of 16.

The length of time spent in the institutions is only relevant in relation to the adult population since in the three schools visited, children entered in the normal way from the age of five onwards.

So far as the adult population was concerned, the picture was similar to that in the hospitals, a considerable number having entered their present institution at the age of 16 or over. However this may be much less meaningful in the homes since unlike hospitals few homes cater for both adults and children, or, as we mentioned earlier, for adults of both sexes, so that it is necessary to transfer at some time during adolescence. This may present very real problems for parents who have to make alternative provisions when their children leave either a school or a children's home, when the transition may be from a community-orientated school or home setting to the more isolated environment of the subnormality hospital. In this respect 'village communities' may offer considerable advantages, since the children can progress from school to training and thence to work whilst remaining in an environment with which they are familiar. One residential home visited transferred only the very physically disabled children to hospital at the age of 16, the remainder were cared for in the households of the nearby 'village community' run by the same organization.

Physical Disabilities In Chapter 4 we drew attention to the relatively small proportion of patients in hospital who suffered from severe physical disabilities. The situation in homes was even more striking: three-quarters of the sampled patients suffered from no physical handicap at all; over 90 per cent were fully ambulant, and fewer than ten per cent were spastic or epileptic; only approximately 12 per cent were incontinent. Amongst those in homes who *do* suffer from physical handicaps, with two important exceptions, there was little difference between the proportion of adults and the proportion of children. The exceptions relate to incontinence where, as might be expected, one-third of the children were moderately or severely incontinent, compared with approximately 8 per cent of the adults sampled. The other difference related to physical handicaps which were symptomatic of subnormality (hydrocephalus, mongolism, etc.): here the proportion of children was double that of adults.

Furthermore, if the situation in homes is compared with that in hospitals purely on the basis of *type* of disability, there was virtually no difference for such items as speech defects, deafness, blindness, etc. However, whereas the proportion of patients in hospitals suffering from a physical handicap symptomatic of subnormality was 4·2 per cent of the sampled population, the proportion in homes was almost 17 per cent. We think that this may be accounted for partly by the fact that staff in homes were able to devote more time to completing the research questionnaires, and our interviewers were able to probe more intensively and to extract more detailed information. Furthermore, with fewer patients in the homes, it was easier to identify those selected in the sample and to discuss their disabilities with the staff. It is possible too that by virtue of being in small units, staff had a greater knowledge about the patients in their care, though this would be difficult to substantiate because even in the very large hospitals senior staff, in particular, tend to stay on one ward for many years and get to know their patients very well. Two other major differences between hospitals and homes related to those suffering from severe paralysis and those suffering from motor handicap; in both cases the proportion of such patients in homes was markedly less than in hospitals.[1]

Probably the major reason for the limited amount of physical disability amongst patients in homes lies in the pattern of selection for admission to homes as compared with hospitals. Only one home visited accepted all types of patient; a very high proportion (over 60 per cent of patients) were in residential homes which excluded non-ambulant patients as well as those suffering from behaviour disorders, and those requiring medical care (including those suffering from severe epilepsy). Even nursing homes often excluded patients on medical grounds if they were non-ambulant. Schools were even more selective and apart from excluding those they thought unsuitable on educational grounds, they also excluded children on medical grounds, or if they were non-ambulant. Children's homes were less selective, excluding mainly on grounds of behaviour disorder, though some would not accept cases requiring medical treatment, or those who were non-ambulant.

Intelligence The staff in homes frequently referred to patients being severely subnormal though interviewers were struck by the fact that compared with many of the patients seen in hospitals, those in homes appeared to be much less seriously handicapped. Similarly

---

[1] Although 17 per cent had a handicap symptomatic of subnormality, the fact that 90 per cent of patients were fully ambulant indicates that the symptoms were not usually of such a severe nature as to require constant nursing.

we thought it probable that many patients described as subnormal may have been borderline cases who might be expected to have IQs of 70 or more. Unfortunately it was not possible to substantiate these impressionistic findings, since the data on IQs was almost totally lacking. In one school we were told specifically that the patients had identical IQ scores with those found in hospitals, but that because of the more individual treatment methods used the children in the school were said to be educable, though in the respondent's view they would have been 'written off as ineducable' in a hospital. In fact 25 children were sampled in this home, of whom only five were untestable and the majority had IQs of 70 or more. These figures certainly present a very different picture from that obtained in most hospitals.[1]

In only 24 per cent of cases was any estimate of the patient's IQ score available; bearing in mind this limitation, of those about whom we have information, 32 per cent had IQs of less than 50, 52 per cent came within the range 50–79 and 16 per cent scored 80 or more.

Even in the schools, test results were known by staff in less than one-third of the cases, such tests having been carried out before admission by the Local Authority. These were considerable differences in the amount of testing carried out in residential homes and registered nursing homes. In the former, where visiting psychologists were employed, 40 per cent of the patients had been tested, whereas in the latter, where regular medical staff were in attendance, the number of patients tested was only 8 per cent.

Schools

Ninety per cent of children of school age in homes attended full-time education. As has been indicated, three institutions visited were recognized schools and as such were inspected by the Department of Education and Science. In addition, six of the homes visited provided schooling for children in their care.

Two of the schools were based upon Rudolf Steiner principles of education,[2] having their own particular methods of teaching, although their staff would not be recognized as having state qualifications. The members of the research team were in no way qualified to comment on the methods used, though one feature of these schools which appeared to us extremely positive, was the extent of parental involvement. On the other hand in some National Health Service hospitals, as well as in other homes, there was some criticism of the fact that Rudolf Steiner schools were extremely selective in their

[1] See Chapter 4, Table 4.4, p. 67.
[2] Rudolf Steiner developed his own teaching of what he called 'anthroposophy'. His aim was to develop the faulty cognition latent in ordinary people and to bring men back into touch with spiritual reality from which he considered they had become estranged. He sought to work out the consequences of this spiritual knowledge in medicine, education, etc. *Chambers Encyclopaedia*, Vol. XIII, Pergamon Press (1967).

choice of pupils and that their methods did not train children to live outside in the wider community.

The third school visited employed exclusively qualified teachers in a full-time capacity, giving a staff/pupil ratio of approximately 1:13. So far as schools within the homes were concerned, only two of the six had full-time qualified teaching staff, though in addition one small home employed a part-time teacher with NAMH diploma, but no formal teaching qualification.

One registered nursing home had an extremely well-equipped domestic science block. This catered almost exclusively for high-grade epileptics, and the most promising of these were subsequently sent to a college of education for further training.

There was a general feeling of satisfaction among staff in all the schools – including those in the homes – regarding the equipment provided and the amount of contact with outside educational bodies. But in the homes, school provision was often considered by the research workers to be unsatisfactory; three in particular were very overcrowded and the accommodation seemed quite unsuitable for the purpose.

The staff in two schools said that if behaviour became too disturbed the child was either removed by the parent or sent to a subnormality hospital; the fact that the others made no special arrangements for such children may reflect the careful pattern of selection prior to admission to which we referred earlier.

Occupation

Adult patients in homes were occupied differently from those in hospitals. Although the figure for those who did not work at all was almost identical in both cases – approximately 31 per cent – of those who had some occupation, 50 per cent in homes did utility or domestic work in the home or its grounds compared with rather fewer than 24 per cent of working patients in hospitals. The position with regard to occupational or industrial training is also reversed – whereas about 22 per cent of hospital patients were so engaged, in homes the figure was only about 12 per cent. Only 2·4 per cent of patients in homes worked outside on daily licence; if we are correct in believing that patients in homes are less severely physically and mentally handicapped than the majority of hospital patients (or possibly may have to some extent become less so) it seems likely that a considerably higher proportion would be able to work in the community, or would at any rate benefit from training with a view to doing so at a later date.

Ten homes catering for 53 per cent of all the patients[1] in the homes visited offered some form of occupational or industrial therapy ranging from 12 adults (out of a population of 27) putting corks into

[1] Unweighted figure.

bottle tops, to approximately 90 adults (50 per cent of the population) blending and packing incense. One nursing home for approximately 120 women had an extensive programme of occupational therapy, including cooking, basketry, weaving, dressmaking, musical activities, art, etc. Almost all patients took part in these activities.

Only rarely were there purpose-built buildings for work or training, and accommodation generally was of a low standard. There were many complaints about difficulties in getting work, due to lack of suitable industry in the area. One matron claimed that 50 per cent of the women were engaged on occupational therapy, but our interviewer saw little evidence of any materials being available in the shed at the bottom of the garden which had been allocated for this purpose.

Four of the homes employed a full-time qualified occupational therapist and two had a part-time one, but the vast majority of staff working in occupational or industrial therapy had no professional or specialist qualifications (this includes nursing). Nine of the homes had farms or small-holdings ranging from 152 acres of dairy farming to two and a half acres used for poultry. Produce was usually for domestic consumption and only occasionally sold on the open market. The number of patients working on the farms and small-holdings or gardens was generally extremely small, with the exception of one home where a third of the patients were so employed. Those patients who worked outside seemed to enjoy it greatly and it was felt by the staff to be of considerable therapeutic value. This may have been enhanced by the fact that the staff/patient ratio in this type of work was very high; in some cases there were more staff than patients, and in many instances one staff member worked with only two or three patients.

It seems relevant to ask why so many more patients in homes than in hospitals do domestic or utility work and by contrast why so few do any form of occupational or industrial training. In many homes we were told that the fee barely covered the outgoing expenses, so that they could not afford to employ outside domestic help. At the same time this precluded the employment of specialist staff and made it difficult to buy equipment and materials for occupational training.

In the village communities, a feeling of self-sufficiency is consciously fostered, and outsiders (in the form of specialist staff) would not be seen as necessary. In the case of religious organizations the sense of vocation amongst the staff had much the same effect, though many of the nuns and priests had trained in recognized schools of nursing or teaching, whereas the village communities' staff had a specialized form of training which would not necessarily be accepted in the wider community.

One other factor which might account for this situation was that most of those who ran smaller homes seemed to feel that the function of the establishment as a 'homely place' was reinforced by the patients doing household or utility tasks around the house. Finally it must be remembered that many of the patients in homes are paid for by relatives and it may be that they are satisfied that the patient be occupied on domestic duties, this being the kind of activity in which they would be engaged were they living at home.

Reward money Not only was the pattern of occupation different as between homes and hospitals but the reward money patients received was also different. Whereas only 5 per cent of adults in hospitals received no money or were paid in kind, the figure for adults in homes was approximately 59 per cent of the working population. Furthermore considerably fewer patients in homes were able to earn sums exceeding five shillings. This may, in some cases, have been due to the fact that the patients were fee-paying and provided for by their relatives, but the ethos of the village communities was that they should be self-supporting and no one (staff or patients) was paid individually for work done. The communities' funds were divided up and handed out to the households each month in cash. An article in the *Manchester Guardian* (8 December, 1959) described the situation in a typical village community:

> Great stress is laid on the use of cash; the leaders of the community feel that it is essential to teach the young people that there is a relationship between the work they do and their standard of living, and that food, shelter, and clothing do not fall into their laps without being earned. This helps them to feel that their work is needed and to guide them towards adult responsibility.

It was this sense of community and the stress on sharing which some critics felt prevented patients from living a normal life outside the sheltered environment of the village community.

Pocket money In addition to reward money patients could receive pocket money, although in fact 27 per cent received none, and a further 10 per cent of patients received it only in special cases. Again there were important differences between types of home: for example two-thirds of patients in nursing homes received between ten shillings and one pound and a further 28 per cent between five shillings and ten shillings. This figure is well in excess of the amount received in residential homes, where most received nothing (51 per cent) and 19 per cent received under five shillings. In schools about one-third received under five shillings and two-thirds received none; in children's homes it was given only in special cases.[1]

[1] Unfortunately no information was obtained as to the source of pocket money. In the National Health Service subnormality hospitals it is the responsibility of the Hospital Management Committee, and subnormal patients in general hospitals are given pocket money by the Ministry of Social Security. No such arrangements appear to exist for patients in nursing homes and residential homes and we therefore believe that a considerable amount of the money received by patients comes from relatives and solicitors.

Parole

There was a striking difference between the number of patients confined to the ward in hospitals (42 per cent) and those in homes (10 per cent). The majority of patients in homes (54 per cent) were allowed to walk freely around the home and its grounds (the comparable figure for hospitals being 31·9 per cent). However it is interesting that the number allowed outside the home unaccompanied was the same in both types of institution – nearly 18 per cent. The difference between hospitals and homes in terms of parole status may reflect the differences in degrees of mental and physical handicap to which we referred earlier, and this in turn may account for the fact that in the homes there was much less emphasis on a purely custodial function.

Contact with families

Information about families was normally much more readily available in homes than had been the case in hospitals. This may have been largely a question of size, making it possible for there to be a much closer contact between the staff and patients' relatives.

Of all the sampled patients in homes only 7·5 per cent were known to have no relatives, as compared with over 13 per cent in hospitals; but so far as children were concerned, the position differed only very slightly: 2 per cent of those in homes had no known relatives as compared with 3·6 per cent of those in hospitals.

Any overall comparison with hospitals concerning the number of patients who go home is invalidated by the fact that three of the homes sampled were in fact boarding schools from which the children returned to their own homes in the normal school holiday. However, even amongst adults the difference is striking – half the patients went home as compared with approximately one-quarter of those in hospitals. Furthermore whereas in hospitals roughly the same proportion went on holidays whether organized by the hospital itself or by relatives, in homes many more went with relatives. Few special arrangements were in fact made by schools or children's homes, possibly because there was little need for this; on the other hand nursing homes appeared to make such arrangements far more frequently than residential homes and it is difficult to see why this should be the case.

There also seemed to be much more visiting of patients by relatives than was the case for hospital patients. Whereas approximately 42 per cent of hospital patients had received no visits in the preceding year, the figure for patients in homes was approximately 27 per cent. Furthermore in the homes visits were more likely to have taken place recently and there was less likelihood of their declining in frequency associated with length of stay. There were, of course, exceptions, and those in charge of some homes complained bitterly that parents became virtually uninterested once the child was admitted.

It is difficult to account with any certainty for the greater degree of contact between patients and relatives in homes than in hospitals. There are a number of factors which *may* be relevant, but much more evidence would be required before any definite statement could be made. It is possible that the better physical and mental condition of the patients in homes makes it easier for families to accept their subnormal relatives, and in particular to care for them for short periods at home. If they are contributing financially for the patient's care they may feel more inclined to ensure that the treatment he or she receives is adequate. But it is also likely to depend partly on the attitude of the home itself. Visiting hours were generally less restrictive than in hospitals and most kept formalities prior to leave to a minimum, except where Court cases were concerned, when the authorities had to be informed. In a number of homes we were told that arrangements were made for the relatives to be visited first where it was thought advisable.

Again the attitudes of staff towards relatives may make a considerable difference to the amount of visiting, and in homes these appeared to be much less ambivalent than in hospitals. Eighty per cent of patients were in homes where relatives were invited and actively encouraged to visit before admission (in hospitals the figure is approximately 38 per cent). Furthermore in most cases relatives responded to this invitation, though it was suggested in at least one instance that it was the paying patients whose relatives were most likely to do so. Type of home was important here: for example in schools parents almost always visited before admission, even where the child was being paid for by the Local Authority. On the other hand in residential children's homes only just over half the parents were invited, and this was not done by the staff of the home itself, but through some other agency. Again there was a difference between residential homes and nursing homes, the latter being considerably less involved in contacting relatives.

This more positive attitude towards parents was not always sustained after admission, and in some cases relatives were excluded for periods of up to three months. The medical officer in one school for some 60 children advised the parents not to visit for two or three months: 'This allows the child to settle in peace, undisturbed by emotional disturbances'. In another home, children admitted from other institutions were isolated whilst routine checks for dysentery were carried out.

Parents' associations

Only six homes had a Parents' Association, three of these being schools; in one case the Association arranged lectures and talks for parents, but for the most part they were concerned to provide material comforts and to raise funds. Nevertheless they were more generally active and supportive to other parents than appeared to be the case in hospitals, and in two homes the Management Committee was largely drawn from members of the Parents' Association who were therefore closely concerned with the administration of the home.

Management committees

Forty-four per cent of patients were in homes having no Management Committee or Board of Governors. Where they existed, most of the committees seemed primarily concerned with administration and played little part in the community life of the home. Some were said to be very understanding *and* very active, this situation often arising either in a home run by a religious Order, where the whole ethos was designed to express interest and concern, or where the Management Committee was elected from the membership of the Parents' Association.

There was in fact a marked difference in the attitudes of staff towards Management Committees as between hospitals and homes. In the latter, even where they were criticized for failing to understand the needs of the home, or for lack of activity, there was by no means the same degree of generalized hostility as was found in the hospitals; there was no suggestion, for example, that members of the committee were there simply for political purposes or to enhance their social status.

Staff

Many of the homes visited were run by religious Orders where charitable service to the community is expressed in many forms, thus caring for the subnormal was an integral part of their life's work. A somewhat similar situation pertained in the village communities where the ideal of service predominated. In some of the smaller homes the people in charge had themselves a subnormal relative; others had previously run homes for different kinds of patients and had sometimes been asked by the Local Authority to take more subnormal patients. The three schools visited were run by people having a specific interest in the educational aspects of subnormality.

In terms of the day to day administration, the most noticeable difference between the homes and the hospitals was the virtually complete autonomy of the person in charge of the former, be they principal, matron, Mother Superior, etc., and an unquestioning acceptance of this situation by other staff members. As in the hospitals the power structure was hierarchical, but within one chain of command rather than being split into the three hierarchies of medical, nursing and administrative staff. Even in village communities which

v

were broken up into a number of individual households, with house parents having a high degree of managerial autonomy, the overall direction was clearly vested in the hands of a principal or director.

There appeared to be a number of different ways by which this was achieved with a minimum of friction. Where there was a religious ethos supporting the organization, there was a sense of shared beliefs and purpose which included an acceptance of an hierarchical system. For different reasons this system was accepted in schools, where they followed a traditional pattern differing little from schools catering for normal children.

Some homes were run by individual members of a family on a commercial basis, though this was usually combined with a concern to care for less fortunate members of society. Staff in such homes usually performed domestic tasks, and the relationship was one of employer/employee. Alternatively, a Board of Governors might appoint a matron to run a home, she was then responsible for employing the necessary staff; again such staff were usually employed in a domestic capacity rather than being directly concerned with the daily care and training of patients.

Medical and ancillary staff Most of the larger homes received regular visits from general practitioners, generally on a weekly basis; the remainder called in a general practitioner as they felt necessary.

We referred earlier to the fact that three homes mentioned psychiatric treatment as part of their function. Two of these were religious communities, closely linked with National Health Service hospitals; they received visits from psychiatric consultants and most of their staff were in fact qualified in mental nursing. In the third case the home was run jointly by a husband and wife, both registered nurses; they catered predominantly for mongols, many of whom they felt might subsequently fulfil a useful role in the community. They hoped to extend their premises to include a farm in order to provide further training for the patients. This home was also visited regularly by a consultant psychiatrist from a nearby subnormality hospital. One school which mentioned the value of psychiatric treatment did not in fact employ any staff trained in psychiatry or in mental nursing, either full- or part-time, nor was there a visiting psychiatrist. Schools and village communities had the services of a paediatrician available to them as required.

The position with regard to dentistry and other ancillary services was by no means so satisfactory. In urgent cases we have no doubt that contact was made with the local hospital, but for the most part there was no regular form of inspection that would bring to light any cases requiring attention. For example, in one residential home for 17 subnormal children under the age of 16 the matron commented: 'Never needed a dentist, I suppose we would get one in if needed. They can't speak, so can't tell us. Some have very bad teeth, but nothing is done. Anyway, you wouldn't get them to a dentist'. It was noticeable that village communities and schools appeared to be better provided for in terms of auxiliary medical staff such as oculists, speech therapists and physiotherapists. Unfortunately, even where establishments for such staff existed, national shortages often resulted in the posts remaining unfilled.

We feel that in some of these homes patients may be too easily 'written off' by those running them, and that in particular the children might have benefited from education and training as well as from speech therapy and physiotherapy. For example, the children referred to in the home above were described by the matron as 'ineducable' as well as being unable to talk. In fact our interviewer observed that at least six out of 17 children could talk, and when completing our questionnaire the matron described only one child as hydrocephalic and two as mildly spastic, the remainder suffering from no physical handicap. However no therapy or education of any kind was offered to the children, whose lives consisted of playing with toys and going for walks.

Nursing staff It was only in the schools that there was a widespread feeling that staff needed to be specially trained to look after subnormal patients. This view was shared to a limited extent by those in registered nursing homes, but in residential homes and children's homes it was generally felt that personality and aptitude were more important than specialized training.

We pointed out earlier that under the Mental Health Act (1959) one of the factors which distinguished nursing homes from residential homes was the availability of nursing and medical staff in the former. However in two of the largest nursing homes visited, only one member of the staff was qualified. Furthermore, in one of the residential homes, claiming in its prospectus to have a full nursing staff, no one had such training at the time of our visit – not even the matron.

The registered nursing homes visited had an overall staffing ratio of 1:4·9 patients[1] (trained and untrained) though this average conceals very wide variations between homes ranging from 1:3 to 1:17. With one noticeable exception it was usually the smaller nursing homes that had the better staff/patient ratio.

It seems, therefore, that in terms of numbers the staffing ratio in nursing homes is comparable with that found in hospitals (1:4·7), but in terms of patient care the situation in homes may be rather better because of the greater number of patients suffering from severe physical and mental handicap in hospitals, and who may therefore require more nursing and supervision.

---

[1] This includes all nurses and house parents concerned with the daily care of patients, but excludes teachers, training staff and domestic workers. Part-time staff have been counted as working half-time.

So far as residential homes are concerned, staffing ratios were almost the same, the overall figure being 1:4·5, though here too the variation was wide (from 1:3 to 1:13)[1] and again there was a tendency for the smaller homes to be more generously staffed. Furthermore, all but five of the 14 residential homes employed some qualified nursing staff, suggesting that there may be relatively little difference in terms of nursing qualifications between nursing homes and residential homes.

The availability of nursing staff at night varied as between type of home, for example in nursing homes and children's homes almost 60 per cent of patients lived in conditions where a member of staff was on duty at night. In residential homes the figure was 12 per cent and in schools 31 per cent, perhaps reflecting the different needs of the different type of patient. Elsewhere a member of staff was on call when required.

Staff discussions It will be remembered that in the hospitals relatively little meaningful discussion took place either between medical and nursing staff or between staff at various levels. In the homes there was little contact with medical staff, and it became evident from our pilot study that in denominational homes the question as it related to staff generally seemed meaningless because there was the implicit assumption that communication flowed freely among all members of the community. Nor was the question relevant in very small family units where the only staff employed were domestic. Thirty-eight per cent of sampled patients lived in one or another of these types of home.

So far as the remainder were concerned, all the homes claimed that there were adequate opportunities for informal discussion, but there appeared to be some distinctions made between the amount of confidential material made available to trained and untrained staff in those homes which employed both. Even in homes where all staff were said to be involved in discussions of this kind, only just over half were said to be familiar with the patients' background and history. In defence of this one superintendent, who was a qualified nurse, said he thought it unwise to allow untrained staff to have access to confidential records.

Contact with the Medical Officer of Health

Those running homes appeared to have very little contact with the Medical Officer of Health except in a few instances where they were personal friends. Sixty-five per cent of patients were in homes where there was only 'official' contact and 7 per cent in homes where there

[1] In one case the ratio was 1:26 but this home was run as a boarding school and there were seven full-time teachers who supervised the children during the day and six of these were residential. In the two other schools the ratios were 1:3 and 1:6.

was no contact at all. In almost 14 per cent of cases the contact was described as very good and frequent and in a further 11 per cent, good but infrequent, usually consisting of no more than an annual visit and occasional telephone calls. It would seem that the amount of inspection afforded to these homes is quite minimal, and bearing in mind the fact that a high proportion of patients are in homes which have neither a Management Committee[1] nor a Board of Governors, this would seem to be a matter of considerable concern, and suggests that registration may be a pure formality. Such inspection as takes place at the moment seems simply to ensure that minimum standards are met, but there would appear to be a case for regular visits from the staff of the Mental Health Department in order to see that patients receive preventive treatment (for example, dentistry, chiropody, physiotherapy, etc.) as well as to ensure that those patients who seem able to transfer to hostels or even to work outside, are found suitable employment.

Contact with the community

Most of the heads of homes visited expressed a desire for more voluntary help and more contact with the wider community. The matron of one small children's home commented:

> We found so many people had strange ideas about our home, children in chains, etc., so we have an Open Day and now the village has a better understanding. The local newspaper reporter didn't come for three years because of what he might see; he apologized after he visited us. We refer to our children as 'backward' because the word 'mental' upsets people.

One school which had a scout troop endeavoured to integrate this with a local group, but the superintendent commented wryly: 'You couldn't say the local scouts took an active interest in the school'. Not all the homes want any interest taken in their activities: in one home for approximately 18 adult females the matron said the parents wouldn't like outside bodies to take an interest: 'We had a small fête last year, just between ourselves, but they (parents) wouldn't let us advertise it and bring anyone in from outside'. This home was founded by a group of relatives who now administer it.

Summary

We have in this chapter described some of the most obvious ways in which homes tend to differ from hospitals. There were clearly advantages and disadvantages in both types of care. As was discussed in Chapter 2,[2] it is difficult to define the concept of 'need', or to

---

[1] See p. 271 *supra*.
[2] See, for example, p. 41 ff.

measure the provision of services, so that as in the case of hospitals we can only endeavour to relate the objectives of the home to what appeared to be their achievements. This is not easy because of the wide variety of types of home sampled, the only thing they all had in common being a degree of independence from the state system, and for those with contractual arrangements such independence was often purely nominal.

In general, life in the homes appeared to be more comfortable and less regimented than in state hospitals and staff were almost invariably motivated by a desire for service which transcended the simple question of caring for the patients or being paid. Enthusiasm and aptitude may well have compensated for any lack of professional qualifications. Because of the organizational structure of the hospitals, as well as the poor conditions of work, overcrowding, etc., hospital staff were frequently disenchanted with the job and there were often major conflicts both within the hierarchical systems and between them. However, the lack of any active system of inspection and the lack of trained staff (and particularly of specialist staff) did seem to us a major disadvantage in homes.

At first sight the choice facing the relatives of a mentally subnormal patient seeking residential care may be between a more institutional setting with some opportunities for training and therapy, or more comfortable living conditions, where other facilities are limited. However the choice may be more apparent than real, partly because many homes are fee-paying, and where the fees are wholly or in part paid by the Local Health Authority or Regional Hospital Board, the question of choice may be largely removed from relatives. Furthermore the question may not arise because homes of all kinds operate a discriminatory selection process which excludes a wide range of the most severely disturbed and physically handicapped patients. If the majority of such patients are obliged to seek care in *hospitals* it is perhaps not surprising that even with more specialist staff, a high proportion of patients in hospitals are unable to benefit from these services because the demand is so great and the availability of staff relatively small. In other words the homes, by being more selective, are faced with a much less difficult task; whilst it is true that hospitals have a high proportion of patients who are not severely disabled, either physically or mentally, they also have a minority who *are*, and the difficulty exists in trying to meet the needs of all types of patient.[1]

Patients in homes probably received more individual attention and had a closer personal relationship with the staff than was the case in hospitals. This was reflected, for example, in their leisure activities: in hospitals there was a tendency for patients to spend a great deal of

---

[1] This situation is not inevitable; in one home visited on the pilot study there were a great many chronic patients and the Mother Superior in fact commented that the Regional Hospital Board seemed to select such patients for this home.

time watching television (a relatively unsupervised activity) whereas in homes this was not encouraged and indoor games, country dances, parties and entertainment, etc., were more common.[1]

In most cases the homes were well run and the physical needs of patients were provided for within the limitations of the facilities available. However only in isolated cases did we feel that the psychological implications of subnormality, or the special needs of this type of patient were fully met, or even understood. By this we mean that the homes might equally well have been caring for the elderly, the physically disabled, or any other group of disprivileged persons needing residential care.

At the beginning of this chapter we drew attention to the uncertainty and confusion experienced by staff in National Health Service subnormality hospitals as the emphasis on care changes from custody to training and education. We feel that this problem does not exist in the homes, partly because of a difference in administrative structure, but more importantly because they mostly operate outside the mainstream of current thinking about the treatment of subnormality (there are, of course, important exceptions and schools, for example, could not be included in this generalization). This is linked closely with the second point we raised about hospitals, namely their isolation from the wider community. Again the situation in homes is different, and it is complex: in some ways they are certainly less isolated than hospitals, but this tends to be at a purely social level, for example both staff and patients tend to have more contact with the local community and more patients go home and on holiday. But as institutions they are in other ways even *more* isolated than hospitals. Because they rarely see representatives of the Local Health Authority and have virtually no contact with psychiatrists, psychologists, educationalists, etc., they have little or no opportunity for development and growth. In hospitals the idea of rehabilitation and return to the community relates to few patients, in most homes it is doubtful whether the idea exists at all.

---

[1] We were often told by staff in hospitals that dances had become less popular since the advent of television, but it was not clear whether patients were ever asked to express a preference.

Part Three
DISCUSSION

Chapter 12

THE IDEOLOGY OF TREATMENT

THE Oxford Dictionary defines treatment as 'a mode of dealing with a person or thing'; it is perhaps in this sense that the word is particularly applicable in the institutional care of subnormal patients. Yet in a hospital setting 'treatment' more usually has a medical connotation; the fact that a person is in hospital implies that he is there because he is 'ill', and the use of the term 'patient' to refer to the inmates of all hospitals whether general, psychiatric, geriatric or subnormality, reinforces this idea. But as we have suggested earlier, the subnormal patient, like the senile patient or the tractable psychotic, may be less in need of medical treatment *per se* than of physical or social care.

There is a need to distinguish between *illness*, requiring actual physical care, and *sickness*, as an overall condition which is relevant in terms of the allocation of a social role. The person who is ill is seen as having physical needs which must be met by treatment; if he is not to suffer pain or somatic deterioration then something needs actually to be *done* to and for him. 'Sickness' on the other hand, because it relates to role definition, implies a limited tolerance of the person's behaviour and a consequent redefinition of attitudes towards him.

As far as the mentally subnormal are concerned it is 'sickness' rather than 'illness' which is most relevant; by no means all of them need to be treated by doctors. Sickness is more in the nature of a blanket euphemism for deviance and abnormality, and because our culture is most ready to accord tolerance to those who are defined as being in some way ill, the subnormal person is most readily accommodated by the convenient fiction that he is, first and foremost, in need of some medical attention. Hence what may be no more than an institution for the residential containment of the subnormal is defined as a 'hospital', although its doctors may operate in a way more common to general practitioners than to housemen.

Types of patients and their needs

At a practical level it is suggested that the subnormality hospital has to provide three main services: firstly the physical care of a small group of severely subnormal patients who are unable to look after themselves. Secondly, and the great majority of patients will fall into this category, it must provide treatment and training for those whose physical and mental condition may be ameliorated, but whom it is unrealistic to suppose will ever achieve a sufficient degree of independence to enable them to live unsupervised in the community. And thirdly the hospital must provide training for a small group of those who can benefit to the extent that they may play some role in the life of the community, at least for a certain period in their lives.

But any consideration of hospital services for the subnormal cannot satisfactorily be divorced from consideration of community provisions, and within the second and third of these broad categories, there will be many subdivisions of people requiring really intensive and specialized treatment programmes – both medical and educational – at specific periods in their lives. Such treatment might, for example, be particularly valuable for young children over a period of a few years, and might enable them to return home and make a satisfactory adjustment if suitable sheltered workshops were available in the community. Similarly, adolescents might benefit from a period away from home at a stage in life when it is recognized that there are additional emotional strains even for those not handicapped by subnormality. Again, those who have managed to lead a reasonably independent life in the community might need to be admitted as they get older and find competitive life too difficult. Clearly this latter group will require neither constant care nor specialized training, but simply a sheltered environment which enables them to remain occupied and retain contacts with the outside community.

Thus a wide variety of different *kinds* of service may be needed to meet the differing needs of patients both in terms of their handicap and in terms of the stage they have reached in their life cycle. As suggested by Grad,[1] family situations change, and the possibility of full- or part-time residential care may ease the burden of caring for the child at home, but nevertheless avoid the present situation where the separation, once initiated, is virtually total. At the same time it must be accepted that hospitals cannot change their role until alternative sheltered provisions for accommodation, work and training are made by local authorities in the community; the burden cannot be allowed to fall exclusively upon the families.

The provision of services

The provision of physical care in some way illustrates the less usual meaning of the term 'nurse' in the English language. In former days the nurse in a private household was as much a personal body servant as a medical aide, particularly where children were con-

[1] Grad, J.: 'Social Work with Families of the Mentally Subnormal', paper read to Congress of the *Royal Society of Health*, 1964.

cerned.[1] The elderly, like the very young, may be in similar need of personal service in dressing, performing their toilet and taking exercise. For a large part of the time the nurse in the subnormality hospital performs these tasks not because the patient is 'ill' but simply because he is unable to perform them himself (or does not do them sufficiently quickly or efficiently), either because of his disability, or because he has never been taught to do so.

Furthermore just as the children's nurse must see that her charges do not get into mischief, so the subnormality nurse must exercise some custodial surveillance, backed up by drugs, and in certain circumstances by a system of punitive sanctions.[2]

Treatment and training, on the other hand, imply at least a minimum level of technical skill and a capacity to provide for the patient when he is in need of specific attention. Where subnormal patients are concerned, one of the nursing skills which is important is the capacity to *identify* the patient who is physically ill and to distinguish this from mental disturbance; when the patient ceases to move about in the usual way it may mean no more than a disinclination to pursue his normal pattern, but it may, on the other hand, mean that he is unwell, yet unable to communicate the fact.

Clearly, the changes which have taken place in what might be called the formal ideology of treatment, stem from a recognition of some of these facts, and the Ministry of Health circular *Improving the Effectiveness of the Hospital Service for the Mentally Subnormal*,[3] issued at the end of 1965 was the first official recognition that new considerations should apply to subnormality hospitals.

The Royal Commission on Mental Health (1957) which classified subnormal patients under the general heading of 'mentally disordered persons' argued for a re-orientation of the mental health services as a whole, stressing the need to move away from institutional containment towards community care. The Ministry's circular makes it clear that this is now official policy, and also stresses one other very crucial point, namely the importance of education, training and vocational facilities.

Nevertheless the intention of the circular appears in certain respects to be ambiguous; the emphasis in the early part is still very clearly on a combination of nursing care, supervision and control. The stated criteria for admission seem to imply that the hospital ought to be regarded as a last resort, although section vii covers 'patients who normally live at home but require short-term care'. The emphasis in the latter part of the circular differs however; it stresses the need for an expansion of education and training within the hospitals (paras. 16 and 21 in particular). There seems to be some

[1] Even today the 'mother's help' or 'au pair' girl is at one end of a continuum which includes the pram-pushing uniformed nurse.
[2] See Chapter 8, p. 173 ff.
[3] HM (65) 104.

contradiction here since if under ideal conditions only those requiring nursing care or supervision and control are to be housed in hospitals (para. 6), this will mean that hospitals are left with a residue of severely subnormal and physically handicapped patients who will need much nursing and medical care, and the mentally ill who will require psychiatry.

Barriers to change

Whether change is in the direction of increased medical or psychiatric treatment or towards community care, or an increasing recognition of the importance of education, training and vocational facilities, very far reaching changes in the work of the subnormality hospitals will undoubtedly be involved. The organizational implications of this will be discussed in the next chapter, but it is perhaps worth noting here that two of the main findings of the research appear to place severe limitations upon the extent to which a treatment and training ideology can be implemented in an effective way and can replace the present curative/custodial ideology. These are firstly the degree of isolation within which the hospitals function, and secondly the acute lack of adequate specialist staff and training facilities for patients, and the low status afforded to those engaged in such work.

(a) *The isolation of the hospital* In the past the policy was to isolate the hospital physically, its site being rural and removed from the main centres of population. Partly as a consequence of this, and partly because of the nature of the work, the staff have tended to be cut off, sometimes acutely, from the wider community.

Whilst the *social* effect of this may be most noticeable in respect of nursing staff, since they more often live in the grounds and have little life away from the hospital, the medical and specialist staff are *professionally* isolated from similar work in other fields. The custodial function with which the subnormality hospital is often burdened is one which was similarly borne by the mental hospital, but advances in modern chemo-therapy have tended to break down the walls of the mental hospital and to allow the development of outpatient psychiatric care. Such developments have made very little impact on subnormality; it is true that advances in the field of bio-chemistry have begun to show that the severity of certain forms of sub-normality can be reduced,[1] and in another field psychologists have offered convincing evidence that many subnormal patients respond dramatically to training and education, given the right environment

[1] This raises an interesting point: to what extent are community resources likely to be made available to cater for the special needs of those who, in the past might have been institutionalized for life, but who are now able to function in the community provided certain medical and social supports are available? An example of this would be the recent developments in the treatment of spina bifida.

and stimulation. But these findings have barely touched the sub-normality hospitals as yet, though the implications of the work done by psychologists in particular should have an important bearing on their future development.

A further factor which perpetuates the isolation of these hospitals lies in the fact that whereas there have been changes in the attitude of the public towards mental *illness*, these are not paralleled in the field of *subnormality*.[1] Improvements in public knowledge have, if anything, sharpened the distinction between the mentally ill and the subnormal who were once seen as belonging to the same broad category of problematic individuals. Nowadays mental illness is often seen as curable and responsive to a variety of treatments. These treatments, moreover, benefit from the immense prestige which has accrued to physical medicine through the development of 'wonder' drugs and surgical gadgetry. Subnormality, in contrast, is still seen as a tragedy, as something 'final', 'absolute', or 'incurable'. But whereas other types of 'absolute damage' such as limb loss, blindness and deafness can now be modified by medical technology, nothing can be wrought from metal alloys or powered by transistors that will assist the mongol or the ESN.[2] The 'accommodation' possibilities that exist for other groups of handicapped persons seldom exist for the sub-normal, possibly because attitudes towards them go so deep into the human unconscious. Nursery tales still number dwarfs and change-lings among their *dramatis personae*, and the mongol child is a living representation of the monster to which the young expectant mother fears she may give birth. The child which 'turns out' to be subnormal in a hitherto 'normal' family is indeed the 'changeling' left by the evil spirit. And whereas so many of the physically handicapped were once quite whole, and mentally they still are so, the subnormal have always been subnormal and are likely to remain so.

Furthermore the position of the subnormal may be particularly acute because their appearance is often disturbing to lay people, and since they often have a somewhat uninhibited way of approaching strangers this too may be quite frightening. Thus the physical isola-tion of the hospital is reinforced by the reluctance of the community to accept persons who may both look 'odd' and may behave in a strange way.[3]

Yet another element contributing to isolation relates to the fact

---

[1] One might ask to what extent it is realistic to expect the general public to accept a person so different from themselves when our school system accustoms us to segregating from the earliest formative years the exceptionally able, the normal, the slow, the ESN and the physically handicapped.

[2] It could be argued that one marginal benefit from the thalidomide tragedy is that a vast segment of public opinion now accepts that certain forms of gross physical deformity can have chemical origins.

[3] An area of research which appears to be neglected relates to the extent to which subnormal persons are aware of the rejection of society or aware of the deprivations and punishments they receive in hospital.

that unlike other types of hospital patient, and unlike prisoners, many subnormal patients know little about the world outside the hospital, so that they are not motivated to leave the safety of what they have come to regard as their 'home'. Furthermore, the fact that they are there at all suggests that for medical or social reasons family and friends have found the burden of looking after them too great, so that they may not readily be welcomed home other than for short periods. This raises a complex issue – parents are often in a situation where they can no longer 'cope' with a retarded child (or adult) and so they try to get the patient admitted to a hospital. But the parents' guilt at so doing may be reinforced by the fact that in our culture institutionalization, particularly of children, is a negation of family life. We institutionalize those whom we cannot contain, and to that extent the subnormality institution is the functional antithesis of the family. Whereas the family aims at the socialization of the child in order that he can participate in the dynamic cycle of social continuity, the institution must in many cases do no more than contain his helplessness in a static situation that may not significantly change as he moves from chronological childhood to physical maturity and old age.

Our data suggests that once in the institution, little effective effort is made to encourage the maintenance of family ties.[1] This situation has repercussions beyond that of the relationship between individual parents and their children, since the attitude of 'keep out' appears to extend to parents' associations and friends of the hospital.[2] We believe that an increasing attempt to broaden the activities of such groups, and to encourage them to act as pressure groups, might be an important function of the National Society for Mentally Handicapped Children.

Much could undoubtedly be done by the hospitals themselves, not only to encourage contact with parents, but also to make the general public more aware of the work being done by the hospitals. Greater encouragement could be given to voluntary workers who would almost certainly be willing to do far more than at present if they were made to feel useful. They could, for example, help feed and dress patients, could take them out shopping or invite them to their homes for a visit; they could teach them elementary tasks such as how to use a telephone, or to do simple sewing; alternatively they could play games with them. Closer contact between community and hospital would help to create in the public mind a more realistic understanding of mental subnormality. At present, apart from an annual Open Day most hospitals appear to do nothing to encourage public interest at a *personal* level,[3] though this is less true in some of the ancillary units.

---

[1] See Chapter 9, p. 196 ff.
[2] See Chapter 9, p. 205 ff.
[3] Gifts of money, toys, equipment, etc., are always sought after, but personal service is rarely given much encouragement.

Clearly it will be necessary for any plans such as these to be carefully worked out with the full co-operation of hospital staff since the latter may well feel anxious and threatened by the presence of 'outsiders'; nor may they know how to make satisfactory use of their services. It should be possible, however, for each hospital to have a joint committee of parents, friends of the hospital and staff (to include specifically charge nurses and sisters who are responsible for the patients on their wards) who would work out some satisfactory arrangements whereby voluntary workers could be encouraged to offer effective services on a regular basis, either to help in the hospital setting or to take patients out into the community.

(b) *The lack of specialist and training staff* At present a high proportion of patients receive little that could be described as active treatment; they suffer from living in an atmosphere of inertia where lack of facilities, overcrowding and shortage of specialist staff result in stagnation if not deterioration.

The suggestion made by one eminent psychiatrist that 'little active treatment is known to be of practical value for many of their (the hospitals') present patients', combined with the suggestion that higher grade patients should be treated in a therapeutic community attached to the general hospital,[1] appears to do little more than 'write off' those patients who remain in the subnormality hospitals as unworthy of skilled help. It *may* simply be that little active help is known to be of value simply because although there has in *theory* been a move away from custodial care to therapeutic treatment based on improved clinical and psychiatric knowledge, for the majority of patients only the first of these steps had so far been taken, namely the move away from custody. The second stage, that of replacing it with active treatment has not, we believe, generally been tried, largely through lack of suitable facilities, though undoubtedly due also to such factors as inertia and the bureaucratic structure of the hospitals.[2]

Our research data suggest that even in those hospitals where experimental units or practices have been set up within the organization, what actually goes on often diverges very considerably from what the superintendent believes to be the case, a situation which is linked with poor communication and organization procedures.

The argument that because the great majority of patients are not physically handicapped they do not therefore require the organiza-

[1] Pilkington, T. L.: 'Hospital Services for the Subnormal', *The Lancet*, 9 November, 1963, pp. 992–3. One might compare this view with Goffman's discussion of the 'tinkering-services model', Goffman, E.: *Asylums*, p. 340, *et seq.*

[2] While the application of greater resources in, for example, the fields of speech therapy and physiotherapy can only improve the possibilities for patients to communicate or move around it is far from clear at what point such improvements are likely to be limited by the law of diminishing marginal returns. Nevertheless on humanitarian grounds alone there is a case for arguing that no human being ought to be permitted to retreat to 'vegetable' status.

W

tional complexities of hospital life is by no means universally accepted by staff. There are those who feel that it ignores an important aspect of the problem, namely that the mentally subnormal may benefit from the kinds of skills offered by the psychiatrist and the psychiatric nurse, in conjunction with other specialist services such as educationalists, psychologists, occupational therapists, physiotherapists, social workers, biochemists, etc. It could be argued that if we were solely concerned with the physical handicap of these patients it would be pointless to have psychiatrists heading the medical team. We suggest that it is the ambivalence of those working in the field, of the Ministries concerned, and of the general public, about the type of treatment we are seeking to offer, which results in the debate regarding where and by whom care should be given.

This ambivalence is reflected by those responsible for medical training, who provide virtually no instruction on the subject of subnormality for psychiatrists. As one medical superintendent put it: 'psychiatry is a medically unmentionable subject and subnormality is non-existent'. A number of younger doctors referred to the urgent need for increasing recognition to be given to the psychiatric aspects of mental subnormality. This view is typified by one doctor who commented: 'Their psychiatric manifestations should be *treated*; mental subnormality should not be a backwater to psychiatry, but closely linked'. If the emphasis on psychiatric aspects is to increase, then clearly it must start by a growing recognition that the problem exists, and that subnormal patients have a right to be treated for their neuroses and psychoses in the same way as any other human being. Medical treatment may therefore be necessarily specific, and appropriate to the individual patient, but it needs to be organizationally distinct from the provision of what can be termed 'accommodation-adjustment programmes'.

Accommodation possibilities exist for other groups of handicapped persons; for example certain occupations, such as lift attendants, are to a large extent reserved for the physically disabled, just as some janitorial tasks are reserved for the elderly. The Remploy organization is a significant recognition of the right to work of those who cannot otherwise compete in the open market. What is demanded of the handicapped person in exchange for these offers of accommodation is that he should in some way adjust to a role which is a publicly visible expression of social benevolence.

But for the subnormal such possibilities seldom exist and they have a long way to go before they can achieve parity in this respect with the limbless and the blind. That they *can*, in many cases, benefit from accommodation and adjust to it is no longer seriously in doubt.[1]

---

[1] Note for example the type of work performed by 'villagers' in the village communities discussed in Chapter 11. At the same time it must be recognized that these patients appear to be generally speaking less physically or mentally handicapped than most of those in hospitals.

Colour-coded wires and ingeniously constructed jigs enable the subnormal person to perform tasks such as soldering which might be beyond the unskilled man in the street. But work situations, particularly of this kind, require a degree of stimulus and persistence that many of the custodial features of the regime of the subnormality hospital do little, if anything, to develop when educational and training facilities are at a minimum.

To develop and extend such facilities will require a considerable amount of re-education amongst those working in the hospitals. Any increase in professional or specialist staff will certainly be seen as a threat to the *status quo* and will involve working out new roles for existing staff, particularly the nurses. For the most part institutions such as the subnormality hospitals are characterized by a degree of structural inertia that derives largely from the fact that the maintenance of the *status quo* is one of the surest ways of achieving smoothness in day-to-day operations. Continuity is achieved by routinization and disrupted by innovation, while examination of objectives and the assessment of daily activities against them, are certain ways of producing dissatisfaction.[1]

Treatment and the nurse

We suggested earlier that the term 'nurse' in the subnormality context bears a closer resemblance to the personal body servant than to the starched and blue-caped nurse in evidence in our general hospitals. The contrast becomes even more marked when the subnormal patient is reasonably ambulant and does not need the treatments of physical medicine. Nevertheless the whole of the nursing profession has been influenced to a greater or lesser degree by the nineteenth-century revolution in general nursing, so that professionalism is now intermingled with the concept of vocation. The fact that the subnormality nurse in the Health Service is a pay-roll employee is the one which enables the most ready distinctions to be drawn between those who work in hospitals and those who work in those private or voluntary homes run by religious bodies.

Savoca[2] writes: 'Most families will more easily accept placement in a Catholic institution (regardless of their religion) . . . because nuns are seen as dedicated by vocational choice to serving their fellow-men'. The findings of our survey support very strongly the vocational orientation of most private care, though as we pointed out in Chapter 11 there was relatively little consideration of the patients as specifically subnormal, they could equally well have been any other group of disprivileged persons needing residential care. In all of the

---

[1] For a discussion of routine as opposed to contingent activities see Morris T., and P.: *Pentonville*, Routledge & Kegan Paul (1963), pp. 106–8.

[2] Savoca, R.: 'Family Counselling for the Retarded' in Nicholds, *In-Service Carework Training*, Columbia University Press (1966).

homes run by religious organizations care is a voluntarily assumed responsibility for which the costs are not really counted. In the homes run by what might be termed quasi-religious organizations (certain schools, village communities, etc.) there is also a high degree of vocational ideology although the cost, both financial and social, of individual care is high and by no means available to all.

In overall terms this situation may be contrasted with the hospitals where public provision is made at social and economic cost, but we think it would be a great mistake to underestimate the extent of vocational orientation on the part of most of the staff working in these hospitals, particularly the nursing staff who retain a great sense of vocation despite the many frustrations from which the service suffers and which result in poor staff morale.

The majority of subnormality nurses work in a job which is held in low esteem by many, including others in the nursing profession. Nevertheless, most of them are deeply concerned for the patients in their care; if there are frustrations and difficulties these are more than matched by the satisfactions they derive from their daily contacts with patients – the evident joy they experience in seeing them learn, however slowly, and for those patients who are discharged, the pride experienced in hearing from them about the adjustment they have made to life in the community. The vocational ideology which embodies the notion of personal sacrifice implies that the nurses will see some result, but the many frustrations which they suffer can well lead to a lowering of morale and a dilution of vocational enthusiasm. One method of meeting such a threat to their investment in the job is for the objectives to be lowered, in this way conserving physical and emotional energy and reducing vulnerability to criticism by superiors.

The need for flexibility

At present hospitals are overcrowded and understaffed; the mass treatment of patients demanded by bureaucratic administration is reinforced by the fact that more individualized treatment could not be offered in many cases because of the existing physical conditions in the hospitals.

In our present state of knowledge, and bearing in mind that large new resources are unlikely to be made available in the near future, either for hospital or community care of the subnormal, it would seem important to maintain a high degree of flexibility in determining the type of patient to be admitted and the type of care to be offered. What seems important is to avoid a situation whereby the subnormality hospital becomes merely a receptacle for those who cannot be provided for in the community. The criteria for admission set out in the Ministry circular seem to us rather too rigid, and they assume that admission to hospital is rationally determined. It may well be that hospital patients exhibit a degree of chronicity which implies all these problems, but it may be equally true that the selection of the hospital population is the result of inadequate or non-existent provision of alternative services in the community. Nor does it follow that in terms of the actual nature of the treatment regime, the care at present provided will necessarily be oriented in the directions indicated by the circular. Indeed the evidence of our study seems to suggest that a substantial proportion of hospital activity is exclusively confined to physical care in its various manifestations. To this extent the subnormality hospital is, more often than not, a negative solution to the problem of accommodation-adjustment, rather than a positive device for effecting it.

Chapter 13

ORGANIZATIONAL CHARACTERISTICS OF THE SUBNORMALITY HOSPITAL

The model of the total institution

THE model of the 'total institution' has tended to be used in a somewhat undifferentiated way; monastries, boarding schools, prisons, army units and mental hospitals have all been referred to under this 'umbrella' description. Yet the dissimilarities between such institutions may be greater than would at first appear. Although they are structurally similar, there are important differences in their objectives: just as the context in which the teacher, the prison officer and the nurse exercise power varies, so does their avowed purpose and so does their role.[1]

In so far as their encompassing, or total, character is symbolized by the barrier to social intercourse with the outside world, the two types of institution which appear to approximate most closely to the 'ideal type' are, we suggest, prisons and mental subnormality hospitals.[2] In both cases the life of the staff tends to be almost as confined as that of the inmates or patients, and the subnormality hospital has the added disadvantage of an extremely low patient turn-over.[3] We believe that our empirical data illustrates very clearly the degree and extent to which subnormality hospitals are isolated not only geographically and socially, but also from the mainstream of both medical and educational advances.

It is suggested that this degree of isolation is an important obstacle to change. The role of the Management Committee could be crucial here, in that they represent the outside community but, as we believe emerges from our research, the present arrangements for the selection of committee members and their lack of professional knowledge, tends severely to limit the role they are able to play within the institution.[4]

---

[1] Street, Vinter and Perrow: *Organization for Treatment*, Collier-Macmillan (1966) refer to such organizations as 'people changing' and suggest that differences are related to the extent, direction and difficulty of the change pursued.

[2] It could be argued that religious retreats are equally isolated from the outside world, but unlike prisons and subnormality hospitals, their inmates chose to enter them voluntarily.

[3] It should be noted that an exceptionally high turnover, as in many prisons, creates problems of a different order.

[4] The difficulties of the Hospital Management Committee in discovering what

Furthermore, since so few patients return to live in the community, there is little feed-back of information to the hospital of the sort which might enable managers and hospital staff to evaluate their work; thus 'success' tends to be measured largely by the degree to which the institution is quiet and apparently well ordered.

Another important difference between subnormality hospitals and other types of total institution lies in the fact that subnormality imposes a child-like dependency upon patients, so that unlike mental hospitals where patients are *re*habilitated, or prisons, where they may be *re*socialized, in subnormality hospitals training often has to be directed towards *primary* socialization. In this they have more in common with boarding schools, yet they differ from these in so far as they operate on the assumption that all inmates will live virtually throughout the year in the institution. Unlike school children, hospital patients are not prepared for membership of a family outside, nor for independent living, and to this extent their dependency is reinforced – they are regarded as children for ever.[1]

Blau and Scott[2] have classified organizations in terms of 'who benefits'; one might expect that hospitals of all kinds would come within the classification 'service organization', i.e., an organization created to serve its clientele who are the main beneficiaries; but it is our contention that mental subnormality hospitals could be said to come within the classification of 'commonweal organization', society being the beneficiary, in so far as it is thereby protected from the social misfit. To the extent to which this is true, subnormality hospitals are functionally more closely linked to other forms of 'containment' institutions such as prisons than they are to general hospitals. This contention is based upon the belief that the power structure, and the resultant pattern of communication, is so hierarchically structured as effectively to neutralize the curative function of the hospitals, in much the same way as the reformative function of prisons is neutralized.[3]

However, in institutions for the subnormal, we believe the consequential features of the social structure to be much more pervasive

---

[1] For references to the way in which nurses tend to reinforce dependency roles, see also Chapter 6, p. 116.

[2] Blau, P. and Scott, W.: *Formal Organizations: A Comparative Approach*, Routledge & Kegan Paul (1963). The authors suggest that in service organizations (e.g., hospitals) failure to serve the welfare of clients is probably a more prevalent problem than is becoming subservient to them.

[3] Julian, J.: 'Compliance Patterns and Communication Blocks in Complex Organizations', *A.S.R.*, June 1966, Vol. 31, No. 3, studied the nature and scope of compliance patterns in five hospitals and the relationship between different compliance patterns and communication blocks. General hospitals tended to be normative and custodial hospitals coercive, but none of the hospitals studied was for the mentally ill or subnormal.

---

goes on in a hospital are referred to by Professor Abel-Smith, 'Administrative Solution: A Hospital Commissioner?', in *Sans Everything*, ed. Robb, Nelson (1967).

than is the case in the prisons because of the type of inmate. With very few exceptions all inmates of prisons receive a determinate sentence and, as suggested earlier, most are there for a relatively short period.[1] The majority remain in contact with family or friends outside, both through visits and correspondence. In respect of the mentally ill, new discoveries in the use of drugs have resulted in a somewhat similar situation arising in mental hospitals, though it is recognized that there remain a substantial minority of chronic patients who will never leave hospital and have little or no contact with the outside world. In subnormality hospitals this latter group constitute the vast majority of patients; unless there are dramatic changes in medical knowledge or in the provision of community services outside the hospital, most patients, once admitted will never leave. The longer they remain the fewer will be their contacts with the outside world, and perhaps most significant of all, their powers of communication, if they ever existed, will be eroded by the institutional experience.[2]

At the time the research was carried out, important administrative changes were being initiated. In describing these changes as 'important' we do not mean to imply that they involved a major rethinking of the principles of the administrative system. They were important in so far as they threatened the *status quo* and thereby had major repercussions within the hospitals. From an administrative point of view they were little more than an attempt to switch from medical to administrative control;[3] in the past the hospitals had been dominated by the medical superintendent – sometimes acting autocratically, sometimes paternalistically – but with the increasing intervention of government in the planning and management of hospitals, there was a move away from the medical emphasis and a trend towards control by the administration. It is important to note that this change has also coincided with rumblings of change in treatment ideology, moving away from a custodial regime with basic reliance on the hospital, to one more concerned with education and training, and more directly oriented towards the community.[4]

[1] In 1966, 72 per cent of males and 85 per cent of females received into prisons in England and Wales were sentenced to periods of six months or less. *Report on the Work of the Prison Department*, HMSO, Command 3494 (1967). This picture may well change with the introduction of suspended sentences under the 1967 Criminal Justice Act.

[2] See, for example, Tizard, J.: *op. cit.*

[3] See particularly Chapter 3, p. 52 ff. and Chapter 10, p. 233 ff. Note that in Brown, G. and Wing, J.: 'A Comparative Clinical and Social Survey of Three Mental Hospitals', *The Sociological Review Monograph*, No. 5 (1962), the authors point out that many progressive regimes in mental hospitals were pioneered in institutions where the Medical Superintendent had the power and influence to carry them through. See also Bowen, W. A. L., 'Need for Inspection (or Survey) of Psychiatric Hospital Services' in *Psychiatric Hospital Care*, ed. Freeman, Bailliere, Tindall and Cassell (1965).

[4] For a discussion of such changes, see particularly Chapter 12.

The degree to which such changes had been initiated by the Regional Hospital Boards and accepted by the Hospital Management Committees and staff generally, varied considerably in the institutions visited. In some regions the changeover had been completed, medical superintendents had become medical or clinical directors, and the hospital secretary was rapidly becoming the chief executive. In other regions the change had taken place in some hospitals but not in others, and in yet other regions the change was seen by the staff as only a distant threat.[1] It is therefore not possible to assess the extent to which the new system will, in the long run, modify the disadvantages of the past. Certainly as we observed it, those hospitals having component organizational sectors operating with the highest degree of functional autonomy (i.e. those with the most diffuse system of administration) were generally those which were marked by either a high degree of apathy or a high degree of conflict, but this may have been a reflection of the transitional period.

The impact of current administrative policy

Under the present system there are three corps of line and staff – medical, nursing, and lay administration, theoretically reflecting a division of labour, but in practice having overlapping concerns which may be a constant source of friction. In formal terms the medical superintendent (or director) has the ultimate responsibility for 'determining the nature, scale, co-ordination and method of functioning of the therapeutic services of the hospital'.[2] But although the chief administrator responsible for these therapeutic services, he has no authority over the other consultants as regards patients, so that his position, except in relation to his own particular patients, demands *managerial* rather than medical skills. The fact that other staff groups now have greater autonomy has tended to block, rather than extend, channels of communication and in particular to limit the effectiveness of communications between superintendent and the lower levels of both nursing staff and lay administration. Information can now be distorted or blocked by the higher ranks of these administrations, with the result that the lower levels (and this is particularly relevant in the nursing hierarchy) tend to have a stereotypical image of the medical superintendent which emphasizes the social distance between them.

Other medical staff are in a somewhat different position with regard to the nursing staff because without their advice there is at present no way of knowing which patients need treatment. For unlike

---

[1] Change of any kind may be seen by staff as threatening, to the extent that it involves uncertainty and insecurity, but in this context it was probably the medical staff who felt most threatened.

[2] Circular HM (56) 51.

the role of the doctor in the general hospital, his role in the sub-normality hospital is ill-defined; apart from regular routine examinations, the doctor will normally see only those patients whom the sister or charge nurse draws to his attention.[1] Here the nurse is in an advantageous position *vis-à-vis* the doctor, although such a situation is confused by what might be termed 'traditional' attitudes of deference.

Traditionally the roles of doctor and nurse have been complementary but unequal in status, but in the subnormality hospital the situation cannot be like this; doctors do not go round wards administering treatment because most patients are not in bed, the majority are not 'ill', and for many there is no treatment.[2] Where there is a bias towards physical methods of treatment, mainly drugs, doctors tend to regard training and education as being outside their sphere of responsibility or concern. Generally speaking they have very little contact with training staff, psychologists, or other specialist services. In some instances they appear to be jealous of their authority and loath to share it with specialists from other departments. From our data, conflict between doctors and training staff appears to be very frequent.[3]

The situation amongst the second group, the nursing staff, is complicated by two important factors; firstly the division into two autonomous hierarchies, male and female,[4] and secondly, the large proportion of male nurses, a group who have always endured relatively low occupational status in society. Furthermore, a large part of the role of the nurses in the subnormality hospital is not a nursing role at all, but rather a quasi-maternal/domestic one, in which they are expected to relate to their patients in much the same way as foster parents relate to the children in their care at various stages of development.[5]

Members of the third hierarchy in the hospital, the lay administration, are at a disadvantage because, whilst some may possess superior managerial skills, as a group their professionalism is still very embryonic and they are acutely lacking in the security which stems from belonging to a nationally organized and recognized group. We

[1] See also Chapter 6, p. 120 ff. where the position of patients in ancillary units is discussed in relation to the very limited amount of contact they have with either the medical staff of the hospital or with general practitioners.

[2] Most patients receive maintenance doses of an appropriate drug and these tend to be changed only if the nurse draws the doctor's attention to the fact that the response to the drug is in some way unsatisfactory.

[3] For details of this situation see in particular Chapter 7, p. 131 ff.

[4] This situation is already changing with the appointment of chief and principal nursing officers.

[5] See discussion in Chapter 6, p. 118 ff. See also Caudill, W., 'Around the Clock Patient Care in Japanese Psychiatric Hospitals', *Amer. Soc. Review*, 26 (1961), pp. 204–14, where he refers to the use of *tsukisoi* ('a motherly servant for psychiatric patients').

believe the presence of an autonomous lay administration reinforces the difficulties of the doctors' role (and particularly that of the medical superintendent). Reference was made earlier to the fact that the nature of the patient population circumscribes the doctors' opportunities to deploy his medical skills; we suggest that the autonomy of the lay administration threatens the other acceptable area of doctor behaviour, namely administration. Traditionally the organization has centred round the relationship between the medical and nursing staff, where at the lower levels the doctor made decisions and nurses carried them out. At the higher levels the doctors organized the hospital and the administrator likewise carried out decisions.

There is, however, a fourth group of staff, though they can scarcely be said to represent a hierarchy. These are the training, educational, and welfare staff who remain virtually in 'limbo', officially responsible to the medical superintendent, and enjoying a certain degree of ascribed status (most noticeable when associated with membership of a professional organization), although exerting virtually no power.[1]

When specialized personnel want to become concerned with individual patients and to make a direct contribution to rehabilitation, the resentment of nursing staff is likely to increase. This is partly because it will be seen to interfere with the traditional lines of authority – where do these 'outsiders' fit in a tripartite system? – and partly because it will be thought to deprive nurses of yet another aspect of their role as nurses in subnormality hospitals.[2] Because these specialist staff do not fall easily within any of the three hierarchies, their position is further weakened by lack of support, and they are confused because their aims often appear to conflict with those of other staff members.

Changes which threaten the vested interests of other staff members, such as the introduction of professional personnel, will undoubtedly meet with resistance, and the tendency towards traditionalism and a custodial role may well be reinforced. Since there are few formal channels of communication between specialist and medical or nursing staff, these problems are unlikely to be resolved.[3] Thus the power

---

[1] Note how religious officials, educators and social workers are in a similar position in prisons. See also discussion of the reduction in decision making by treatment experts in prison, and the increasing importance of the 'bureaucrats' as decision makers in Matheisen, T.: *The Defences of the Weak*, Tavistock (1965).

[2] We referred earlier to the fact that they are deprived of much of the traditional nursing role.

[3] Stanton, A. and Shwartz, M.: *The Mental Hospital*, Basic Books (1954), and Caudill, W.: *The Psychiatric Hospital as a Small Society*, Harvard University Press (1958); both indicate how staff conflicts within an organization affect the treatment of patients, and they suggest that such conflict must become overt before it can be resolved.

structure of the hospital functions as an effective bulwark against attempts at teamwork (joint medical, nursing and training teams) in the treatment of patients. It seems likely that increased functional autonomy has increased status-consciousness, and this in turn breeds conflict amongst departments who are competing for both power and for scarce resources.

Adjustment to administrative changes We believe that the response of the medical superintendents to the administrative changes taking place, largely determines the attitudes and responses of other staff members. It appeared to us that the patterns of response fell into three broad categories:[1]

(a) Hospitals where the medical superintendents have become increasingly apathetic and/or uninterested; believing that as doctors or psychiatrists they have little to contribute in the field of sub-normality, they now see even their managerial function being eroded, and they respond by withdrawal. The reduction of interest and concern shown by these superintendents may be reflected in a similar attitude on the part of other medical staff, and the daily care and control of patients thus passes almost exclusively into the hands of senior nursing administrators.[2] In such situations contact between medical and nursing staff may be minimal, and the quality of care is likely to become very dependent upon the personality and skills of the matron and chief male nurse respectively. Where nursing administrators are competent and efficient, lack of contact with medical staff may have relatively little effect on overall nursing performance, but where this is not the case, staff morale may be very low and standards of care on the wards may vary widely. In this situation the authoritative position of the lay administration is reinforced, and in conjunction with the Chairman of the Management Committee they perform an active managerial role, the superintendent and senior nursing staff playing a relatively minor role in the decision-making processes.

(b) Hospitals where the medical superintendents have, as in category (a) above, conceded the effective exercise of administrative and managerial powers to the lay administration. Nevertheless, there remains an important difference between the two categories, since in this group the superintendents have retained a very real interest in

---

[1] For purpose of this analysis we recognize that we are over-simplifying the situation; there is in fact a considerable element of overlap, and the response of medical and nursing staff is undoubtedly more complex than we have suggested here. More detailed study would certainly expand and/or modify these categories of response.

[2] In at least one such hospital the situation was reinforced by the existence of an active local authority mental health department, which reinforced the superintendent's view that subnormality hospitals would eventually be replaced by a combination of local authority hostels and integration with general hospitals.

the medical and psychiatric aspects of their work. Consequently they retain contact with other medical staff, who are thereby encouraged to show an active interest in the work, as well as with administrative nursing staff on whom they are largely reliant for ensuring that treatment programmes are carried out. Unfortunately, because the interest of these doctors tends to be confined to strictly medical matters, a situation which may be encouraged by nursing administrators, social aspects of patient care are often not included; thus, for example, the punishment of patients for being 'naughty', and rigid control of their leisure activities, are not regarded as within the sphere of medical treatment, but are the concern of nursing staff, many of whom have little or no contact with medical staff. As a result, some of the advantages of therapeutic treatments devised by doctors may be lessened, due to the less satisfactory social care of patients.

(c) A third group of medical superintendents could perhaps best be described as 'charismatic' figures. In some instances this quality is a purely personal one, in others it is based rather upon 'expertise'. In both cases the incumbent remains very much the traditional superintendent, although individuals tend to exercise power in different ways, positioning themselves on a continuum ranging from despotism to benevolent paternalism. In the case of the 'experts', these men are highly regarded in the field of subnormality and in consequence may spend a considerable amount of time away from the hospital advising, lecturing and attending conferences. Their status outside the hospital results in their position within the hospital remaining unchallenged. Most superintendents in this category pay 'lip-service' to a tripartite administration, whilst a few ignore the change and continue to behave as before; either way it makes little difference since administrative staff are for the most part willing to allow authority to remain in the hands of the medical superintendent whose position they view with respect.[1] The power of the Management Committee is circumvented by the authority of the superintendent, supported by other medical members of the committee who defer to his presumed superior competence. Nursing staff remain traditionally deferential. In other words, the existence of tripartitism is acknowledged by the superintendents, but remains virtually meaningless in practice so long as they retain their position of authority.

Personality factors in the organizational system

We have so far stressed the importance of organizational factors, and the adaptation of the organizational leader to the role he is expected

---

[1] Only one important exception to this was noted by the research. In this case there was overt conflict between the superintendent and the lay administration.

to play. But it is our belief that not only will institutions differ to the extent that they house different kinds of inmate,[1] but they will also vary with the personalities of those who hold positions of authority either at ward, departmental or administrative level.

In Chapter 2 we suggested that interpersonal relationships were at least as important as physical conditions in determining the kind of care given to patients. There is not *necessarily* any direct connection between the quality of nursing care, or the educational and training facilities, and the decrepitude and unsuitability of many of the buildings, although the relationship needs to be investigated systematically. Support is lent to our views by Bowen[2] who, commenting on the variation in the performance of different hospitals even within the same area writes: 'The regional survey . . . left me, after the initial shock, with the impression that the difficulties which were encountered were due to inter-personal relationships at least as much as they were due to obvious material shortcomings'.

In ancillary units the personality of senior nursing staff may be even more important than in the main hospitals since there is less diversity within the staff structure, and the role of medical staff is often very limited.[3] Furthermore, the increased organizational responsibilities falling on the nursing staff reduce the possibilities of personality factors being neutralized as they might be in the more complex structure of the main hospital. It appears to us that persons in charge of ancillary units may even, to a considerable extent determine the goals of the particular unit, though clearly these will also be affected by other factors such as the type of patient, the attitudes of the doctors who visit, and the availability of resources.

The sociological rather than psychological bias of this research precludes us giving any hard data to support these suggestions, nor are we able to determine the *extent* to which personality factors can account for pockets of 'good' or 'bad' within the same institution. We think it important, however, that such factors be taken into consideration when planning for change.

The need for change

The major failing of many complex organizations is that the bureaucratic technique can, as a result of pre-occupation with administrative problems, become an end in itself. In other words, far from being a means to an end, i.e. to meet the needs of the patient, bureaucratic procedures are justified in order to run the hospital. Where, as in many subnormality hospitals, the needs of the patients are ambiguous

---

[1] See, for example, earlier discussion in this chapter on the difference between prisoners and mentally subnormal patients.

[2] *op. cit.*

[3] See Chapter 6, p. 120 ff.

or ill-defined,[1] there is a greater likelihood of administration being the focal concern of the hospital, rather than the patient.[2]

We suggest that the adoption in subnormality hospitals of organizational features which may be appropriate to other types of hospital neglects to consider a number of important factors. Firstly, the subnormality hospital is regarded as a discernible socio-legal entity by the Mental Health Act, whereas in reality the social differences between organizations that are collectively described as hospitals can be enormous. Thus there is all the difference in the world between a 2,000-bedded hospital and a 300-bedded one; equally there are real differences between the very large hospitals themselves – some are concentrated on one or two sites near each other, others are divided into a plethora of small subsidiary units separated by considerable distances, occasionally as much as 90 miles from the main administrative centre.[3] Even more than is the case with general and mental hospitals, the subnormality hospital is a product of the patch-work of sporadic public provision and random philanthropy dating from far more recent times than almost any other type of hospital.

Secondly we think that adopting the same organizational structure as general hospitals neglects to consider that there is a ratio between energy spent on *treatment* and energy spent on *care*, and this ratio varies considerably according to the type of hospital. Where more time and effort is spent on treatment, and care is a secondary feature, there needs to be a high mobilization of medical and nursing effort. Where, however, care rather than treatment receives priority (as in the present subnormality hospitals) there will be a relatively inert situation relating to medical and nursing skills, and the institution will be much less like a hospital. This may require a different kind of organizational structure geared towards a socio-therapeutic regime.[4]

Thirdly, and closely linked with the other two factors, in the attempt to reduce the power of the medical superintendent, the power of the lay administration was increased, following the model of the general hospital. But whereas in general hospitals treatment objectives are clear and administrative efficiency is vital both from

---

[1] This has, we suggest, different implications from, say, the prison situation where the aims tend to be clearly defined but conflicting.

[2] Blau and Scott, *op. cit.*, refer to certain types of bureaucratic organization where a 'succession of goals' may be observed rather than the displacement of goals to which we draw attention here. They explain this in terms of the organizations' relation to its environment; where the latter supplies stimulating challenges this will give support to the organization and allow flexibility and a succession of goals to develop. As we believe is clear, in the case of mental subnormality institutions, the high degree of isolation from the community prevents this happening.

[3] See Appendix F.

[4] We think this term may be more appropriate for subnormality institutions than a 'therapeutic community'.

the point of view of technical economy and in order to maximize efficiency in the allocation of medical and treatment resources, the position in subnormality hospitals is, we believe, very different. Apart from medical and nursing care the most important aspect of the work is (or should be) concerned with education and training (in its broadest sense) and the need here is to raise the status of *this* aspect of hospital care. Administrative efficiency is always important to the smooth running of an organization, but in subnormality hospitals where the patient population is of a very different order, we suggest that it should have lower priority than in other types of hospital. Although it would be unrealistic to make too close a comparison with the homes included in our sample, since these are considerably smaller in size, it is nevertheless noticeable that administration appears to play a relatively small part in the life of these establishments, all of which are markedly less bureaucratized than the N.H.S. hospitals which are, in any case, larger.

Organizational differences between hospitals and homes

Because of the wide variation in the *types* of home visited, as well as important differences in size, we wish to mention only one other aspect of organizational structure in relation to homes, namely, the high degree of autonomy vested in the person running the establishment, and by contrast the limited amount of external supervision. To this extent homes are administratively more comparable with the ancillary units of hospitals, but the remarks made earlier regarding the importance of the personality of the person in charge have, perhaps, even greater significance, both because of the lack of alternative controls, and because there is virtually no diversity within the staff structure.

Many of the homes have no Management Committee or Board of Governors, no parents' association, and very little contact with the local health authority. We noted earlier that Management Committees were not normally very effective as representatives of the outside community, nevertheless they are formally charged with safeguarding the interests of patients, and they act as a channel of communication with Regional Hospital Boards. The power accruing to persons in charge of a home with no Management Committee is almost total – the possibility of intervention by parents being virtually the only form of external control. This in itself is not a satisfactory alternative since although parents may be in a position to complain about particular abuses,[1] they cannot so effectively replace the function of a good Management Committee whose atten-

---

[1] In practice parents are likely to complain only in exceptional circumstances since alternative accommodation may be difficult to find and they may also fear that the staff will 'take it out' on the patient.

tion should be directed towards the operation of a positive/constructive regime.

Suggestions for organizational change

As will have been apparent from the foregoing discussion, the present tripartite system in hospitals is essentially a modification of the traditional power structure. It is a system designed to take into account the growing professionalization of nurses and administrators, but it ignores the important changes in treatment ideology towards an educative and rehabilitative function.

The report of the King Edward's Hospital Fund *The Shape of Hospital Management in 1980* (1967) envisages hospitals being run by a small board of management with a general manager, together with directors of the main hospital services – in other words, an industrial type management structure.[1]

Hunter[2] and Strauss[3] have proposed a system of 'negotiated order', a 'locale' or 'arena' where professionals work together in an atmosphere of give and take. A general manager sits at the centre of a communications system and a committee acts as a mediating structure between the 'arena' of the hospital and the wider society outside.

But are either of these alternatives desirable for the mental subnormality hospital where patients are likely to remain for very long periods, and where there is little clarity of objectives beyond that of 'caring'? So far as the former suggestion is concerned, we do not believe that conditions applicable to the industrial world, and more appropriate to large business corporations or factories, have any relevance to the requirements of a socio-therapeutic community. With regard to the latter, it may be that a scheme such as the 'arena, implies a higher degree of active participation by the patients in the arena than could be expected of those mentally subnormal patients who are in hospitals.[4]

Whilst far-reaching changes of this nature may be relevant for general hospitals, we are not convinced that they are suitable for mental subnormality hospitals. Nor do we think it realistic to expect such major changes to occur within the foreseeable future, there being too many vested interests in the *status quo*.

---

[1] Their suggestions refer more specifically to the projected District Hospitals.

[2] Hunter, T.: 'Hierarchy or Arena: The Administrative Implications of a Socio-Therapeutic Regime' in *New Aspects of the Mental Health Services*, ed. Freeman and Farndale, Pergamon Press (1967).

[3] Strauss, A. (*et al.*): *Psychiatric Ideologies and Institutions*, The Free Press, Glencoe, III (1964).

[4] Although some patients would certainly be able to participate, and if the training function of the hospital were successful this number might increase, we think it unlikely that many would be able to participate in any meaningful way.

x

However, the suggestions we put forward below should not preclude experiment with other forms of care for these patients; at most we are suggesting an alternative organizational structure which makes use of existing facilities and might be thought of as transitional until resources are available for new purpose-built hospitals and hostels for the subnormal. It might be argued that hospitals have no place in the future care of subnormal patients and that local authority provision in the form of small homes and hostels, together with day centres, would cater for all such patients. If this were true it would clearly be futile to make alternative suggestions for the organization of these hospitals, but we believe that even with improved educational and training facilities, many severely subnormal adults will not be able to function adequately without a very considerable degree of medical supervision and nursing care, as well as the provision of auxiliary medical services. Many of the suggestions for new forms of residential care[1] have concentrated largely, though not exclusively, on provisions for *children*. It will nevertheless be necessary to provide residential care for many of these children when they reach adulthood, as well as for those who at present do not enter institutions until they reach the age of 16 or over, and who, it will be remembered,[2] constitute the largest number of admissions.

There seems no reason why a start should not be made in the drastic re-organization of Management Committees. Whilst many individual members of such committees undoubtedly perform their task with conscientious enthusiasm, our evidence suggests[3] that the situation is so structured that the committee as a whole is virtually unable to perform one of its primary responsibilities, namely, the administration of the hospitals in the best interests of the patients. Nor is it desirable that the power of the committee should be vested so exclusively in the hands of the Chairman, as seems largely the case at present. A greater sense of involvement by all members would be desirable in order to counteract the present situation whereby decisions tend to be made by the permanent members of the hospital staff and 'rubber-stamped' by the committee, who have little knowledge of the day-to-day workings of the hospital.

If their management functions are to be adequately performed, their penetration of the hospital world needs to be intensified and they should be required to visit the hospital both formally and informally instead of, as at present, being taken round the wards by senior nursing and/or administrative staff. There is a need to recruit younger people who might serve for a maximum period of, say, five

---

[1] See, for example, Kushlik, A.: 'A Method of Evaluating the Effectiveness of a Community Health Service': *Social and Economic Administration*, Vol. 1, No. 4, October 1967.

[2] See Chapter 3, p. 49, and Chapter 4, p. 62.

[3] See in particular Chapter 9, p. 191 ff., and Chapter 10, p. 212 ff.

years, and reimbursement for expenses and loss of earnings might well be extended to this sphere of voluntary work. Finally there is a strong case for a representative from the field of education, as well as the local authority on all such management committees. The daytime meetings of most Committees also make it difficult for younger people in full-time occupations to serve, and this is a potential loss to the system.

Secondly, in order to support new treatment ideologies, we would envisage three levels of care: those severely subnormal patients requiring constant medical and/or nursing care, the non-ambulant, the severely disturbed, and those received into an admission unit for assessment, might all be housed in the main units of the present hospitals,[1] where they would receive intensive medical, psychiatric and nursing care to meet their particular needs.

The great majority of patients would not, however, require this high degree of supervision and care, and for these we would envisage turning parts of the existing hospital complex into more informal hostel-type homes, from which patients would travel daily to the main hospital centre for treatment, education and occupational facilities. Thus the hospital 'core' would be not only a residential unit for chronic cases and for investigation and diagnosis, but would become a day centre offering positive therapy to those needing a sheltered environment, but having little need of medical and nursing services. For the time being these patients might be housed in the existing ancillary units,[2] though the structure of these would need to be changed in order to accommodate both male and female patients, and ideologically they would be 'community oriented' rather than 'hospital oriented'. In the long run such units might become the responsibility of the local authority welfare department, to correspond with the anticipated restructuring of local authority social work.[3]

Since it is anticipated that improved treatment and training facilities in the day hospital centre would result in a higher proportion of patients being able to live in hostels or foster homes, we would envisage a third level of care, dependent upon the development of local authority hostels providing living units of, say 20 or 30 patients, situated in small urban areas. Such patients would work in the community as far as possible, but would retain close links with the hospital centre, so that any deterioration or change of circumstance could be noted and if necessary the patient could be moved, possibly

---

[1] The fact that the total number of patients living in such hospitals would be greatly reduced by such an arrangement would leave ample scope for re-designing the existing wards.

[2] In some cases this would obviously prove impracticable because of the distance from the main hospital.

[3] Viz., the report of the Seebohm Committee which, at the time of writing, is still awaited.

temporarily, to the more sheltered conditions provided by the 'homes', or even to the main hospital for intensive care.

Such changes would necessitate a considerable reorganization of staffing arrangements. There would need to be an increasing emphasis on training (including education, work, leisure activities and community contacts) and an expansion of auxiliary clinical services (psychology, physiotherapy, speech therapy, etc.). Not only would it mean *more* staff, but also an expansion of their sphere of operation. The two aspects of treatment – medico-psychiatric and training should be functionally autonomous but of equal status. We would envisage the former under a medical director and the latter under a director of training, possibly an educationalist, and both would be serviced by an administrative department.

Not all the nursing staff would need to be trained as they are at present since, as we have seen, much of the care of subnormal patients does not require nursing skills.[1] We suggest that there should be a staff of nurses trained in psychiatric and subnormality nursing who would come within the orbit of the clinical team. A skeleton staff of trained nurses might live with each group of patients in the 'homes' and be responsible for the nursing care of those patients, though if they became seriously ill they would probably need to be transferred to a sick bay at the main hospital centre. Trained nurses would also be responsible for supporting doctors and other clinical staff in their treatment programmes at the main hospital, and would ensure that such programmes were continued if necessary in the patients' living unit.

A second group of staff would be 'social therapists' who would be attached to the training section. They would be responsible for the patients' non-medical care in the living unit, would accompany patients to school and work, and would actively involve themselves in training under the supervision of specialist staff. In addition they would be concerned to encourage patients to remain in touch with the outside community, and where this could not be done adequately in conjunction with relatives and friends, the social therapists would themselves take patients out.

Finally, we suggest that much of the domestic work should be contracted to outside firms, though some might usefully be done in the living units by patients and social therapists as a form of training. Each living unit would also employ residential cook-housekeepers, and a non-resident gardener/handyman who would have patients working with him.

A plan of this kind would aim to ensure that all but the most seriously handicapped and bedfast should leave their living unit every weekday and travel to a hospital centre which would provide adequate

[1] See O'Hara, J. O.: 'The Role of the Nurse in Subnormality: A Re-appraisal', *J. Ment. Sub.*, Vol. XIV, Part I, No. 26 (1968).

medical, educational and training facilities.[1] Treatment staff would be able to visit the wards of those unable to attend the centre because they would be virtually in the same building and would be few in number.[2] It is worth noting that much can be done even for those who are bedfast; for example, the Dutch Red Cross have a hospital boat, with large windows, on which bedfast patients are taken for holiday cruises on the canals. The boats stop at various small towns and villages where they are serenaded by the town band and the inhabitants are encouraged to go aboard and talk to patients. Whilst many of our own canals may be too narrow for this purpose, the river Thames would seem eminently suitable.

From an organizational point of view, the fact that medical and training staff would be working in parallel might provide greater opportunities for communication and staff involvement in treatment. Clearly, however, such an arrangement as is suggested above will not of itself eliminate conflict, nor necessarily reduce it, since the proposal allows for two heads of equal status, a situation in which structurally induced conflict may be endemic. Nevertheless the presence of two complementary but competing systems may represent productive competition and to this extent conflict may be functional in so far as it may attack and overcome resistance to change.[3] Conflict as manifested at present appears to be largely dysfunctional since blocked channels of communication prevent it resulting in innovation.

Clearly these are not the only possible solutions to the problems facing subnormality hospitals, and as was mentioned earlier, experimentation with different forms of organization would be desirable and there may still be a need for small specialist units to cater for specific groups of patients. In particular, the use of existing subsidiary units as 'living units' is at best a makeshift arrangement, since they are often too large, too structurally unmanageable and too far from the main hospital. Nor do all the subnormality hospitals have such ancillary units. Consideration might be given, therefore, to the possibility of selling off hospital land, much of which appears to be uneconomically used,[4] as well as selling off some of the more unsuitable houses which are at present used as ancillary units, and with the proceeds buying up smaller houses in the local communities nearer the main hospital. Whatever methods are tried it seems

[1] Assuming the data obtained from our sample to be representative of subnormality hospitals generally, the bedfast and seriously incapacitated account for approximately 17 per cent of the patient population. A high proportion of the remaining 83 per cent might be expected to live in hostel-type accommodation, providing varying degrees of supervision, or in foster homes.

[2] This point would need to be carefully watched in order to ensure that the condition of such patients was not allowed to deteriorate as a result of doctors and therapists not visiting wards.

[3] See Coser, L.: *Continuities in the Study of Social Conflict*, Part I, 'The Functions of Social Conflict Revisited', Collier-MacMillan, 1967.

[4] This matter was not sufficiently investigated to enable any proper assessment to be made.

important to adapt the existing structure to meet the needs of the new treatment ideologies, for there is a danger that these will only be effective if both the physical setting within which the patient lives is changed, and the 24 hour a day 'control' by nursing staff gives way to a more open society, with expectations that the majority of patients will spend a considerable part of each day away from the place in which they live, or in separate occupational therapy units, schools, or sheltered workshops.

Chapter 14

SUMMARY AND CONCLUDING COMMENTS[1]

THIS study has aimed to examine the range and quality of institutional provisions for the mentally subnormal; for example, the physical setting of hospitals, the kinds of patient to be found in them, the staff who care for the patients, the life of the community and its contact with the outside world. At the same time we were concerned with certain broad aspects of the organizational structure of these institutions, and in particular with the following:

1. To discover the stated objectives of policy as seen by those inside the organization, as well as by the policy makers outside, and where there was no *explicit* statement of objectives, to discover what they were thought to be.
2. To examine the extent to which treatment generally accorded with these objectives.
3. To explore the possibility that certain unintended consequences followed from attempts to execute the objectives of policy, i.e. of there being an element of both latent and manifest function within the institution.

The research has been carried out during a period of transition. Changes are taking place both in the administrative structure of the hospitals and in treatment ideology. The supremacy of the medical superintendent is being questioned, and a tripartite system is emerging, theoretically giving autonomy to the medical staff, the nursing staff and the lay administrators. At the same time existing concepts of care based primarily upon a custodial regime are being challenged, with the new emphasis focussing on education and training, and oriented towards the wider community rather than the hospital.

But if the philosophy of treatment is changing, our findings clearly indicate that this is not paralleled by similar changes in the provisions available for subnormal patients. A review of these findings necessarily over-simplifies the situation and throughout the report we have stressed the danger of this – there are wide differences not only between hospitals but between units of the same hospital.

[1] These remarks refer exclusively to the National Health Service hospitals For a summary of our findings in relation to voluntary homes and hospitals see Chapter 11, p. 275 ff.

Generally speaking, however, it would be true to say that a high proportion of patients live in buildings which are dilapidated and decrepit, two-thirds of which were put up before 1900, originally to house the sick, the destitute and the aged. Inside these barrack-like edifices, over one-third of the patients sleep in dormitories of 60 or more, often with only a few inches between the beds and with no room for any other furniture. Patients are not encouraged to have personal possessions; there is nowhere to keep or display them. Physically the day rooms are in rather better condition, but most are too large to be 'homely' and few have sufficient arm-chairs or settees to enable all patients to sit comfortably at the same time. Provisions in sanitary annexes are often extremely rudimentary, being deficient in lavatories and baths, as well as totally lacking in opportunities for privacy.

Whilst there is no general shortage of clothing, only rarely is it provided on an individual basis. Items supplied from a communal pool may be ill-fitting, and styles tend to be dull and unimaginative, so that patients are not encouraged to take a pride in their personal appearance.

Living conditions and clothing are generally speaking better in the smaller hospitals, though size is not *necessarily* a relevant factor, and in the ancillary units much depends upon the interest taken in these matters by the matron or chief male nurse.

Only 12 per cent of the hospital population are under the age of 16, a high proportion being adults who may enter an institution for social rather than medical reasons, or because of the shortage of hostels and occupation centres in the community.

By virtue of being defined as 'ill' and housed in a hospital, there has been a tendency to assume that all patients require skilled medical and nursing care. That this assumption is in fact wrong is perhaps one of the most striking conclusions of this research. Our findings indicate that over 80 per cent of patients are fully ambulant, and apart from epilepsy, the amount of serious physical or mental illness amongst them appears to be small, though this is less true in the case of children.

We were able to obtain only very limited and unreliable data regarding the IQ of patients. Whilst there has been considerable criticism of the use of intelligence tests as a means of classifying subnormal patients, it is nevertheless virtually the only procedure currently used. Yet relatively little use appears to be made of such tests in hospitals for the subnormal; even where an initial assessment is carried out, the information is seldom made available to those members of the nursing staff most closely concerned with the patients' day to day care, nor is it normal for subsequent tests to be carried out with any regularity. Furthermore, no alternative methods of assessing capacity (e.g. tests of physical functioning) are applied in these hospitals. This lack of any adequate classificatory system may reinforce the tendency which exists in any large-scale bureaucracy for uniform methods of treatment to be used, rather than devising programmes designed to meet diverse particular needs. It must also necessarily limit the extent to which attempts can be made to evaluate the treatment provided.

There appears to be little concensus regarding treatment objectives, either within the hospital service as a whole, or within individual institutions. Staff perceptions of the function of subnormality hospitals varies with status positions in the formal hierarchy, as well as with the role they perform. The views of medical superintendents tend to be highly generalized in conception and somewhat idealistic; they see the hospital as having different goals for different groups of patients. Some of the senior nursing staff share these views of the hospital fulfilling a differentiated function, but our findings suggest that this is a somewhat over-optimistic picture of what actually goes on. For the vast majority of patients the objective consequences of hospitalization are those of containment and the relief of familial incapacity to provide care. The use of terms such as 'hospital', 'treatment', 'training', remains, we suggest, in the realm of wish-fulfillment. Our findings indicate that as many as 48 per cent of adult patients spend a large part of every day on the ward doing virtually nothing, yet as we have seen, very few of them are physically incapacitated. Because they receive little stimulus and training they remain in a state of childlike dependency, reinforced by the fact that they are constantly referred to by the nursing staff as 'children', and by the extensive use of such sanctions as are normally reserved for small children, in order to maintain a quiet and orderly regime.[1]

For the most part nurses tend to conceptualize their role in terms of what they aim to achieve for the particular group of patients in their care. Most frequently this is defined as 'nursing and care', though much of it is generally speaking little more than the exertion of social control; in the overcrowded, poorly staffed wards which are so prevalent, nurses need to give priority to the maintenance of order, since the situation can so easily deteriorate to one of generalized disorder. Whilst the differentiation between male and female nurses should not be exaggerated, the 'expressive' (caring) objective of female nurses can be contrasted with the 'instrumental' (social training) objective of many male nurses.[2]

Lack of a satisfactory classificatory system is not the only barrier to individualized treatment. Where units of 40, 50 or 60 are dealt with on one ward and share perhaps one day room, the needs of the individual must almost inevitably be submerged in the hurly-burly of

---

[1] Pocket money may be stopped, patients may be sent to bed early and privileges may be withdrawn (see Chapter 8, p. 173 ff).

[2] It is important to stress that these are differences in expressed *goals*, there is not necessarily any difference between male and female nurses with regard to patients' daily care and treatment.

ward routines. Under such circumstances and with an average of one nurse on duty to every sixteen patients, there is a tendency for the resources of nursing staff to be exclusively directed towards those in greatest physical need – those who have to be dressed, fed and generally supervised. Nor, according to the staff, is there time to teach patients to do these things for themselves – it is quicker and more efficient for the nurses to do them. As a result those patients who are in need of training, or who might benefit from greater social activity either within the hospital or outside in the community, may be prevented from sharing in them because there is no one with time to make the necessary arrangements or to accompany them.

It is debatable whether this situation might be improved if there were more homogeneity amongst the patients on different wards – without systematic experiment it is impossible to know, for example, whether lower grade patients talk more under the stimulus of higher grade patients in the same ward, or whether the latter deteriorate if kept with lower grades. All that might be argued is that *heterogeneity* provides opportunities for social stimulus and the means of informal care systems, though at present little use is apparently made of such opportunities.

Even had a more active treatment ideology been dominant in the hospitals, our findings suggest that the available facilities would have been sadly deficient. Most hospitals suffer from an acute shortage of trained specialist staff, both in terms of auxiliary medical services and education and training facilities. Such provisions as do exist are most often to be found only in the main units of the hospitals. Yet almost one-third of the patients live in relatively small ancillary units at some distance from the main hospital. In these units, conditions may often be more 'homely', but opportunities for treatment and training may be minimal.

Partly as a result of an absolute shortage of specialist facilities, only a relatively small number of patients are able to benefit from them. But other factors contribute to this situation: probably one of the most significant is the constriction of channels of communication within the hospital. There appears to be virtually no cross-fertilization of ideas between medical, nursing and specialist staff, with the result that senior medical and nursing staff who might be responsible for stimulating a demand for specialist services, are often unaware of the extent to which patients might be helped by alternative forms of treatment and/or training. This lack of communication not only stunts the development of knowledge and skill amongst nursing staff in particular, but also results in strong feelings of frustration and dissatisfaction among specialist staff, who feel their position within the institution as of peripheral importance. Such feelings are further reinforced by their sense of professional isolation from similar work both in the outside community and in other types of hospital.

The isolation of most subnormality hospitals is virtually total.

Geographically they tend to be situated in rolling countryside far from the nearest town or village. Their physical remoteness helps to maintain the barrier to communication with the outside world: most of the nurses (and many of the doctors) live in the grounds of the hospital, and whilst the doctors are often married and have a social life away from their workplace, this is less true of nurses whose whole life, both professional and social, may be centred round the hospital.[1]

For the patients the isolation of the hospital, and the lack of public transport serving it, not only prevents easy access by friends and relatives (in practice most visiting appears to be by private car), but also makes it difficult for the patients themselves to maintain links with the local community.

But the barrier is not solely physical; to a certain extent it is erected and maintained by the attitude of the hospital staff who make little or no attempt to encourage communication with the wider community. 'Outsiders', be they relatives, friends, voluntary organizations or interested individuals, are not really welcomed as visitors, and there is little opportunity for them to offer personal service to the hospital. Whilst most patients do in fact have living relatives, more than one-third of them had not been visited nor gone home during the twelve months preceding the research visit. Contact with the outside world may be seen by staff as disruptive of the smooth running of the organization, and as a consequence will be regarded as a threat to its efficient working.

The hospital is not only remote from informal contacts with the community, but to a large extent it is socially cocooned, lacking relationships even with formal organizations. For example, considerable bitterness is expressed by medical superintendents at the way in which policy is imposed from above, without prior discussion. Even in those hospitals where consultation with the Regional Hospital Board does take place, the resultant decisions are said to bear little relationship to the discussion. Even greater dissatisfaction is expressed with regard to the Hospital Management Committees: both superintendents and administrative nursing staff are highly critical of the way they perform their role, and to a considerable extent their interest in the activities of the hospitals is discouraged.

But it would be a mistake to see the picture of subnormality hospitals as wholly painted in greys and black. Despite the appalling conditions in some places, despite the overcrowding and the lack of specialist services – in particular education and training facilities – the staff are fundamentally very concerned about their patients as individuals. This is particularly true of some of the older, more senior staff in charge of wards, who have often spent a lifetime in subnormality hospitals, often the same one. They may be sceptical of new ideas and changes in treatment ideology, but their concern for

[1] In the case of male nurses, marriage is more usual, but their wives often work as nurses too.

the patients cannot be doubted. It is true, too, of many of the more recently trained younger sisters and charge nurses who would like to do more for their patients, but who feel frustrated by a system which provides little scope for their training and abilities, and uses them more like ward orderlies. Such nurses, especially the men, tend to move on, either to obtain training in general nursing or in administration, hoping to become the principal nursing officers of tomorrow. In a world where patients are deprived of almost everything which most human beings take for granted in a modern industrial society – freedom, a home, marriage and children, opportunities for choice in work and leisure – who is to criticize the nurses if they treat their patients like children, and in the process of 'caring' remove the remaining vestiges of independence? Until such time as more positive and effective treatments are available, it is as well for society that some people at least are willing to devote their lives to looking after a group whom society finds it so difficult to accommodate.

Nevertheless change must come. The Ministry of Health circular 'On Improving the Effectiveness of the Subnormality Hospital' (1965) has now set out the official policy objectives and it remains to be seen how quickly these will be implemented. But changes will not be achieved without major alterations in administration and in the type of staff required in institutions for the subnormal. Most, if not all of these changes have been suggested elsewhere in this report, but we believe that the following points should be borne in mind in attempting to put any of them into practice:

1. These are not hospitals in the true sense of the term and staff appointments must be built up in areas other than medical and nursing.
2. There is a need to integrate the hospitals with the wider community both professionally and physically, and this must involve both staff and patients.
3. The present internal conflicts amongst staff appear to be incapable of resolution without more effective communication and drastic modification to the hierarchical structures.

As a transitional measure we have suggested that the existing hospitals perform two functions: firstly they should provide living accommodation and treatment for the bedfast and those requiring constant medical and nursing care; secondly they should become day centres providing outpatient medical and psychiatric treatment, education, training and occupation for the great majority of patients who would live in a more informal hostel-like system (housed in the present ancillary units until proper 'homes' could be made available and from which they would journey to the day centre. In due course such homes might become the responsibility of the local authority social work services, meanwhile we would envisage a very few trained nurses in each home, the remaining staff being social therapists who would work closely with the treatment and training staff at the day hospital, and be responsible for the social and leisure activities of patients in the homes. Cook-housekeepers, maintenance men and gardeners would be responsible for the domestic running of the homes, assisted by the patients as seemed appropriate.

Within the main hospital there would be expanded training programmes, as well as the development of auxiliary medical services, facilities for research and for diagnosis and assessment. The two aspects of treatment – medical and training – would be functionally autonomous, and serviced by an administrative department. The total number of trained nurses would be considerably reduced, since so much of the care of subnormal patients requires skills of a quite different order.

But major changes in policy and ideology cannot occur overnight, nor, unless much more money is made available, is it likely that there will be important developments in building or staffing programmes. Possibly certain modest short-term changes could be initiated with a minimum of delay and without much additional cost, and it is to be hoped that the findings of this survey will assist hospital administrators to discover ways in which the existing services can be modified and improved.

Nevertheless, it is important to bear in mind that most of the short-term and transitional suggestions we have put forward are no more than 'tinkering'. The truth of the matter lies in the fact that the National Health Service is itself in competition for scarce resources, and within the health service the problems of the subnormal remain at the bottom of a long scale of priorities. Much more needs to be done to bring about a change in public attitudes; at present the public is ignorant and apathetic, and whilst the idea of social euthanasia is theoretically outmoded, few are prepared to bring the problem out into the light of public scrutiny if it means spending money on people who are looked at furtively and with a degree of embarrassment. The Mental Health Act of 1959 provided for the community care of the mentally subnormal, but as the Ministry's own figures show, relatively few patients are in residential care provided by the local authorities, whilst the number in hospital has remained virtually static. There are many things wrong with our subnormality hospitals; conditions in some places are Dickensian and grotesque; in a few cases there is certainly unnecessary unkindness; but for the most part these patients are looked after by people who *care*, however misguided this form of treatment may be in the light of new knowledge about the possibilities of training the subnormal. The staff in the subnormality hospitals badly need better instruction and guidance, as well as more time to devote to fewer patients, but it should not be forgotten that in one important sense many of them accept those whom society chooses to reject.

APPENDIX A

Sample Design for the Study of National Health Service Hospitals for the Subnormal

As described in Chapter 2 (p. 28 ff), the definition a of National Health Service hospital for the subnormal was taken to be a group of subnormal patients and their staff, whether housed together in a single complex or not, under the charge of a single Medical Superintendent or his representative. The first stage of the sample design was to prepare a list of such hospitals in Great Britain (see pp. 28–29). Eighty-two hospitals were identified for this list, but four of these had been contacted for the pilot study and, since it was felt that they should not also be included in the main study, they were removed from the list before the sample was selected. There remained 78 hospitals on the list, from which it was decided to select 35 for the study.

The hospitals varied greatly in size, ranging from those with under 50 occupied beds to those with over 2,000. Since the main unit of analysis was to be the patients, it was considered appropriate to sample the hospitals with probability proportional to number of occupied beds. First the hospitals were divided into four size strata as shown in Table 1:

Table 1

NATIONAL HEALTH SERVICE SUBNORMALITY HOSPITALS IN BRITAIN: SAMPLE DESIGN

(i) Stratum	(ii) Size of hospital: occupied beds	(iii) Total number of hospitals in stratum*	(iv) Total number of occupied beds in all hospitals†	(v) Number of hospitals sampled
I	1,750 or more	8	16,844	8‡
II	1,000 – 1,749	16	20,941	12
III	300 – 999	32	20,941	12
IV	Under 300	22	2,671	3
TOTAL		78	61,397	35

* Excluding four hospitals contacted in pilot survey.

† As indicated by Regional Hospital Boards, October 1964. This figure includes Scottish hospitals but excludes hospitals in the pilot study.

‡ One of these hospitals declined to co-operate with the research (see text).

Columns (*iii*) and (*iv*) of Table 1 clearly show the marked variation in size of hospital. At one extreme over a quarter of the occupied beds but only a tenth of the hospitals are in stratum I; at the other extreme, a quarter of the hospitals but only 4·4 per cent of the occupied beds are in stratum IV. In view of their large size, all of the hospitals in stratum I were automatically included in the sample. Within each of the other three strata, the hospitals were grouped by Regional Hospital Board and the Boards were ordered geographically, starting with those in the south and ending with those in the north. The sample of hospitals within a stratum was then selected by sampling systematically with probability proportional to size, the number of hospitals selected being given in column (*v*). The ordering of hospitals and the systematic selection within the strata were adopted in order to obtain some regional stratification.

The number of patients selected within each hospital was determined in order to give each patient, over both stages of selection, an equal chance (one-in-twenty) of appearing in the sample. Thus, in terms of the sampled patients, the design is self-weighting. In stratum I the number of sampled patients per hospital varied between 90 and 126, depending upon the size of the hospital. In strata II and III the number of sampled patients per hospital was approximately 87. In stratum IV, where less than a quarter of the hospitals contained more than 150 patients, a smaller sub-sample was needed and in this stratum the number of sampled patients per hospital was approximately 45. Within a selected hospital the patients were selected by a systematic sampling procedure from a random start. Some problems encountered with the lists of patients within the hospitals are described on p. 34.

While the design is self-weighting for the sampled patients, it is not self-weighting for the staff, e.g. Superintendents, heads of specialist departments, and nurses, nor is it self-weighting for *all* patients in the sampled hospitals. Thus, except in the case of the analysis of sampled patients, weighting has been necessary to allow for the varying selection probabilities of the hospitals.

Two hospitals selected for the sample declined to co-operate with the research. One was in stratum II, and in order to give correct weight to the stratum, a substitute hospital was included. The other hospital was in stratum I where it was not possible to provide a substitute since all hospitals were already included in the sample. An alternative procedure would have been to take a higher sampling fraction in each of the other hospitals, but as most of them had been visited before it was finally known that this particular hospital would not co-operate in the research, this plan was considered unsuitable because of the high cost involved in re-visiting the hospitals. The situation was dealt with at the analysis stage by duplicating the punch cards of 94 of the sampled patients in stratum I to represent the patients who would have been sampled from that hospital. While these procedures for dealing with the two non-co-operating hospitals give each stratum full representation in the sample, this is all they achieve: they do not, of course, solve the non-response problem. The sample remains biased to the extent that the non-co-operating hospitals differ from the other hospitals within their own stratum.

As a result of the method of treating the problem of the non-co-operating hospital in stratum I, only 34 (not 35) hospitals and their ancillary units were actually visited in the research.

APPENDIX B

Sample Design for the Study of Residential Homes and Nursing Homes

The sample design for the study of residential homes and nursing homes is similar to the one employed for the study of the National Health Service Hospitals for the Subnormal. Again the first step was to prepare a sampling frame but, unlike that for the hospitals, this frame did not prove easy to compile (see p. 30). It was decided to exclude the very small homes from the study, and therefore homes with less than five patients were removed from the sampling frame. The final list comprised 127 homes with five or more patients.

These homes were then separated into five strata and listed systematically within strata. The details are as follows:

Stratum A This stratum was defined as homes recorded as having 200 or more patients. In the event it contained only one home, a nursing home.

Stratum B This stratum consisted of nursing homes for adults, or adults and children, recorded as having between 30 and 199 patients. The homes were listed in three groups in the following order: first, homes for both male and female adults: second, homes for female adults only; third, homes for adults and children. (There were no homes in this stratum for male adults only.) Within the groups the homes were listed in order of their recorded numbers of patients.

Stratum C This stratum consisted of residential homes for adults, or adults and children, recorded as having between 30 and 199 patients. The homes were listed in four groups in the following order: first, homes for both male and female adults; second, homes for male adults only; third, homes for female adults only; fourth, homes for adults and children. Within the groups the homes were listed in order of their recorded numbers of patients.

Stratum D This stratum consisted of nursing and residential homes for children, recorded as having between 30 and 199 patients. Residential homes were listed first, followed by nursing homes. Within these two groups homes were listed in order of their recorded numbers of patients.

Stratum E This stratum consisted of homes recorded as having between five and 29 patients. The homes were listed in four groups in the following order: first, nursing homes for adults, or adults and children; second, residential homes for adults, or adults and children; third, nursing homes for children; fourth, residential homes for children. Within each group homes were listed in order of their recorded numbers of patients.

The sample design was planned to give each patient an equal (one-in-eight) chance of selection. The home in Stratum A was included with certainty in the sample, and a one-in-eight systematic random sample of its patients was selected.

Since the homes in Strata B, C and D varied considerably in size, sampling with probability proportional to recorded size was employed in these strata. In each case a systematic selection procedure from the ordered list was used to obtain some further stratification. By this means seven of the 17 homes in Stratum B, four of the 12 homes in Stratum C, and five of the 17 homes in Stratum D were selected. Within each selected home a systematic random sample of about 24 patients was to be taken.

In Stratum E, where the homes were recorded as having only a small number of patients, the homes were selected with equal probability. Again, a systematic selection procedure from the ordered list was used to obtain some further stratification. A one-in-eight sample of homes led to the selection of ten of the 80 homes in the stratum. Within each selected home all the patients were to be included in the sample.

Some difficulties were encountered when this sample design was put into practice. First, although the recorded size of the homes had been thought to be reasonably accurate estimates of the actual size, for a number of the selected homes the two figures were found to differ considerably. It would still have been possible to maintain a self-weighting design but this would have necessitated very large samples of patients in some homes (thus placing an undue burden on the staff), and small samples in other homes. Therefore the self-weighting aspect of the design was sacrificed and weights were allocated to the sampled patients. Since some of the discrepancies between the recorded and actual sizes were very large, the weights differed widely and as a result the sample design is less efficient than it would have been had the initial information regarding size been correct.

The second difficulty arose because five of the 27 selected homes were found to have closed or to be no longer taking mentally subnormal patients. In order to keep the sample to 27 homes, substitute homes of a similar type were selected to replace these five. This problem drew attention to a further deficiency in the sampling frame: on finding many of the homes to be impermanent, at least in the function of caring for the subnormal, the out-of-dateness of some of the lists from which the sampling frame was compiled becomes a major drawback. It is also likely that many new homes for the subnormal may have opened since the lists were prepared, which means that the sampling frame may have been seriously incomplete. Thus it cannot be claimed that the sample is fully representative of all the homes in Britain.

A third difficulty was that one home declined to co-operate with the research (see p. 31) and a substitute home was therefore included as a replacement.

Since not all the homes were selected with equal probabilities, weights are needed in analyses of the staff. The same weights are required also in analysis relating to *all* patients within the selected homes. However, these weights, which depend on the selection probabilities of the homes, are not the same as those used in analyses of the *sampled* patients.

APPENDIX C

Copy of Letter sent to
Superintendent of Hospital

Dear Dr ———,

The University of Essex department of Sociology (Chairman Professor Townsend), has been given a research grant by the National Society for Mentally Handicapped Children and I believe you have been approached by the ——— Regional Hospital Board at the request of the Ministry of Health, with regard to this.

The aim of this study is to undertake a national survey of the residential provisions for the mentally handicapped, the information to be obtained from a random sample of hospitals and nursing homes provided both within the National Health Service and by Voluntary and Private agencies. It is hoped to evaluate the extent to which these provisions meet the needs of the patients in relation to their physical and mental handicap.

Your hospital is one of those selected in the sample, and I am now writing to enquire whether you would be willing to help by allowing us access. It is a little difficult to be sure at this stage, just how long the work will take, but I would estimate that two people working together for approximately ten days would be sufficient. Naturally, we would try to finish in as short a time as possible, and would do our best to avoid disrupting the work of the staff.

In order to give you a rough idea of our plan, I attach a sheet showing what we hope to achieve during this period; if it were convenient, and you are willing to allow the research to be undertaken in your hospital, we should very much like to start work on ———. I should like to stress that all information obtained on this survey will be treated in the strictest confidence, and there is no obligation upon any member of your staff to co-operate if they prefer not to do so.

We hope, however, that the research will be seen as a positive contribution towards the future planning of hospitals and homes for the retarded, rather than a negative attempt to look for what is wrong.

If you have any queries you would like to raise, please do not hesitate to get in touch with me.

I look forward to hearing from you soon, and hope very much that you will be willing to help us carry out this research.

Yours sincerely,

COPY OF LETTER SENT TO
VOLUNTARY HOSPITALS AND HOMES

Dear ———,

Financed by the National Society for Mentally Handicapped Children and with the co-operation of the Ministry of Health, we are undertaking a national survey of the residential provisions for the mentally retarded in this county.

In order to carry out this work, a random sample of homes and hospitals has been selected and ——— is one of the homes selected in this sample.

I am now writing to enquire whether you would be willing to help by allowing a research worker to come and visit your home in order to interview you personally, and any senior staff you may have. We should also like to look round the home and obtain information about the patients in your care. This will not mean interviewing them since we can learn all we need to know from the staff concerned with their care.

If you are agreeable to this, I wonder whether it would be possible for our worker, ———, to come to the home on ———, or alternatively, ———. If neither of the two dates suggested are convenient, we would be very glad if you could kindly let us know as soon as possible.

Your help would be very much appreciated.

Yours sincerely,

PLAN OF WORK TO BE CARRIED OUT IN EACH HOSPITAL

1. Before arrival, we would like to send a very short questionnaire to the hospital secretary, to obtain information regarding numbers of patients, type of patient, buildings, etc. This can be returned to the office or collected when we come to the hospital whichever is most convenient.

2. On arrival, we would like to meet the Medical Superintendent and be introduced to Senior Staff members, so that our presence in the hospital is formally known and in order to obtain a clear idea of the layout and administration of the hospital.

3. If possible, we would like a meeting with all nursing staff in charge of wards as soon as possible after our arrival, in order to tell them a little about the research, to ask for their co-operation and to answer any questions they might like to raise. If necessary, this could be done in two shifts.

4. We should like to interview during the course of our stay the following people:

   a. Medical Superintendent
   b. Matron and/or Chief Male Nurse
   c. Nurse in charge of each ward
   d. Person in charge of all Specialist Departments (i.e. Occupational Therapy, Industrial Training, School, etc.)

5. We should like to visit each ward in the hospital, including any subsidiary units, in order to make observations regarding existing facilities. (This would not require the assistance of any staff member, merely permission to be on the ward.) The short interview with the nurse-in-charge referred to in (4c) above would take place at this time.

6. We would like to leave, for completion by the nurse-in-charge a short questionnaire which will cover a sample of patients in the hospital,

distributed between the wards. This form requires only a series of ticks and has been designed to take as little of the nurses' time as possible.[1]

7. We should like to spend time visiting all specialist departments. The short interview with the person in charge referred to in (4d) above would take place at this time.

[1] Although this had been our original intention it was later found more satisfactory to complete these forms with the nurses (see Chapter 2, p. 34).

APPENDIX D

Instructions for Interviewers

Aims of the Inquiry

During the present stage of this inquiry we aim to carry out a national survey of the residential provisions for the mentally handicapped from a sample of hospitals and nursing homes provided both by the National Health Service and by voluntary and private agencies. We hope to evaluate the extent to which these provisions meet the needs of the residents in relation to their mental and physical handicap.

Very little is generally known about the residential care provided for mentally handicapped people. Since the last Mental Health Act much attention has been focussed on the community services and upon rehabilitation schemes, and while we do not doubt that these are of the utmost importance, it is generally recognized that there will always be a proportion of mentally handicapped people who (for social or medical reasons) require some form of residential care.

If we knew more about the residential services which are provided now, it should be easier to plan adequately for the future. It is planned that this will be an extensive and therefore unavoidably superficial survey. We hope that this will lay the foundation for more detailed work in the future.

The information to be collected will be (a) the physical conditions of the hospital, primarily of the wards; (b) the specialist provisions such as school, physiotherapy, etc.; (c) reported accounts of hospital policy in various fields; and (d) the staffing levels. In order to evaluate these provisions it will be essential to know something about the hospital population, so a census will be taken of a sample of patients in each institution.

General Instructions

'The research interviewer is a social reporter, seeking first of all an accurate account of human experience.'

As an interviewer you play a very vital part in the success or failure of a survey. Not only must you be well versed in the technique of interviewing, but you need some insight into your own personality and the part it plays in the interview situation. You also need keen hearing, legible writing, a friendly smile and a wealth of emotional and physical energy.

In this study information will be obtained in three ways:

1. Directly by interview;
2. By observation;

Y*

3. Schedules to be completed by hospital staff members.

The relationships which you establish with the people you will meet, both in the interview situation and informally, are of the greatest importance. The 'perfect interviewer' is flexible enough to take on the role which her informant feels happiest with, but always retains control of the situation.

Bias A great deal has been written about the need for interviewers to be sympathetic receptive and 'interested in people'. This is true, but it is worth while reminding you of the dangers inherent in this attitude. Firstly many of the people you may meet during this survey *may be* in a situation where morale is low and where there is little opportunity to air their grievances. Your sympathy may create a strong bias in the interview and unless you are careful, you may find that you are also getting 'hot under the collar', whereas your aim is to remain detached, in so far as this is necessary to obtain an unbiased and accurate report. Secondly, your experience and impressions from one interview may be carried over into the next and all subsequent interviews, predisposing you towards certain attitudes which again may result in biassed reporting. It will be difficult to avoid feeling strongly about some of the things you will see and hear, you will also probably have some preconceived opinions and attitudes of your own, but do not allow your personal feelings or opinions to influence those of your informant. There are those who say that it is impossible to remain truly neutral and the very fact that you are there, in a receptive role, presupposes a sympathetic attitude. However, some of the people you will meet will presuppose your attitude to be condemnatory and they may consequently be defensive and hostile. All we can do is remind you of the need to be as 'uncommitted' as possible, and certainly never to make any kind of approving or disapproving remark, though it may be necessary on occasion to be supportive.

(b) *Interview Schedules*

1. *General* We have attempted to reduce interviewer bias to a minimum by providing fairly structured schedules. Keep to the order of the questions, and also to the wording on the schedule. There are three types of question:

(i) Pre-coded: Where there are several specified possible answers which may or may not be prompted and where one or more must be ringed.
(ii) Open ended: Where there are specified possible answers and a category for an answer that does not appear in the suggested list, e.g. 'other' (or one which comes in the suggested list but for which fuller information is required). Here you must write down exactly what the informant says.
(iii) Open: Where you will record your information verbatim, probing where necessary.

Never ask a leading question or suggest answers to the informant, unless specified on the schedule – the informant may agree with you for the sake of ease. When probing for facts and for opinions be particularly careful not to suggest ideas to the informant. If you are trying to get more information about a specific point you can probe sympathetically, e.g. 'yes?' (expectantly), 'Would you like to add anything to that?' etc. If the informant does not appear to have understood the question you should repeat it slowly and clearly, only if he still does not understand may you re-word it (*and record that you have done so*). On no account should you attempt to clarify by giving examples of answers.

Where 'PROMPT' appears in the instruction column on the schedules, make sure that the answer is recorded verbatim *before* using the prompts provided. Then make sure that all prompts are used, allowing your informant to select the appropriate ones, and make sure that you ring the relevant numbers. Be careful when you prompt not to put undue emphasis on any of the possible answers. This can easily happen after you have got into a routine and are expecting certain replies to some question.

Be careful of paraphrasing: this easily leads to an inaccurate account of what the informant said. Write down the reply *verbatim* whenever possible. This does not of course include all the 'ers', but we want to know exactly what the answer was, and not the interviewer's idea of the answer. It is obviously important therefore that you should listen carefully, and that if you do not understand the meaning exactly you should probe until you do.

2. *Census Forms* Form A1 is to be completed by the nurse in charge of each ward. It consists of a series of questions which have been carefully worded and coded so that only the briefest of answers is necessary. This sometimes consists of a code number to be ringed, or a yes/no answer, and in one or two cases a figure is required. Each patient in the sample is allotted a column on this form – there are six columns per form. Sometimes you will be collecting information for fewer than six patients in a ward in which case leave the remainder empty. The blank column at the end is for office use only. Detailed instructions on selecting the sample will be given for each hospital. You will be responsible for showing the nurses how to complete this form so please make sure you are well acquainted with it yourself.

Specific Instructions

(a) *Programme and Organization:* Mrs X will be the office organizer of the survey. She will be responsible for co-ordination and for sending you supplies of schedules. If you are not returning to Colchester between visits, completed schedules should be sent to her.

(b) *Visits:* It is proposed that a sample of hospitals and homes should be visited. For ease of sampling a hospital is defined as 'the hospital(s) and annexes which are supervised by one medical superintendent'. Many of the hospitals may therefore consist of several units, all of which have to be visited. We envisage that visits to large hospitals which will be undertaken by two people at a time, will take anything from ten days to two weeks. Small homes may be completed by one person in two to three days.

The normal delegation of responsibility in a hospital catering for both sexes would be: Hospital secretary who is head of the clerical and financial department; Medical superintendent; matron and chief male nurse who run the male and female nursing services at the main hospital, and possibly those at subsidiary units also. If the nursing service at any of the subsidiary units is independent there will, of course, be another matron and/or chief male nurse. In a small home or hostel which is not attached to a bigger hospital, there may only be one person responsible for all branches of administration. This person may be called the Matron, Warden, Superintendent, etc.

In each hospital (home) the medical superintendent, the chief male nurse and the matron will be interviewed. Every ward, day room and sanitary annexe will be visited and a schedule completed. All specialist departments will be visited and the supervisors interviewed. Detailed instructions on all the interviews follow.

Appointments will always have been made in advance for your visit and the superintendent will have been told about the programme you will follow (a typical letter to a superintendent is attached for your information). If there are specific instructions about your time of arrival and to whom you should report, Mrs X will see that you get these.

Schedule C3 (yellow) will have been sent in advance to the hospital secretary for completion, and you should collect this as soon as possible during your visit since some of the information it contains will be useful to you.

Where two research workers are visiting a hospital, it is advisable that you split the ward visits between you so that one does the female side and interviews Matron, and the other visits the male wards and interviews the chief male nurse. Split the remainder of the work as you wish.

It is probable that you will meet the superintendent when you arrive and it may be necessary to refresh his memory about the aims of the research and the methods of work. Be prepared also for some probing and searching questions such as 'What do you think you are going to get out of this survey?' 'What do you think you are going to find?': 'What have you found at other hospitals?'; and so on. Obviously we cannot give you a set of answers to this type of question, but can only warn you not to fall into the trap of revealing information about any other specific hospital, and not to be 'on the defensive' about your work. Simply admit that you cannot really know what will come out of the survey until it is done and remain as friendly and relaxed as you are able. Conversely you may more probably be led into revealing information about another hospital by an informant who appears sympathetic and helpful. This situation must be avoided at all costs except in the most general of terms. This advice is of course applicable to all your contacts with members of the hospital staff.

You will probably be asked on your first day when you want to interview the superintendent, matron and chief male nurse, and when you wish to visit the subsidiary units. You should make it quite clear that the interviews can be arranged at the convenience of the interviewee. Visits to subsidiary units should be arranged towards the end of your stay. You should also find out whether it has been possible to arrange for you to meet the senior nursing staff, and when these meetings are to take place. If possible they should have been arranged for your first day.

Nurses' Meetings

We have asked for you to meet the nursing staff in charge of wards as a group because it is very important to secure their co-operation if this survey is to be at all successful. *Do not worry if this is not possible and in particular do not attempt to force the issue* since you will meet them all as you go round the wards anyway. The purpose of the meeting is principally to explain the aims and methods of the survey. You should do this very simply and clearly and be prepared to repeat yourself as often as necessary. You should invite questions from the nurses at each stage. Emphasize the confidential nature of all information, and that no names will be known to anyone except the research workers. You should then circulate copies of census forms to everyone in the audience (A1) and explain that they will be required to complete these for a small number of patients in their wards and that you would therefore like to explain them. Go through each item carefully and again ask for questions. (You will probably have to go through the form again on each ward, but this preliminary run through may save some time later. You may need to reassure them that you will do this.) Do not forget to ask for these forms to be returned to you at the end of the meeting! End the meeting by emphasizing that you are well aware that nurses in subnormality hospitals are doing a wonderful and devoted job in what are sometimes far from satisfactory conditions and that you hope that more information will lead to improvements.

Ward Schedules: B1 (Orange)

At each ward you should first ask the permission of the senior nurse to wander around. If there has been no nurses' meeting you will have to explain your work briefly, but make it clear that you would like to spend a few minutes with her before you leave the ward, and that you need not take up her time to begin with. Be prepared for a refusal of permission to go round. Be friendly in your initial approach and offer to come back later at a time which would be more convenient to her. If she (he) is completely unco-operative, try to visit the ward later when other staff are on duty.

For each ward you will be required to complete a schedule B1. The instructions are clearly written on the form. Please pay particular attention to the instructions at the top of the sections referring to Day rooms and Sanitary annexes. 'Wards' might also be called 'bedrooms' or 'dormitories'. Day rooms might be referred to as 'sitting rooms, 'dining rooms', 'play rooms', etc. and 'sanitary annexes' refers to all bathrooms, washrooms, showers and lavatories. Where there is a single room or cubicle which is definitely attached to a ward you do not need to fill in a separate sheet for it. The most usual arrangement in these hospitals is that of a ward with its own day room and sanitary annexes and the schedule is designed for this plan, but all rooms must be covered and none must be covered twice, so you will have to use your schedules accordingly.

When you have completed the schedule for wards, day rooms and sanitary annexes you will find that page 5 consists of a series of questions for the nurse in charge. At this stage you should also ask for her help in clarifying any other parts of B1 which you found difficulty in answering. On every 10th ward schedule you will find an extra sheet attached (B2). This deals with clothing and linen and is only to be completed for a sample of wards. Make sure that you keep your uncompleted schedules in the order in which they were given to you so that a B2 will be completed for every 10th ward.

Census Forms

On arrival at the hospital ask if there is an alphabetical list of all patients (if there is only one in order of admission date, use this instead). From this list select the first and every subsequent 20th patient and make a list of the names, hospital numbers and ward numbers of all such patients.

Take a census form for each ward and having inserted the ward number at the top, fill in IN PENCIL at top of column the names (surname in Capitals) and hospital numbers of those patients on your list who are in that particular ward. When you arrive at the ward explain the purpose of the form again, and ask the nurse to complete it and send it to Matron (Chief Male Nurse's) office within the next three days. Make sure that she understands how to complete the form and that she is aware of the need for accuracy. Go through the first column with her if necessary. Please remember in all your contacts with nurses that they are busy people.

Subsidiary Units

You will have the form C3 completed by the hospital secretary from which you will be able to see what other units are attached to the main hospital (generally we shall be able to tell you beforehand but there may be some subsidiaries which we do not know about). If there are several subsidiaries there will almost certainly be two interviewers, so that you can split these visits between you. From Q.10b on Form C3 you will see to what extent these units are autonomous. If a unit shares nursing administration with the main hospital you should attempt to treat it as another ward (or wards). You should of course use a separate schedule B1 for every bedroom or ward just as you have done in the main hospital, but if there is only one nurse in charge of all wards (rather than a nurse on each ward) you complete the nurse's questions on B1 only once and indicate what you have done on the other forms. If there is no tick in column 1 of Q.10b on C3, i.e., nursing administration is not shared with the parent hospital, you should treat this unit separately and complete the matron's interview schedule C1 again.

Interview with Matron and Chief Male Nurse C1 (Pink)

All the advice on public relations given so far applies to your contacts with matron and the chief male nurse. You may have to tread very cautiously indeed, for it is possible that our visit to the hospital may have been agreed without first consulting them. Remember that it is only through their influence that we are likely to secure the co-operation of the nursing staff, and that they are also responsible for allowing us access to the wards. After this initial warning we add that in our experience most matrons and chief male nurses have been only too ready to help.

The schedule for this interview is C1 (pink). The instructions are in the left hand column. Please read these and act accordingly. It is important to remember that you are dealing with one side of the hospital only, and that figures asked for refer only to that side, unless you are in a hospital (home) where there is no division between male and female (such as a children's home, etc.).

Question 4 may need some clarification: 'Senior administrative' staff means the nursing staff in administrative posts, such as matron, deputy and assistant matrons, home sister, and the corresponding posts on the male side. 'Teaching staff' are the nursing staff engaged in teaching student nurses, usually known as Sister Tutors. 'Ward sisters'/Charge nurses' is self explanatory. 'Staff nurses' again refers to trained staff (trained means holding the R.M.N. or S.R.N. certificates). Staff nurses are usually second in command of wards. 'Student nurses' are those nurses who are engaged in training for the R.M.N. certificate. 'Assistant nurses' are those who are untrained and who may or may not be engaged in training for the S.E.A.N. certificate. 'Cadet nurses' are young girls working in the hospital prior to starting nursing training. 'Domestic staff' means those who are employed from the community, i.e. not patients who are doing domestic work. The answers to Q. 39, 46 and 47 may not be known immediately, and matron (C.M.N.) may prefer to let you have this information later.

Interview with Medical Superintendent C2 (Green)

You will almost always have met the superintendent before you interview him, and if you have spent some time going round the hospital he is very likely to ask what you have found and what you think of the hospital. If this happens you should give him a brief but non-commital account of some of your impressions, remembering that it is not his fault if, for example, the hospital is overcrowded. Whenever possible, you will already have completed Questions 1 and 2 before the interview, but do not forget to do so.

Instructions for the remainder of the questions are in the left hand column. Please read these and act on them.

Medical superintendents are notoriously difficult to interview, mostly because they are inclined to wander off the subject. You will find that you are also interested in what they are saying, and it will need all your perseverance and control to keep the situation in hand and to complete the questionnaire. It may be necessary to say something like: 'That is extremely interesting and I wonder if we could come back and discuss it later, but first of all I have to get through this schedule'.

Specialist Departments: D1–6 (Blue)

There are short schedules to be completed for each specialist department. You should visit each department, and try to interview the person in charge. If you have to interview a substitute please record this on the schedule. In each case if the department does not exist please record 'none'.

We expect there to be a school (or teaching provisions) although this might not apply in an institution catering for adults only; occupational therapy department; industrial (or domestic) training; physiotherapy department; psychology department; and social work department. Instructions are in the left hand column in all questionnaires. Please read these and act accordingly.

We shall not make any rules about the hours which you work, but if possible and you are staying near the hospital, you should try to make a few of your ward visits in the evening. You are also encouraged to attend some of the hospital functions, such as the dances or social club.

Conclusion of Visit

On all the schedules you will find that there is room to record any observations you may wish to make as you visit the various parts of the hospital. From these observations you should write a *short* account of your visit under the following headings:

> Food
> Clothing
> Any incidents
> Extent of segregation in the hospital
> Use of institutional language and terminology
> Experimental treatment and training
> Account of any social functions you attend
> Comments on attitude of staff
> General impressions

Before leaving the hospital and indeed after terminating each interview, check through your schedule and make sure that each is completed. You will not be able to make return visits to fill in uncompleted schedules.

Do not leave the hospital without first seeing the matron and chief male nurse and medical superintendent and thanking them for their co-operation and hospitality. You should offer to pay for any meals you have eaten on the premises; do not forget to leave a forwarding address for any census forms which have not yet been returned.

As soon as possible after your visit write your report and send your schedules to Mrs X.

After your visit Mrs X will be responsible for writing to the hospital concerned to thank them for making your visit possible.

APPENDIX E

Number of Patients Suffering from Multiple Handicaps, by Diagnosis*

Diagnosis	Under 16	16 and over
Spastic, epileptic, physical deformity symptomatic of mental subnormality:	2	1
Spastic, epileptic, total paralysis (including severely or completely crippled):	1	12
Spastic, epileptic, total paralysis (including severely or completely crippled), mute:	5	3
Spastic, epileptic, total paralysis (including severely or completely crippled), severe speech defect:	—	2
Spastic, epileptic, partial paralysis, mute:	—	1
Spastic, epileptic, blind:	1	—
Spastic, epileptic, partial paralysis:	12	12
Spastic, epileptic, other deformity:	—	1
Spastic, epileptic, motor handicap:	1	7
Spastic, epileptic, severe ocular condition:	1	4
Spastic, epileptic, severe ocular condition, physical deformity, symptomatic of subnormality:	1	—
Spastic, epileptic, motor handicap, mute:	—	1
Spastic, epileptic, severe speech defect:	9	17
Spastic, epileptic, total paralysis, blind:	1	2
Spastic, epileptic, total paralysis, severe ocular condition:	2	1
Spastic, epileptic, physical deformity symptomatic of mental subnormality, mute:	—	1
Spastic, epileptic, physical deformity symptomatic of mental subnormality, severe speech defect:	3	—
Spastic, epileptic, partial paralysis, severe speech defect:	—	4
Spastic, epileptic, other deformity, blind:	1	—
Spastic, epileptic, other deformity:	2	1
Spastic, epileptic, partial paralysis, deaf mute:	1	—
Spastic, epileptic, physical deformity symptomatic of mental subnormality, mute:	1	—
Spastic, epileptic, cardio-vascular disorder:	—	2
Spastic, epileptic:	—	18

* No distinction is made here between severe and moderate forms of epilepsy and spasticity.

APPENDIX E (Contd.)

Diagnosis	Under 16	16 and over
Spastic, mute:	1	—
Spastic, physical handicap symptomatic of mental subnormality:	1	3
Spastic, total paralysis:	16	42
Spastic, total paralysis, mute:	3	2
Spastic, total paralysis, severe speech defect:	5	3
Spastic, total paralysis, blind:	—	1
Spastic, partial paralysis:	17	42
Spastic, motor handicap:	2	14
Spastic, motor handicap, mental illness:	—	1
Spastic, other deformity:	—	3
Spastic, cardio-vascular disorder:	1	3
Spastic, cardio-vascular disorder, mental illness:	—	1
Spastic, blind:	—	3
Spastic, severe ocular condition:	—	2
Spastic, severe deafness:	—	1
Spastic, total paralysis, deaf mute:	—	2
Spastic, partial paralysis, mental illness:	—	1
Spastic, motor handicap, severe speech defect:	—	1
Epileptic, mute:	7	11
Epileptic, severe speech defect:	5	8
Epileptic, severe deafness:	1	4
Epileptic, physical handicap symptomatic of mental subnormality:	6	6
Epileptic, total paralysis:	3	5
Epileptic, motor handicap:	4	21
Epileptic, blind:	2	4
Epileptic, severe ocular condition:	—	4
Epileptic, deaf mute:	—	3
Epileptic, cardio-vascular disorder:	—	2
Epileptic, partial paralysis:	3	16
Epileptic, physical handicap symptomatic of mental subnormality, metabolic disorder:	—	1
Epileptic, physical handicap symptomatic of mental subnormality, mute:	2	—
Epileptic, physical handicap symptomatic of mental subnormality, severe ocular condition:	1	—
Epileptic, total paralysis, mute:	1	2
Epileptic, total paralysis, severe speech defect:	—	1
Epileptic, other deformity:	2	12
Epileptic, other deformity, mute:	1	1
Epileptic, mental illness, mute:	1	—
Epileptic, motor handicap, mute:	1	—
Epileptic, motor handicap, severe speech defect:	2	2
Epileptic, motor handicap, severe ocular condition:	1	—

Diagnosis	Under 16	16 and over
Epileptic, severe speech defect, metabolic disorder:	1	—
Epileptic, infectious illness:	—	2
Epileptic, partial paralysis, blind:	—	1
Epileptic, partial paralysis, severe ocular condition:	—	1
Epileptic, mental illness:	—	2
Epileptic, metabolic disorder:	—	1
Severe ocular condition, metabolic disorder:	—	1
Physical handicap symptomatic of subnormality, mute:	—	2
Physical handicap symptomatic of subnormality, severe speech defect:	—	4
Physical handicap symptomatic of subnormality, blind:	—	3
Physical handicap symptomatic of subnormality, mental illness:	—	1
Physical handicap symptomatic of subnormality, severe ocular condition:	2	—
Total paralysis, mute:	—	4
Total paralysis, blind:	—	2
Partial paralysis, severe speech defect:	2	—
Partial paralysis, mental illness:	1	—
Motor handicap, mute:	1	—
Cardio-vascular disorder, mute:	1	—

APPENDIX F

Description of Buildings

Hosp. No.	Total No. of pts.*	No. of sites	Description of buildings
0	2,147	2	Main building (1875), 12 ward blocks 3 storeys high with central offices, etc. Three detached wards. Annexe buildings containing 7 wards. Three villas, chapel, various ancillary buildings. Hostel.
1†	2,516	11	Administrative block and 26 villas. One large house used mainly for geriatric patients. One house. One mansion with 3 villas. One old farm house. One old house. Six villas. Geriatric hospital containing 2 villas for subnormals. One geriatric hospital containing one villa for subnormals. Small converted convalescent home. One large house. One new unit with renovated buildings.
2	1,715	2	Two main blocks (1880), central corridor down length of each with wards leading off. Group of cottage homes (1900).
3	1,803	2	Victorian mansion in centre of H-shaped complex of wards. Two detached villas plus ancillary buildings. Hostel.
4	2.066	1	Complex of storeyed and bungalow villas, nucleus is a central 'square' formerly an Inebriates Reformatory (1902–4) housing administration block,

* Information derived from interviews with matrons and chief male nurses since where units of the same hospital did not all share the same secretary, the former provided a more reliable source of information.

† Including 82 psychiatric patients since no distinction is made between the mentally subnormal and the mentally ill in living arrangements.

APPENDIX F (Contd.)

Hosp. No.	Total No. of pts.	No. of sites	Description of buildings
			remainder erected between 1932–40, 'village' type structure, including all facilities for staff.
5	1,706	5	Complex of villas and blocks (1911–56) of which nineteenth century mansion forms nucleus. Eleventh century tower used as ward. Mansion (1660). Mansion (1814). Two residential type houses used as hostels.
6	1,715	15*	Mansion (1877) plus various villas and blocks. Large house (1930) plus villas. Converted Anglican convent. Old residence with modern wings. Three Victorian houses. Former workhouse with annexe. Large residence (undated). Detached Victorian residence. Farmhouse. Pair of converted farm cottages.
7†	—	—	—
8	1,568	5	Fifteen detached villas (1939), other miscellaneous buildings including administrative block. Four other subsidiary hospitals on different sites.
9	1,185	3	Main block comprising 15 wards, offices, etc., 4 villas and various outbuildings. Two small hostels for working patients (different sites).
10	1,691	8*	Administrative block with villas (1930–64), chapel. Old detached house with old annexe. Mansion with one modern villa. Victorian residence. Former workhouse with series of barrack-like blocks. Large house in own grounds.
11	1,014	6	Former workhouse (1830, with 4 villas and 1 bungalow (1930s). Georgian residence with detached block. War-time

* Including holiday home not visited.
† Not visited.

APPENDIX F (Contd.)

Hosp. No.	Total No. of pts.	No. of sites	Description of buildings
			single storey hut used as hostel. Two former workhouses (1860). Complex of former U.S. war-time huts providing 6 wards, with old mansion used for staff residence.
12	1,383	9	Complex of villas (1932) with additional unit (1954). Mansion (1890) pre-1914 villas. One pair semi-detached Victorian houses. Old house with extension (undated). Three detached Victorian houses with extensions. Eighteenth-century town house with 2 wings. Eighteenth-century detached house.
13	1,416	2	Complex of detached blocks and villas (1912–38). One house (undated).
14	1,405	4	Mansion (1850) with 6 E-shaped villas and various outbuildings (1929–30s). One block consisting of 4 wards. Georgian house used as hostel. Complex of detached blocks (date unknown).
15	1,124	2*	Mansion (18th century) with modern wing, 22 2-storeyed villas and houses (c. 1900). One large residence with outbuildings.
16	1,342	6	Mansion (undated) with villas (1935). Former boarding-school (1898) with houses (1902–49) spread over a radius of 7 miles.† One large concrete building (undated). One long, low wooden building. One house used as hostel.
17	1,019	1	Victorian mansion (1868) built as institution for subnormal patients by public subscription, with complex of villas and blocks (1881–1965), one detached house (1964) used as hostel.

* Four villas are each about one mile from the hospital, but these have been included with the main site.

† Not included in this table as separate sites.

APPENDIX F (Contd.)

Hosp. No.	Total No. of pts.	No. of sites	Description of buildings
18	1,656	3	Complex of villas ('village' system) centred round mansion (1880), school (1964). Two old mansions (undated) on different sites, one due for demolition.
19	1,020	6	Two mansions (1750) with villas (1936–60) and outbuildings. Former workhouse (1860) comprising 3 brick blocks. Former workhouse (1802) plus various detached more recently built blocks. Former workhouse (undated). Two detached houses used as hostels.
20	451	2	Mansion (1898) with storeyed and bungalow villas and usual outbuildings (1898–1964). Large mansion (undated).
21	736	3	Mansion (undated) with villas (1945–64). War-time emergency huts attached to an older main block. Former chest hospital (one block, date unspecified).
22	830	5	Mansion (1720) plus villas (1927) and converted war emergency huts (1942). Former workhouse (1840). Former workhouse (1848). Old hospital building (1850). Former workhouse (1838) built in 2 wings.
23	764	8	Mansion (undated). Former workhouse (1860). Large Victorian residence. One block of a general hospital. Stately farmhouse with outbuildings (undated). Two former workhouses (undated). Large, former private residence (undated).
24	445	3	Former workhouse (1856) with modern extension. Two main buildings (undated). Large detached Victorian house.
25	914	7	Mansion (1850) plus villas (1930) and various outbuildings. Mansion (1699) with various outbuildings, 2 villas (1937), 1 single-storey villa (1964) and 1 hutted single-storey villa (1954). Workhouse (1837 – modernised). Victorian mansion

APPENDIX F (Contd.)

Hosp. No.	Total No. of pts.	No. of sites	Description of buildings
			(date unknown) converted to Approved School and then hospital usage (1956). Large Georgian house (undated) used as Approved School and converted to hospital usage (1957). Large Victorian house in residential district used as hostel. Temporary hutted buildings (1940) originally used for War Agricultural Committee, converted to hospital usage (1948).
26	652	8	Administratively centred on Regional Mental Hospital, but no subnormal patients housed there. Former workhouse (undated). Four mansions (mid-eighteenth century c.). Mansion (eighteenth century). Two small residential type houses.
27	747	4	Mansion (1900) with complex of villas. Victorian town house with one detached block. Detached Victorian mansion. One block in complex of hospitals for geriatric and psychiatric patients (undated but probably Victorian).
28	975	8	Administrative block with 10 villas. Five blocks joined by covered corridors. Former workhouse in 2 sections (nineteenth century). Three large houses. One mansion. Converted army huts.
29	727	5	Mansion (nineteenth century) with 3 villas (1930s), one villa (1950). Nineteenth century annexe with ward (1930) and various outbuildings. Nineteenth century residence with villas. One large pre-fab building used as hostel (former land army usage). One large house (1938) with 4 villas. One large Victorian house used as hostel.
30	398	1	Two small mansions (pre-1860) with 8 villas (1920–39) and 5 villas (1940–65).
31	536	2	Mansion (undated) with villas (1923–58). Mansion (1881).

APPENDIX F (Contd.)

Hosp. No.	Total No. of pts.	No. of sites	Description of buildings
32	119	2	Administered from local mental hospital (no mentally subnormal patients). Large house (undated). One house with hutted annexe (part of General Hospital).
33	100	1	Administered from local mental hospital (no mentally subnormal patients). Mansion (1860).
34	210	2	Mansion (1870) with annexe. Mansion (1829) with villa (1962).

Distance Separating Units from Administrative Centre*

Hosp. No.	Total No. of pts. in hosp.†	Ancillary units	No. of pts. in unit	Approx. mileage from main hosp.
0	2,147	a	12	8
1	2,516	a	101‡	30
		b	12	31
		c	177	38
		d	202	15
		e	175	52
		f	15	30
		g	106	30
		h	148	41
		i	20	36
		j	115	43
2	1,715	a	65	10
3	1,803	nil	—	—
4	2,066	a	5	3

* This is defined, for purposes of this table, as the centre to which the Medical Superintendent and consultant psychiatrists are attached.
† Information obtained from matrons and chief male nurses.
‡ Only 19 are subnormal patients.

APPENDIX F (Contd.)

Hosp. No.	Total No. of pts. in hosp.	Ancillary units	No. of pts. in unit	Approx. mileage from main hosp.
5	1,706	a	557	3
		b	215	3
		c	24	5
		d	200	5
6	1,715	a	156	25
		b	47	9
		c	8	4
		d	63	9
		e	12	9
		f	536	4
		g	59	15
		h	108	90*
		i	21	90*
		j	31	65
		k	15	20
		l	100	16
		m	19	4
7	—	—	—	—
8	1,568	a	249	5
		b	21	30
		c	21	30
		d	15	4
9	1,185	a	33	3
		b	22	3
10	1,691	a	70	30
		b	73	26
		c	71	15
		d	343†	20
		e	24	5
		f	75	15
11	1,014	a	65	22
		b	16	12
		c	306	53
		d	175	32
		e	32	2

* These two units are adjacent and could be treated as one unit from the point of view of psychiatric supervision.

† Although administered from the main hospital 20 miles away, this unit is under the supervision of a Deputy Medical Superintendent.

APPENDIX F (Contd.)

Hosp. No.	Total No. of pts. in hosp.	Ancillary units	No. of pts. in unit	Approx. mileage from main hosp.
12	1,383	a	30	5
		b	32	3
		c	27	36
		d	55	13
		e	19	13
		f	48	13
		g	424	5
		h	43	3
13	1,416	a	21	8
14	1,405	a	735	3
		b	247	24
		c	26	4
15	1,124	a	224	8
16	1,342	a	445	10
		b	147	15
		c	162	20
		d	17	20
		e	17	10
17	1,019	nil	—	—
18	1,656	a	83	8
		b	120	25
19	1,020	a	139	36
		b	171	24
		c	217	46
		d	30	30
		e	26	19
20	451	a	67	9
21	736	a	219	50
		b	39	25
22	830	a	176	43*
		b	43	48*
		c	176	33
		d	139	36

* These units are administered as one although separated by 5 miles.

APPENDIX F (Contd.)

Hosp. No.	Total No. of pts. in hosp.	Ancillary units	No. of pts. in unit	Approx. mileage from main hosp.
23	764	a	146	75
		b	157	68
		c	73	35
		d	66	48
		e	58	50
		f	17	17
		g	71	48
24	445	a	107	20
		b	29	30
25	914	a	121	7
		b	64	4
		c	228	5
		d	40	9
		e	20	3
		f	21	4
26	652	a	60	5
		b	14	3
		c	63	6
		d	114	3
		e	60	5
		f	20	3
		g	103	10
27	747	a	51	23
		b	65	27
		c	123	29
28	975	a	259	35
		b	39	30
		c	14	20
		d	24	25
		e	142	36
		f	33	40
		g	73	25
29	727	a	152	20
		b	26	20
		c	26	3
		d	32	3
		e	175	20
30	398	nil	—	—

APPENDIX F (Contd.)

Hosp. No.	Total No. of pts. in hosp.	Ancillary units	No. of pts. in unit	Approx. mileage from main hosp.
31	536	a	316	16
32	119	a	58	6
33	100	nil	—	—
34	210	a	115	12
TOTAL	38,097		12,426	21·8 (mean distance)

INDEX

The International Library of
Sociology
and Social Reconstruction

Edited by W. J. H. SPROTT
Founded by KARL MANNHEIM

ROUTLEDGE & KEGAN PAUL
BROADWAY HOUSE, CARTER LANE, LONDON, E.C.4

CONTENTS

PRINTED IN GREAT BRITAIN BY HEADLEY BROTHERS LTD
109 KINGSWAY LONDON WC2 AND ASHFORD KENT

GENERAL SOCIOLOGY

Brown, Robert. Explanation in Social Science. *208 pp. 1963. (2nd Impression 1964.) 25s.*

Gibson, Quentin. The Logic of Social Enquiry. *240 pp. 1960. (3rd Impression 1968.) 24s.*

Homans, George C. Sentiments and Activities: Essays in Social Science. *336 pp. 1962. 32s.*

Isajiw, Wsevelod W. Causation and Functionalism in Sociology. *165 pp. 1968. 25s.*

Johnson, Harry M. Sociology: a Systematic Introduction. *Foreword by Robert K. Merton. 710 pp. 1961. (5th Impression 1968.) 42s.*

Mannheim, Karl. Essays on Sociology and Social Psychology. *Edited by Paul Keckskemeti. With Editorial Note by Adolph Lowe. 344 pp. 1953. (2nd Impression 1966.) 32s.*

Systematic Sociology: An Introduction to the Study of Society. *Edited by J. S. Erös and Professor W. A. C. Stewart. 220 pp. 1957. (3rd Impression 1967.) 24s.*

Martindale, Don. The Nature and Types of Sociological Theory. *292 pp. 1961. (3rd Impression 1967.) 35s.*

Maus, Heinz. A Short History of Sociology. *234 pp. 1962. (2nd Impression 1965.) 28s.*

Myrdal, Gunnar. Value in Social Theory: A Collection of Essays on Methodology. *Edited by Paul Streeten. 332 pp. 1958. (3rd Impression 1968.) 35s.*

Ogburn, William F., and **Nimkoff, Meyer F.** A Handbook of Sociology. *Preface by Karl Mannheim. 656 pp. 46 figures. 35 tables. 5th edition (revised) 1964. 45s.*

Parsons, Talcott, and **Smelser, Neil J.** Economy and Society: A Study in the Integration of Economic and Social Theory. *362 pp. 1956. (4th Impression 1967.) 35s.*

Rex, John. Key Problems of Sociological Theory. *220 pp. 1961. (4th Impression 1968.) 25s.*

Stark, Werner. The Fundamental Forms of Social Thought. *280 pp. 1962. 32s.*

FOREIGN CLASSICS OF SOCIOLOGY

Durkheim, Emile. Suicide. A Study in Sociology. *Edited and with an Introduction by George Simpson. 404 pp. 1952. (4th Impression 1968.) 35s.*

Professional Ethics and Civic Morals. *Translated by Cornelia Brookfield. 288 pp. 1957. 30s.*

Gerth, H. H., and **Mills, C. Wright.** From Max Weber: Essays in Sociology. *502 pp. 1948. (6th Impression 1967.) 35s.*

Tönnies, Ferdinand. Community and Association. (*Gemeinschaft und Gesellschaft.*) *Translated and Supplemented by Charles P. Loomis. Foreword by Pitirim A. Sorokin. 334 pp. 1955. 28s.*

3

SOCIAL STRUCTURE

Andreski, Stanislav. Military Organization and Society. *Foreword by Professor A. R. Radcliffe-Brown. 226 pp. 1 folder. 1954. Revised Edition 1968. 35s.*

Cole, G. D. H. Studies in Class Structure. *220 pp. 1955. (3rd Impression 1964.) 21s. Paper 10s. 6d.*

Coontz, Sydney H. Population Theories and the Economic Interpretation. *202 pp. 1957. (3rd Impression 1968.) 28s.*

Coser, Lewis. The Functions of Social Conflict. *204 pp. 1956. (3rd Impression 1968.) 25s.*

Dickie-Clark, H. F. Marginal Situation: A Sociological Study of a Coloured Group. *240 pp. 11 tables. 1966. 40s.*

Glass, D. V. (Ed.). Social Mobility in Britain. *Contributions by J. Berent, T. Bottomore, R. C. Chambers, J. Floud, D. V. Glass, J. R. Hall, H. T. Himmelweit, R. K. Kelsall, F. M. Martin, C. A. Moser, R. Mukherjee, and W. Ziegel. 420 pp. 1954. (4th Impression 1967.) 45s.*

Jones, Garth N. Planned Organizational Change: An Exploratory Study Using an Empirical Approach. *About 268 pp. 1969. 40s.*

Kelsall, R. K. Higher Civil Servants in Britain: From 1870 to the Present Day. *268 pp. 31 tables. 1955. (2nd Impression 1966.) 25s.*

König, René. The Community. *232 pp. Illustrated. 1968. 35s.*

Lawton, Denis. Social Class, Language and Education. *192 pp. 1968. (2nd Impression 1968.) 25s.*

McLeish, John. The Theory of Social Change: Four Views Considered. *About 128 pp. 1969. 21s.*

Marsh, David C. The Changing Social Structure in England and Wales, 1871-1961. *1958. 272 pp. 2nd edition (revised) 1966. (2nd Impression 1967.) 35s.*

Mouzelis, Nicos. Organization and Bureaucracy. An Analysis of Modern Theories. *240 pp. 1967. (2nd Impression 1968.) 28s.*

Ossowski, Stanislaw. Class Structure in the Social Consciousness. *210 pp. 1963. (2nd Impression 1967.) 25s.*

SOCIOLOGY AND POLITICS

Barbu, Zevedei. Democracy and Dictatorship: Their Psychology and Patterns of Life. *300 pp. 1956. 28s.*

Crick, Bernard. The American Science of Politics: Its Origins and Conditions. *284 pp. 1959. 32s.*

Hertz, Frederick. Nationality in History and Politics: A Psychology and Sociology of National Sentiment and Nationalism. *432 pp. 1944. (5th Impression 1966.) 42s.*

Kornhauser, William. The Politics of Mass Society. *272 pp. 20 tables. 1960. (3rd Impression 1968.) 28s.*

Laidler, Harry W. History of Socialism. Social-Economic Movements: An Historical and Comparative Survey of Socialism, Communism, Co-operation, Utopianism; and other Systems of Reform and Reconstruction. *New edition. 992 pp. 1968. 90s.*

Lasswell, Harold D. Analysis of Political Behaviour. An Empirical Approach. *324 pp. 1947. (4th Impression 1966.) 35s.*

Mannheim, Karl. Freedom, Power and Democratic Planning. *Edited by Hans Gerth and Ernest K. Bramstedt. 424 pp. 1951. (3rd Impression 1968.) 42s.*

Mansur, Fatma. Process of Independence. *Foreword by A. H. Hanson. 208 pp. 1962. 25s.*

Martin, David A. Pacificism: an Historical and Sociological Study. *262 pp. 1965. 30s.*

Myrdal, Gunnar. The Political Element in the Development of Economic Theory. *Translated from the German by Paul Streeten. 282 pp. 1953. (4th Impression 1965.) 25s.*

Polanyi, Michael. F.R.S. The Logic of Liberty: Reflections and Rejoinders. *228 pp. 1951. 18s.*

Verney, Douglas V. The Analysis of Political Systems. *264 pp. 1959. (3rd Impression 1966.) 28s.*

Wootton, Graham. The Politics of Influence: British Ex-Servicemen, Cabinet Decisions and Cultural Changes, 1917 to 1957. *316 pp. 1963. 30s.*
  Workers, Unions and the State. *188 pp. 1966. (2nd Impression 1967.) 25s.*

FOREIGN AFFAIRS: THEIR SOCIAL, POLITICAL AND ECONOMIC FOUNDATIONS

Baer, Gabriel. Population and Society in the Arab East. *Translated by Hanna Szöke. 288 pp. 10 maps. 1964. 40s.*

Bonné, Alfred. State and Economics in the Middle East: A Society in Transition. *482 pp. 2nd (revised) edition 1955. (2nd Impression 1960.) 40s.*
  Studies in Economic Development: with special reference to Conditions in the Under-developed Areas of Western Asia and India. *322 pp. 84 tables. 2nd edition 1960. 32s.*

Mayer, J. P. Political Thought in France from the Revolution to the Fifth Republic. *164 pp. 3rd edition (revised) 1961. 16s.*

CRIMINOLOGY

Ancel, Marc. Social Defence: A Modern Approach to Criminal Problems. *Foreword by Leon Radzinowicz. 240 pp. 1965. 32s.*

Cloward, Richard A., and Ohlin, Lloyd E. Delinquency and Opportunity: A Theory of Delinquent Gangs. *248 pp. 1961. 25s.*

Downes, David M. The Delinquent Solution. A Study in Subcultural Theory. *296 pp. 1966. 42s.*

Dunlop, A. B., and **McCabe, S.** Young Men in Detention Centres. *192 pp. 1965. 28s.*

Friedländer, Kate. The Psycho-Analytical Approach to Juvenile Delinquency: Theory, Case Studies, Treatment. *320 pp. 1947. (6th Impression 1967). 40s.*

Glueck, Sheldon and **Eleanor.** Family Environment and Delinquency. *With the statistical assistance of Rose W. Kneznek. 340 pp. 1962. (2nd Impression 1966.) 40s.*

Mannheim, Hermann. Comparative Criminology: a Text Book. *Two volumes. 442 pp. and 380 pp. 1965. (2nd Impression with corrections 1966.) 42s. a volume.*

Morris, Terence. The Criminal Area: A Study in Social Ecology. *Foreword by Hermann Mannheim. 232 pp. 25 tables. 4 maps. 1957. (2nd Impression 1966.) 28s.*

Morris, Terence and **Pauline,** assisted by **Barbara Barer.** Pentonville: A Sociological Study of an English Prison. *416 pp. 16 plates. 1963. 50s.*

Spencer, John C. Crime and the Services. *Foreword by Hermann Mannheim. 336 pp. 1954. 28s.*

Trasler, Gordon. The Explanation of Criminality. *144 pp. 1962. (2nd Impression 1967.) 20s.*

SOCIAL PSYCHOLOGY

Barbu, Zevedei. Problems of Historical Psychology. *248 pp. 1960. 25s.*

Blackburn, Julian. Psychology and the Social Pattern. *184 pp. 1945. (7th Impression 1964.) 16s.*

Fleming, C. M. Adolescence: Its Social Psychology: With an Introduction to recent findings from the fields of Anthropology, Physiology, Medicine, Psychometrics and Sociometry. *288 pp. 2nd edition (revised) 1963. (3rd Impression 1967.) 25s. Paper 12s. 6d.*
The Social Psychology of Education: An Introduction and Guide to Its Study. *136 pp. 2nd edition (revised) 1959. (4th Impression 1967.) 14s. Paper 7s. 6d.*

Homans, George C. The Human Group. *Foreword by Bernard DeVoto. Introduction by Robert K. Merton. 526 pp. 1951. (7th Impression 1968.) 35s.*
Social Behaviour: its Elementary Forms. *416 pp. 1961. (3rd Impression 1968.) 35s.*

Klein, Josephine. The Study of Groups. *226 pp. 31 figures. 5 tables. 1956. (5th Impression 1967.) 21s. Paper 9s. 6d.*

Linton, Ralph. The Cultural Background of Personality. *132 pp. 1947. (7th Impression 1968.) 18s.*

Mayo, Elton. The Social Problems of an Industrial Civilization. With an appendix on the Political Problem. *180 pp. 1949. (5th Impression 1966.) 25s.*

Ottaway, A. K. C. Learning Through Group Experience. *176 pp. 1966. (2nd Impression 1968.) 25s.*

Ridder, J. C. de. The Personality of the Urban African in South Africa. A Thematic Apperception Test Study. *196 pp. 12 plates. 1961. 25s.*

Rose, Arnold M. (Ed.). Human Behaviour and Social Processes: an Interactionist Approach. *Contributions by Arnold M. Rose, Ralph H. Turner, Anselm Strauss, Everett C. Hughes, E. Franklin Frazier, Howard S. Becker, et al. 696 pp. 1962. (2nd Impression 1968.) 70s.*

Smelser, Neil J. Theory of Collective Behaviour. *448 pp. 1962. (2nd Impression 1967.) 45s.*

Stephenson, Geoffrey M. The Development of Conscience. *128 pp. 1966. 25s.*

Young, Kimball. Handbook of Social Psychology. *658 pp. 16 figures. 10 tables. 2nd edition (revised) 1957. (3rd Impression 1963.) 40s.*

SOCIOLOGY OF THE FAMILY

Banks, J. A. Prosperity and Parenthood: A study of Family Planning among The Victorian Middle Classes. *262 pp. 1954. (3rd Impression 1968.) 28s.*

Bell, Colin R. Middle Class Families: Social and Geographical Mobility. *224 pp. 1969. 35s.*

Burton, Lindy. Vulnerable Children. *272 pp. 1968. 35s.*

Gavron, Hannah. The Captive Wife: Conflicts of Housebound Mothers. *190 pp. 1966. (2nd Impression 1966.) 25s.*

Klein, Josephine. Samples from English Cultures. *1965. (2nd Impression 1967.)*
1. Three Preliminary Studies and Aspects of Adult Life in England. *447 pp. 50s.*
2. Child-Rearing Practices and Index. *247 pp. 35s.*

Klein, Viola. Britain's Married Women Workers. *180 pp. 1965. (2nd Impression 1968.) 28s.*

McWhinnie, Alexina M. Adopted Children. How They Grow Up. *304 pp. 1967. (2nd Impression 1968.) 42s.*

Myrdal, Alva and **Klein, Viola.** Women's Two Roles: Home and Work. *238 pp. 27 tables. 1956. Revised Edition 1967. 30s. Paper 15s.*

Parsons, Talcott and **Bales, Robert F.** Family: Socialization and Interaction Process. *In collaboration with James Olds, Morris Zelditch and Philip E. Slater. 456 pp. 50 figures and tables. 1956. (3rd Impression 1968.) 45s.*

Schücking, L. L. The Puritan Family. *Translated from the German by Brian Battershaw. 212 pp. 1969. About 42s.*

7

THE SOCIAL SERVICES

Forder, R. A. (Ed.). Penelope Hall's Social Services of Modern England. *288 pp. 1969. 35s.*

George, Victor. Social Security: Beveridge and After. *258 pp. 1968. 35s.*

Goetschius, George W. Working with Community Groups. *256 pp. 1969. 35s.*

Goetschius, George W. and **Tash, Joan.** Working with Unattached Youth. *416 pp. 1967. (2nd Impression 1968.) 40s.*

Hall, M. P., and **Howes, I. V.** The Church in Social Work. A Study of Moral Welfare Work undertaken by the Church of England. *320 pp. 1965. 35s.*

Heywood, Jean S. Children in Care: the Development of the Service for the Deprived Child. *264 pp. 2nd edition (revised) 1965. (2nd Impression 1966.) 32s.*

An Introduction to Teaching Casework Skills. *190 pp. 1964. 28s.*

Jones, Kathleen. Lunacy, Law and Conscience, 1744-1845: the Social History of the Care of the Insane. *268 pp. 1955. 25s.*

Mental Health and Social Policy, 1845-1959. *264 pp. 1960. (2nd Impression 1967.) 32s.*

Jones, Kathleen and **Sidebotham, Roy.** Mental Hospitals at Work. *220 pp. 1962. 30s.*

Kastell, Jean. Casework in Child Care. *Foreword by M. Brooke Willis. 320 pp. 1962. 35s.*

Morris, Pauline. Put Away: A Sociological Study of Institutions for the Mentally Retarded. *Approx. 288 pp. 1969. About 50s.*

Nokes, P. L. The Professional Task in Welfare Practice. *152 pp. 1967. 28s.*

Rooff, Madeline. Voluntary Societies and Social Policy. *350 pp. 15 tables. 1957. 35s.*

Timms, Noel. Psychiatric Social Work in Great Britain (1939-1962). *280 pp. 1964. 32s.*

Social Casework: Principles and Practice. *256 pp. 1964. (2nd Impression 1966.) 25s. Paper 15s.*

Trasler, Gordon. In Place of Parents: A Study in Foster Care. *272 pp. 1960. (2nd Impression 1966.) 30s.*

Young, A. F., and **Ashton, E. T.** British Social Work in the Nineteenth Century. *288 pp. 1956. (2nd Impression 1963.) 28s.*

Young, A. F. Social Services in British Industry. *272 pp. 1968. 40s.*

SOCIOLOGY OF EDUCATION

Banks, Olive. Parity and Prestige in English Secondary Education: a Study in Educational Sociology. *272 pp. 1955. (2nd Impression 1963.) 32s.*

Bentwich, Joseph. Education in Israel. *224 pp. 8 pp. plates. 1965. 24s.*

Blyth, W. A. L. English Primary Education. A Sociological Description. *1965. Revised edition 1967.*
  1. Schools. *232 pp. 30s. Paper 12s. 6d.*
  2. Background. *168 pp. 25s. Paper 10s. 6d.*

Collier, K. G. The Social Purposes of Education: Personal and Social Values in Education. *268 pp. 1959. (3rd Impression 1965.) 21s.*

Dale, R. R., and **Griffith, S.** Down Stream: Failure in the Grammar School. *108 pp. 1965. 20s.*

Dore, R. P. Education in Tokugawa Japan. *356 pp. 9 pp. plates. 1965. 35s.*

Edmonds, E. L. The School Inspector. *Foreword by Sir William Alexander. 214 pp. 1962. 28s.*

Evans, K. M. Sociometry and Education. *158 pp. 1962. (2nd Impression 1966.) 18s.*

Foster, P. J. Education and Social Change in Ghana. *336 pp. 3 maps. 1965. (2nd Impression 1967.) 36s.*

Fraser, W. R. Education and Society in Modern France. *150 pp. 1963. (2nd Impression 1968.) 25s.*

Hans, Nicholas. New Trends in Education in the Eighteenth Century. *278 pp. 19 tables. 1951. (2nd Impression 1966.) 30s.*
  Comparative Education: A Study of Educational Factors and Traditions. *360 pp. 3rd (revised) edition 1958. (4th Impression 1967.) 25s. Paper 12s. 6d.*

Hargreaves, David. Social Relations in a Secondary School. *240 pp. 1967. (2nd Impression 1968.) 32s.*

Holmes, Brian. Problems in Education. A Comparative Approach. *336 pp. 1965. (2nd Impression 1967.) 32s.*

Mannheim, Karl and **Stewart, W. A. C.** An Introduction to the Sociology of Education. *206 pp. 1962. (2nd Impression 1965.) 21s.*

Morris, Raymond N. The Sixth Form and College Entrance. *231 pp. 1969. 40s.*

Musgrove, F. Youth and the Social Order. *176 pp. 1964. (2nd Impression 1968.) 25s. Paper 12s.*

Ortega y Gasset, José. Mission of the University. *Translated with an Introduction by Howard Lee Nostrand. 86 pp. 1946. (3rd Impression 1963.) 15s.*

Ottaway, A. K. C. Education and Society: An Introduction to the Sociology of Education. *With an Introduction by W. O. Lester Smith. 212 pp. Second edition (revised). 1962. (5th Impression 1968.) 18s. Paper 10s. 6d.*

Peers, Robert. Adult Education: A Comparative Study. *398 pp. 2nd edition 1959. (2nd Impression 1966.) 42s.*

Pritchard, D. G. Education and the Handicapped: 1760 to 1960. *258 pp. 1963. (2nd Impression 1966.) 35s.*

Richardson, Helen. Adolescent Girls in Approved Schools. *Approx. 360 pp. 1969. About 42s.*

Simon, Brian and **Joan** (Eds.). Educational Psychology in the U.S.S.R. *Introduction by Brian and Joan Simon. Translation by Joan Simon. Papers by D. N. Bogoiavlenski and N. A. Menchinskaia, D. B. Elkonin, E. A. Fleshner, Z. I. Kalmykova, G. S. Kostiuk, V. A. Krutetski, A. N. Leontiev, A. R. Luria, E. A. Milerian, R. G. Natadze, B. M. Teplov, L. S. Vygotski, L. V. Zankov. 296 pp. 1963. 40s.*

SOCIOLOGY OF CULTURE

Eppel, E. M., and **M.** Adolescents and Morality: A Study of some Moral Values and Dilemmas of Working Adolescents in the Context of a changing Climate of Opinion. *Foreword by W. J. H. Sprott. 268 pp. 39 tables. 1966. 30s.*

Fromm, Erich. The Fear of Freedom. *286 pp. 1942. (8th Impression 1960.) 25s. Paper 10s.*
The Sane Society. *400 pp. 1956. (4th Impression 1968.) 28s. Paper 14s.*

Mannheim, Karl. Diagnosis of Our Time: Wartime Essays of a Sociologist. *208 pp. 1943. (8th Impression 1966.) 21s.*
Essays on the Sociology of Culture. *Edited by Ernst Mannheim in co-operation with Paul Kecskemeti. Editorial Note by Adolph Lowe. 280 pp. 1956. (3rd Impression 1967.) 28s.*

Weber, Alfred. Farewell to European History: or The Conquest of Nihilism. *Translated from the German by R. F. C. Hull. 224 pp. 1947. 18s.*

SOCIOLOGY OF RELIGION

Argyle, Michael. Religious Behaviour. *224 pp. 8 figures. 41 tables. 1958. (4th Impression 1968.) 25s.*

Nelson, G. K. Spiritualism and Society. *313 pp. 1969. 42s.*

Stark, Werner. The Sociology of Religion. A Study of Christendom.
Volume I. Established Religion. *248 pp. 1966. 35s.*
Volume II. Sectarian Religion. *368 pp. 1967. 40s.*
Volume III. The Universal Church. *464 pp. 1967. 45s.*

Watt, W. Montgomery. Islam and the Integration of Society. *320 pp. 1961. (3rd Impression 1966.) 35s.*

SOCIOLOGY OF ART AND LITERATURE

Beljame, Alexandre. Men of Letters and the English Public in the Eighteenth Century: 1660-1744, Dryden, Addison, Pope. *Edited with an Introduction and Notes by Bonamy Dobrée. Translated by E. O. Lorimer. 532 pp. 1948. 32s.*

Misch, Georg. A History of Autobiography in Antiquity. *Translated by E. W. Dickes. 2 Volumes. Vol. 1, 364 pp., Vol. 2, 372 pp. 1950. 45s. the set.*

Schücking, L. L. The Sociology of Literary Taste. *112 pp. 2nd (revised) edition 1966. 18s.*

Silbermann, Alphons. The Sociology of Music. *Translated from the German by Corbet Stewart. 222 pp. 1963. 32s.*

SOCIOLOGY OF KNOWLEDGE

Mannheim, Karl. Essays on the Sociology of Knowledge. *Edited by Paul Kecskemeti. Editorial note by Adolph Lowe. 352 pp. 1952. (4th Impression 1967.) 35s.*

Stark, W. America: Ideal and Reality. The United States of 1776 in Contemporary Philosophy. *136 pp. 1947. 12s.*
The Sociology of Knowledge: An Essay in Aid of a Deeper Understanding of the History of Ideas. *384 pp. 1958. (3rd Impression 1967.) 36s.*
Montesquieu: Pioneer of the Sociology of Knowledge. *244 pp. 1960. 25s.*

URBAN SOCIOLOGY

Anderson, Nels. The Urban Community: A World Perspective. *532 pp. 1960. 35s.*

Ashworth, William. The Genesis of Modern British Town Planning: A Study in Economic and Social History of the Nineteenth and Twentieth Centuries. *288 pp. 1954. (3rd Impression 1968.) 32s.*

Bracey, Howard. Neighbours: On New Estates and Subdivisions in England and U.S.A. *220 pp. 1964. 28s.*

Cullingworth, J. B. Housing Needs and Planning Policy: A Restatement of the Problems of Housing Need and "Overspill" in England and Wales. *232 pp. 44 tables. 8 maps. 1960. (2nd Impression 1966.) 28s.*

Dickinson, Robert E. City and Region: A Geographical Interpretation. *608 pp. 125 figures. 1964. (5th Impression 1967.) 60s.*
The West European City: A Geographical Interpretation. *600 pp. 129 maps. 29 plates. 2nd edition 1962. (3rd Impression 1968.) 55s.*
The City Region in Western Europe. *320 pp. Maps. 1967. 30s. Paper 14s.*

Jackson, Brian. Working Class Community: Some General Notions raised by a Series of Studies in Northern England. *192 pp. 1968. (2nd Impression 1968.) 25s.*

Jennings, Hilda. Societies in the Making: a Study of Development and Redevelopment within a County Borough. *Foreword by D. A. Clark. 286 pp. 1962. (2nd Impression 1967.) 32s.*

Kerr, Madeline. The People of Ship Street. *240 pp. 1958. 28s.*

Mann, P. H. An Approach to Urban Sociology. *240 pp. 1965. (2nd Impression 1968.) 30s.*

Morris, R. N., and Mogey, J. The Sociology of Housing. Studies at Berinsfield. *232 pp. 4 pp. plates. 1965. 42s.*

Rosser, C., and Harris, C. The Family and Social Change. A Study of Family and Kinship in a South Wales Town. *352 pp. 8 maps. 1965. (2nd Impression 1968.) 45s.*

RURAL SOCIOLOGY

Chambers, R. J. H. Settlement Schemes in Africa: A Selective Study. *Approx. 268 pp. 1969. About 50s.*

Haswell, M. R. The Economics of Development in Village India. *120 pp. 1967. 21s.*

11

Littlejohn, James. Westrigg: the Sociology of a Cheviot Parish. *172 pp. 5 figures. 1963. 25s.*

Williams, W. M. The Country Craftsman: A Study of Some Rural Crafts and the Rural Industries Organization in England. *248 pp. 9 figures. 1958. 25s. (Dartington Hall Studies in Rural Sociology.)*
The Sociology of an English Village: Gosforth. *272 pp. 12 figures. 13 tables. 1956. (3rd Impression 1964.) 25s.*

SOCIOLOGY OF MIGRATION

Humphreys, Alexander J. New Dubliners: Urbanization and the Irish Family. *Foreword by George C. Homans. 304 pp. 1966. 40s.*

SOCIOLOGY OF INDUSTRY AND DISTRIBUTION

Anderson, Nels. Work and Leisure. *280 pp. 1961. 28s.*

Blau, Peter M., and **Scott, W. Richard.** Formal Organizations: a Comparative approach. *Introduction and Additional Bibliography by J. H. Smith. 326 pp. 1963. (4th Impression 1969.) 35s. Paper 15s.*

Eldridge, J. E. T. Industrial Disputes. Essays in the Sociology of Industrial Relations. *288 pp. 1968. 40s.*

Hollowell, Peter G. The Lorry Driver. *272 pp. 1968. 42s.*

Jefferys, Margot, with the assistance of Winifred Moss. Mobility in the Labour Market: Employment Changes in Battersea and Dagenham. *Preface by Barbara Wootton. 186 pp. 51 tables. 1954. 15s.*

Levy, A. B. Private Corporations and Their Control. *Two Volumes. Vol. 1, 464 pp., Vol. 2, 432 pp. 1950. 80s. the set.*

Liepmann, Kate. Apprenticeship: An Enquiry into its Adequacy under Modern Conditions. *Foreword by H. D. Dickinson. 232 pp. 6 tables. 1960. (2nd Impression 1960.) 23s.*

Millerson, Geoffrey. The Qualifying Associations: a Study in Professionalization. *320 pp. 1964. 42s.*

Smelser, Neil J. Social Change in the Industrial Revolution: An Application of Theory to the Lancashire Cotton Industry, 1770-1840. *468 pp. 12 figures. 14 tables. 1959. (2nd Impression 1960.) 50s.*

Williams, Gertrude. Recruitment to Skilled Trades. *240 pp. 1957. 23s.*

Young, A. F. Industrial Injuries Insurance: an Examination of British Policy. *192 pp. 1964. 30s.*

ANTHROPOLOGY

Ammar, Hamed. Growing up in an Egyptian Village: Silwa, Province of Aswan. *336 pp. 1954. (2nd Impression 1966.) 35s.*

Crook, David and **Isabel.** Revolution in a Chinese Village: Ten Mile Inn. *230 pp. 8 plates. 1 map. 1959. (2nd Impression 1968.) 21s.*
The First Years of Yangyi Commune. *302 pp. 12 plates. 1966. 42s.*

Dickie-Clark, H. F. The Marginal Situation. A Sociological Study of a Coloured Group. *236 pp. 1966. 40s.*

Dube, S. C. Indian Village. *Foreword by Morris Edward Opler. 276 pp. 4 plates. 1955. (5th Impression 1965.) 25s.*
India's Changing Villages: Human Factors in Community Development. *260 pp. 8 plates. 1 map. 1958. (3rd Impression 1963.) 25s.*

Firth, Raymond. Malay Fishermen. Their Peasant Economy. *420 pp. 17 pp. plates. 2nd edition revised and enlarged 1966. (2nd Impression 1968.) 55s.*

Gulliver, P. H. The Family Herds. A Study of two Pastoral Tribes in East Africa, The Jie and Turkana. *304 pp. 4 plates. 19 figures. 1955. (2nd Impression with new preface and bibliography 1966.) 35s.*
Social Control in an African Society: a Study of the Arusha, Agricultural Masai of Northern Tanganyika. *320 pp. 8 plates. 10 figures. 1963. (2nd Impression 1968.) 42s.*

Ishwaran, K. Shivapur. A South Indian Village. *216 pp. 1968. 35s.*
Tradition and Economy in Village India: An Interactionist Approach. *Foreword by Conrad Arensburg. 176 pp. 1966. (2nd Impression 1968.) 25s.*

Jarvie, Ian C. The Revolution in Anthropology. *268 pp. 1964. (2nd Impression 1967.) 40s.*

Jarvie, Ian C. and **Agassi, Joseph.** Hong Kong. A Society in Transition. *396 pp. Illustrated with plates and maps. 1968. 56s.*

Little, Kenneth L. Mende of Sierra Leone. *308 pp. and folder. 1951. Revised edition 1967. 63s.*

Lowie, Professor Robert H. Social Organization. *494 pp. 1950. (4th Impression 1966.) 50s.*

Mayer, Adrian C. Caste and Kinship in Central India: A Village and its Region. *328 pp. 16 plates. 15 figures. 16 tables. 1960. (2nd Impression 1965.) 35s.*
Peasants in the Pacific: A Study of Fiji Indian Rural Society. *232 pp. 16 plates. 10 figures. 14 tables. 1961. 35s.*

Smith, Raymond T. The Negro Family in British Guiana: Family Structure and Social Status in the Villages. *With a Foreword by Meyer Fortes. 314 pp. 8 plates. 1 figure. 4 maps. 1956. (2nd Impression 1965.) 35s.*

DOCUMENTARY

Meek, Dorothea L. (Ed.). Soviet Youth: Some Achievements and Problems. *Excerpts from the Soviet Press, translated by the editor. 280 pp. 1957. 28s.*

Schlesinger, Rudolf (Ed.). Changing Attitudes in Soviet Russia.
2. The Nationalities Problem and Soviet Administration. Selected Readings on the Development of Soviet Nationalities Policies. *Introduced by the editor. Translated by W. W. Gottlieb. 324 pp. 1956. 30s.*

Reports of the Institute of Community Studies

(*Demy 8vo.*)

Cartwright, Ann. Human Relations and Hospital Care. *272 pp. 1964. 30s.*

Patients and their Doctors. A Study of General Practice. *304 pp. 1967. 40s.*

Jackson, Brian. Streaming: an Education System in Miniature. *168 pp. 1964. (2nd Impression 1966.) 21s. Paper 10s.*

Jackson, Brian and **Marsden, Dennis.** Education and the Working Class: Some General Themes raised by a Study of 88 Working-class Children in a Northern Industrial City. *268 pp. 2 folders. 1962. (4th Impression 1968.) 32s.*

Marris, Peter. Widows and their Families. *Foreword by Dr. John Bowlby. 184 pp. 18 tables. Statistical Summary. 1958. 18s.*
Family and Social Change in an African City. A Study of Rehousing in Lagos. *196 pp. 1 map. 4 plates. 53 tables. 1961. (2nd Impression 1966.) 30s.*
The Experience of Higher Education. *232 pp. 27 tables. 1964. 25s.*

Marris, Peter and **Rein, Martin.** Dilemmas of Social Reform. Poverty and Community Action in the United States. *256 pp. 1967. 35s.*

Mills, Enid. Living with Mental Illness: a Study in East London. *Foreword by Morris Carstairs. 196 pp. 1962. 28s.*

Runciman, W. G. Relative Deprivation and Social Justice. A Study of Attitudes to Social Inequality in Twentieth Century England. *352 pp. 1966. (2nd Impression 1967.) 40s.*

Townsend, Peter. The Family Life of Old People: An Inquiry in East London. *Foreword by J. H. Sheldon. 300 pp. 3 figures. 63 tables. 1957. (3rd Impression 1967.) 30s.*

Willmott, Peter. Adolescent Boys in East London. *230 pp. 1966. 30s.*
The Evolution of a Community: a study of Dagenham after forty years. *168 pp. 2 maps. 1963. 21s.*

Willmott, Peter and **Young, Michael.** Family and Class in a London Suburb. *202 pp. 47 tables. 1960. (4th Impression 1968.) 25s.*

Young, Michael. Innovation and Research in Education. *192 pp. 1965. 25s. Paper 12s. 6d.*

Young, Michael and **McGeeney, Patrick.** Learning Begins at Home. A Study of a Junior School and its Parents. *About 128 pp. 1968. 21s. Paper 14s.*

Young, Michael and **Willmott, Peter.** Family and Kinship in East London. *Foreword by Richard M. Titmuss. 252 pp. 39 tables. 1957. (3rd Impression 1965.) 28s.*

14

The British Journal of Sociology. *Edited by Terence P. Morris. Vol. 1, No. 1, March 1950 and Quarterly. Roy. 8vo., £3 annually, 15s. a number, post free. (Vols. 1-18, £8 each. Individual parts £2 10s.*

All prices are net and subject to alteration without notice

1268 H.B.